Learning Disabilities Sourcebook, 3rd Edition
Leukemia Sourcebook
Liver Disorders Sourcebook
Lung Disorders Sourcebook
Medical Tests Sourcebook, 3rd Edition
Men's Health Concerns Sourcebook, 2nd Edition
Mental Health Disorders Sourcebook, 4th Edition
Mental Retardation Sourcebook
Movement Disorders Sourcebook, 2nd Edition
Multiple Sclerosis Sourcebook
Muscular Dystrophy Sourcebook
Obesity Sourcebook
Osteoporosis Sourcebook
Pain Sourcebook, 3rd Edition
Pediatric Cancer Sourcebook
Physical & Mental Issues in Aging Sourcebook
Podiatry Sourcebook, 2nd Edition
Pregnancy & Birth Sourcebook, 2nd Edition
Prostate Cancer Sourcebook
Prostate & Urological Disorders Sourcebook
Reconstructive & Cosmetic Surgery Sourcebook
Rehabilitation Sourcebook
Respiratory Disorders Sourcebook, 2nd Edition
Sexually Transmitted Diseases Sourcebook, 3rd Edition
Sleep Disorders Sourcebook, 2nd Edition
Smoking Concerns Sourcebook
Sports Injuries Sourcebook, 3rd Edition
Stress-Related Disorders Sourcebook, 2nd Edition
Stroke Sourcebook, 2nd Edition
Surgery Sourcebook, 2nd Edition
Thyroid Disorders Sourcebook
Transplantation Sourcebook
Traveler's Health Sourcebook
Urinary Tract & Kidney Diseases & Disorders Sourcebook, 2nd Edition
Vegetarian Sourcebook
Women's Health Concerns Sourcebook, 3rd Edition
Workplace Health & Safety Sourcebook
Worldwide Health Sourcebook

Teen Health Series

Abuse & Violence Information for Teens
Accident & Safety Information for Teens
Alcohol Information for Teens, 2nd Edition
Allergy Information for Teens
Asthma Information for Teens
Body Information for Teens
Cancer Information for Teens
Complementary & Alternative Medicine Information for Teens
Diabetes Information for Teens
Diet Information for Teens, 2nd Edition
Drug Information for Teens, 2nd Edition
Eating Disorders Information for Teens, 2nd Edition
Fitness Information for Teens, 2nd Edition
Learning Disabilities Information for Teens
Mental Health Information for Teens, 2nd Edition
Pregnancy Information for Teens
Sexual Health Information for Teens, 2nd Edition
Skin Health Information for Teens, 2nd Edition
Sleep Information for Teens
Sports Injuries Information for Teens, 2nd Edition
Stress Information for Teens
Suicide Information for Teens
Tobacco Information for Teens

Women's Health Concerns SOURCEBOOK

Third Edition

Health Reference Series

Third Edition

Women's Health Concerns SOURCEBOOK

Basic Consumer Health Information about Issues and Trends in Women's Health and Health Conditions of Special Concern to Women, Including Endometriosis, Uterine Fibroids, Menstrual Irregularities, Menopause, Sexual Dysfunction, Infertility, Cancer in Women, and Other Such Chronic Disorders as Lupus, Fibromyalgia, and Thyroid Disease

Along with Statistical Data, Tips for Maintaining Wellness, a Glossary, and a Directory of Resources for Further Help and Information

Edited by
Sandra J. Judd

Omnigraphics

P.O. Box 31-1640, Detroit, MI 48231

Bibliographic Note

Edited by Sandra J. Judd

Health Reference Series

Karen Bellenir, *Managing Editor*
David A. Cooke, M.D., *Medical Consultant*
Elizabeth Collins, *Research and Permissions Coordinator*
Cherry Edwards, *Permissions Assistant*
EdIndex, Services for Publishers, *Indexers*

* * *

Omnigraphics, Inc.

Matthew P. Barbour, *Senior Vice President*
Kevin M. Hayes, *Operations Manager*

* * *

Peter E. Ruffner, *Publisher*

ISBN 978-0-7808-1036-5

Library of Congress Cataloging-in-Publication Data

Women's health concerns sourcebook : basic consumer health information about issues and trends in women's health and health conditions of special concern to women, including endometriosis, uterine fibroids, menstrual irregularities, menopause, sexual dysfunction, infertility, cancer in women, and other such chronic disorders as lupus, fibromyalgia, and thyroid disease; along with statistical data, tips for maintaining wellness, a glossary, and a directory of resources for further help and information / edited by Sandra J. Judd. -- 3rd ed.
p. cm. -- (Health reference series)
Includes bibliographical references and index.
Summary: "Provides basic consumer health information about health conditions of special concern to women, along with tips for maintaining wellness. Includes index, glossary of related terms, and other resources"--Provided by publisher.
ISBN 978-0-7808-1036-5 (hardcover : alk. paper) 1. Women--Health and hygiene. 2. Women--Diseases. I. Judd, Sandra J.
RA778.W7543 2009
613'.04244--dc22

2009007211

Printed in the United States

Table of Contents

Visit www.healthreferenceseries.com to view *A Contents Guide to the Health Reference Series*, a listing of more than 14,000 topics and the volumes in which they are covered.

Part II: Breast and Gynecological Concerns

Part III: Sexual and Reproductive Concerns

Part IV: Cancer in Women

Part V: Other Chronic Health Conditions of Special Concern to Women

Part VI: Additional Help and Information

Preface

About This Book

According to the Centers for Disease Control and Prevention, 13 percent of women aged eighteen years and older are in poor, or merely fair, health. More than 12 percent of women face a limitation in their usual activities due to chronic health conditions. In addition, 62 percent of women aged twenty years and older are overweight, a key predictor of future health problems. Moreover, the medical concerns women face often differ from those of most concern to men. Autoimmune diseases strike women three times more often, while depressive disorders afflict two to three times as many women as men. Women are also disproportionately affected by disorders such as arthritis, osteoporosis, and thyroid disease.

Women's Health Sourcebook, Third Edition, provides up-to-date information on the issues and trends in women's health and health conditions of special concern to women, including breast and gynecological concerns, sexual and reproductive concerns, ovarian cancer and other cancers affecting women, and chronic conditions such as autoimmune disease, diabetes, cardiovascular disorders, mental health concerns, and thyroid disorders. Guidelines for maintaining wellness and information about the screenings, checkups, and vaccinations recommended for women are also included, along with a glossary of related terms and a list of resources for further information.

Readers interested in other topics related women's health may wish to consult these additional books within the *Health Reference Series*:

- *Breast Cancer Sourcebook, Third Edition* provides comprehensive information about breast health and breast cancer risk factors, including facts about the types of breast cancer associated with different genes, inflammatory breast cancer, and Paget disease of the nipple.
- *Breastfeeding Sourcebook* discusses the benefits of breastmilk, offers tips for overcoming challenges that breastfeeding women often face, and addresses special situations like multiple births, adoption, and prematurity.
- *Cancer Sourcebook for Women, Third Edition* offers in-depth information about gynecological cancers and other cancers of special concern to women, including cancer of the cervix, fallopian tubes, ovaries, uterus, vagina, vulva, lung, colon, and thyroid.
- *Caregiving Sourcebook* addresses the physical, mental, financial, and legal concerns of patients and their caregivers.
- *Cosmetic and Reconstructive Surgery Sourcebook, Second Edition* provides information about surgical and minimally-invasive procedures used to enhance appearance and diminish the cosmetic effects of aging. It also includes facts about breast prostheses and post-mastectomy breast reconstruction.
- *Depression Sourcebook, Second Edition* describes the most common forms of depression, including unipolar depression, dysthymia, bipolar disorder, seasonal affective disorder, postpartum depression, and other mood disorders.
- *Healthy Heart Sourcebook for Women* tells women why they should be concerned about heart health and what to do to help prevent heart disease.
- *Obesity Sourcebook* discusses obesity-related medical conditions and offers information about setting reasonable goals for weight loss, developing exercise plans, and changing dietary habits.
- *Osteoporosis Sourcebook* helps women identify the important risk factors of osteoporosis and the life-style changes needed to offset them.
- *Pregnancy and Birth Sourcebook, Second Edition* reports on issues related to the prenatal, antenatal, and postnatal periods, and it includes facts for women concerned about high-risk pregnancies and pregnancy complications.

- *Smoking Concerns Sourcebook* provides facts about the health effects of tobacco use, including lung and other cancers, and it offers information about smoking cessation.
- *Thyroid Disorders Sourcebook* offers comprehensive information about thyroid and parathyroid function, related diseases, and their treatment.

How to Use This Book

This book is divided into parts and chapters. Parts focus on broad areas of interest. Chapters are devoted to single topics within a part.

Part I: Issues and Trends in Women's Health provides basic information about how the female body works, guidelines for maintaining wellness, and tips for avoiding risk factors for common health concerns. It details the screenings, checkups, and vaccinations recommended for women, provides a statistical overview of women's health and the health disparities affecting minority women, and discusses lesbian health concerns and the problem of violence against women.

Part II: Breast and Gynecological Concerns describes the conditions affecting women's breasts and reproductive organs, including breast infection and fibrocystic breast disease, premenstrual syndrome, menstrual irregularities, endometriosis, uterine fibroids, vaginal and pelvic infections, sexually transmitted diseases, and pelvic floor disorders. The part concludes with a description of common gynecological procedures and a discussion of the health concerns related to menopause.

Part III: Sexual and Reproductive Concerns discusses sexual dysfunction in women, methods of birth control and their effectiveness, medical and surgical abortion procedures, and infertility. Issues of concern to pregnant women, including prenatal care, staying healthy during pregnancy, childbirth, and pregnancy loss, are also addressed.

Part IV: Cancer in Women details the cancers of special significance to women, including cancers of the breast, cervix, ovaries, uterus, lung, skin, and thyroid. Details about diagnosing and staging the disease, disease progression, and the most effective treatments are provided.

Part V: Other Chronic Health Conditions of Special Concern to Women provides information about such conditions as arthritis, autoimmune diseases, cardiovascular disorders, diabetes, lung disease, anxiety disorders and other mental health concerns, osteoporosis, thyroid disorders, and disorders of the urinary tract. Methods of diagnosis and treatment options are detailed for each.

Part VI: Additional Help and Information includes a glossary of terms related to women's health and a directory of organizations able to provide additional help and support.

Bibliographic Note

This volume contains documents and excerpts from publications issued by the following U.S. government agencies: Agency for Healthcare Research and Quality (AHRQ); Centers for Disease Control and Prevention (CDC); Girlshealth.gov; National Cancer Institute (NCI); National Institute of Allergy and Infectious Diseases (NIAID); National Institute of Arthritis and Musculoskeletal and Skin Diseases (NIAMS); National Institute of Child Health and Human Development (NICHD); National Institute of Diabetes and Digestive and Kidney Diseases (NIDDK); National Institute of Mental Health (NIMH); National Institute on Aging (NIA); National Institute on Alcohol Abuse and Alcoholism (NIAAA); National Institutes of Health, Office of Research on Women's Health; National Women's Health Information Center (NWHIC); NIH Senior Health; U.S. Department of Health and Human Services (HRSA); U.S. Food and Drug Administration (FDA); and the Walter Reed Army Medical Center.

In addition, this volume contains copyrighted documents from the following organizations: A.D.A.M., Inc.; American Academy of Dermatology; American Academy of Family Physicians; American Academy of Orthopaedic Surgeons; American Institute for Cancer Research; American Osteopathic Association; American Pregnancy Association; American Psychological Association; American Thyroid Association; Illinois Department of Public Health; Immunization Action Coalition; MyDR.com.au; NAMI: The Nation's Voice on Mental Illness; Nemours Foundation; Planned Parenthood; Skin Cancer Foundation; Spire Healthcare; University of Michigan Health System; and the University of Rochester/Strong Health.

Full citation information is provided on the first page of each chapter. Every effort has been made to secure all necessary rights to reprint the copyrighted material. If any omissions have been made, please contact Omnigraphics to make corrections for future editions.

Acknowledgements

Thanks go to the many organizations, agencies, and individuals who have contributed materials for this *Sourcebook* and to medical consultant Dr. David Cooke and document engineer Bruce Bellenir. Special thanks go to managing editor Karen Bellenir and permissions coordinator Liz Collins for their help and support.

About the Health Reference Series

The *Health Reference Series* is designed to provide basic medical information for patients, families, caregivers, and the general public. Each volume takes a particular topic and provides comprehensive coverage. This is especially important for people who may be dealing with a newly diagnosed disease or a chronic disorder in themselves or in a family member. People looking for preventive guidance, information about disease warning signs, medical statistics, and risk factors for health problems will also find answers to their questions in the *Health Reference Series*. The *Series*, however, is not intended to serve as a tool for diagnosing illness, in prescribing treatments, or as a substitute for the physician/patient relationship. All people concerned about medical symptoms or the possibility of disease are encouraged to seek professional care from an appropriate healthcare provider.

A Note about Spelling and Style

Health Reference Series editors use *Stedman's Medical Dictionary* as an authority for questions related to the spelling of medical terms and the *Chicago Manual of Style* for questions related to grammatical structures, punctuation, and other editorial concerns. Consistent adherence is not always possible, however, because the individual volumes within the *Series* include many documents from a wide variety of different producers and copyright holders, and the editor's primary goal is to present material from each source as accurately as is possible following the terms specified by each document's producer. This sometimes means that information in different chapters or sections may follow other guidelines and alternate spelling authorities. For example, occasionally a copyright holder may require that eponymous terms be shown in possessive forms (Crohn's disease *vs.* Crohn disease) or that British spelling norms be retained (leukaemia *vs.* leukemia).

Locating Information within the Health Reference Series

The *Health Reference Series* contains a wealth of information about a wide variety of medical topics. Ensuring easy access to all the fact sheets, research reports, in-depth discussions, and other material contained within the individual books of the series remains one of our highest priorities. As the *Series* continues to grow in size and scope, however, locating the precise information needed by a reader may become more challenging.

A Contents Guide to the Health Reference Series was developed to direct readers to the specific volumes that address their concerns. It presents an extensive list of diseases, treatments, and other topics of general interest compiled from the Tables of Contents and major index headings. To access *A Contents Guide to the Health Reference Series*, visit www.healthreferenceseries.com.

Medical Consultant

Medical consultation services are provided to the *Health Reference Series* editors by David A. Cooke, M.D. Dr. Cooke is a graduate of Brandeis University, and he received his M.D. degree from the University of Michigan. He completed residency training at the University of Wisconsin Hospital and Clinics. He is board-certified in Internal Medicine. Dr. Cooke currently works as part of the University of Michigan Health System and practices in Ann Arbor, MI. In his free time, he enjoys writing, science fiction, and spending time with his family.

Our Advisory Board

We would like to thank the following board members for providing guidance to the development of this series:

Dr. Lynda Baker, Associate Professor of Library and Information Science, Wayne State University, Detroit, MI

Nancy Bulgarelli, William Beaumont Hospital Library, Royal Oak, MI

Karen Imarisio, Bloomfield Township Public Library, Bloomfield Township, MI

Karen Morgan, Mardigian Library, University of Michigan-Dearborn, Dearborn, MI

Rosemary Orlando, St. Clair Shores Public Library, St. Clair Shores, MI

Health Reference Series *Update Policy*

The inaugural book in the *Health Reference Series* was the first edition of *Cancer Sourcebook* published in 1989. Since then, the *Series* has been enthusiastically received by librarians and in the medical community. In order to maintain the standard of providing high-quality health information for the layperson the editorial staff at Omnigraphics felt it was necessary to implement a policy of updating volumes when warranted.

Medical researchers have been making tremendous strides, and it is the purpose of the *Health Reference Series* to stay current with the most recent advances. Each decision to update a volume is made on an individual basis. Some of the considerations include how much new information is available and the feedback we receive from people who use the books. If there is a topic you would like to see added to the update list, or an area of medical concern you feel has not been adequately addressed, please write to:

Editor
Health Reference Series
Omnigraphics, Inc.
P.O. Box 31-1640
Detroit, MI 48231
E-mail: editorial@omnigraphics.com

Part One

Issues and Trends in Women's Health

Chapter 1

How the Female Body Works

Chapter Contents

Section 1.1

Breast Anatomy

Women's breasts are made up of fat, nipple, glands (alveoli), and a network of ducts through which milk can pass from the glands to the nipples.

Each breast contains between fifteen and twenty sections called lobes, each of which is composed of many smaller structures known as glands or alveoli. These alveoli produce milk. A system of small tubes known as ducts transports milk from the alveoli to a big central duct that has multiple openings in the nipple. A central duct opens into the nipple from each lobe.

A band of muscle surrounds each gland. This band can contract (squeeze), forcing the milk out of the glands, into the ducts, and through to pools that lie beneath the areola, the brown circle that surrounds the nipple. Eventually, a sucking baby extracts the milk by pressing and pumping it out from these pools through the nipple.

The spaces around the lobes and ducts are filled with fatty tissue and ligaments. The size of a nonlactating breast is largely determined by the amount of fat it contains, as the gland structure is not that well developed.

Underneath the breasts there is fibrous tissue and muscle separating them from the ribs. There is no actual muscle in the breast, but the pectoral muscle passes underneath the breast and connects the chest and the arm. Lying further below the pectoral muscle are the ribs, which are connected by intercostal muscles, which raise and lower the rib cage when breathing in and out.

Deep beyond the ribs is the pleural lining, a thin, moist membrane that lines the chest cavity.

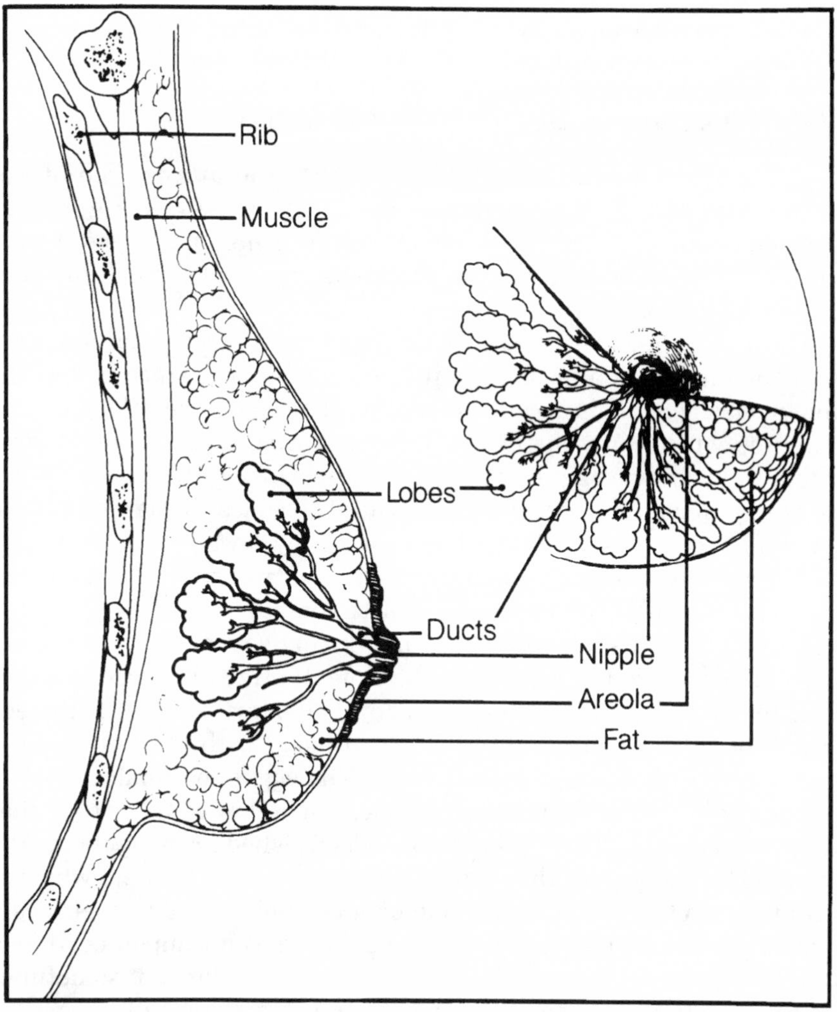

Figure 1.1. *Anatomy of the Breast*

Section 1.2

The Female Reproductive System

Reprinted from "How the Reproductive System Works," Girlshealth.gov, June 18, 2008.

The Reproductive System: On the Inside

The ovaries are two small glands next to the uterus. The uterus (or womb) is like an inside pocket where a baby grows (see Figure 1.2). Ovaries begin to make more estrogen and other hormones during puberty. This sparks the start of the menstrual cycle, which includes a woman's period and other hormonal changes.

The ovaries release or let go of one egg (ovum) about once a month, from the one million or so eggs it has been storing since before the woman was born. This is called ovulation. The egg moves along a fallopian tube, which connects the ovary to the uterus. It takes around three or four days for the egg to get to the uterus. During this time, the lining of the uterus (called the endometrium) becomes thicker with blood and fluid to make itself a better home for a baby. A woman will get pregnant if she has sex with a male, and his sperm fertilizes or joins the egg on its way to the uterus. Barrier birth control methods such as condoms can prevent sperm from passing during sexual intercourse, but these do not work 100 percent of the time. If a fertilized egg attaches itself to the lining of the uterus, a baby may start to grow. If the egg doesn't become fertilized, it will be shed along with the lining of the uterus during the woman's next period. The egg is too small to see.

The vagina, which is made of muscle, is a hollow canal or tube that can grow wider to deliver a baby that has finished growing inside the uterus. The opening of the vagina is covered by the hymen, which is a thin piece of tissue that has one or more holes in it. Sometimes a hymen is stretched or torn when a woman uses a tampon or after a first sexual experience, but this does not always happen; sometimes the hymen stays the same. If it does tear, it may bleed a little bit.

The cervix is the narrow entryway between the vagina and uterus. The opening of the cervix is very small, so a tampon will not slip through here and get lost. At the same time, the muscles of the cervix are flexible so that it can expand to let a baby pass through when she or he is being born.

The Reproductive System: On the Outside

Outside of the body, the entrance to the vagina is covered by the vulva. The vulva has five parts: mons pubis, labia, clitoris, urinary opening, and vaginal opening.

The mons pubis is the mound of tissue and skin just below the stomach. This area becomes covered with hair when a woman goes through puberty. The labia are the two sets of skin folds (often called lips) on either side of the opening of the vagina. The labia majora are the outer lips and the labia minora are the inner lips. The labia minora cover a small sensitive bump called the clitoris, which is at the bottom of the mons pubis. Below the clitoris is the urinary opening, which is where urine leaves the body. Below the urinary opening is the vaginal opening, which is the entry into the vagina.

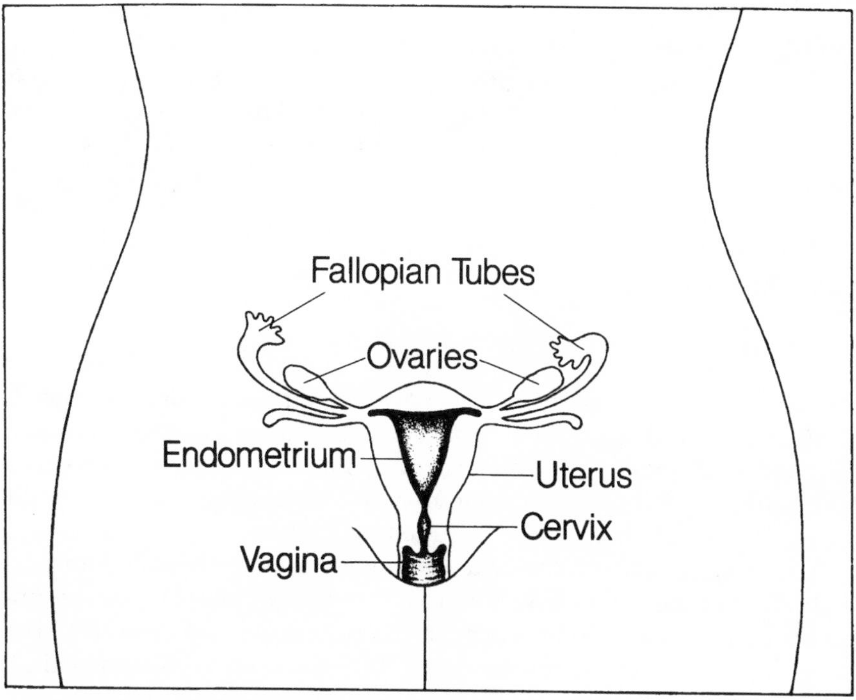

Figure 1.2. *The Female Reproductive System*

Section 1.3

Menstruation and the Menstrual Cycle

Reprinted from "Menstruation and the Menstrual Cycle," National Women's Health Information Center, April 2007.

What is menstruation?

Menstruation is a woman's monthly bleeding, also called a period. When you menstruate, your body is shedding the lining of the uterus (womb). Menstrual blood flows from the uterus through the small opening in the cervix, and passes out of the body through the vagina. Most menstrual periods last from three to five days.

What is the menstrual cycle?

Menstruation is part of the menstrual cycle, which prepares your body for pregnancy each month. A cycle is counted from the first day of one period to the first day of the next period. The average menstrual cycle is twenty-eight days long. Cycles can range anywhere from twenty-one to thirty-five days in adults and from twenty-one to forty-five days in young teens.

Body chemicals called hormones rise and fall during the month to make the menstrual cycle happen.

What happens during the menstrual cycle?

In the first half of the cycle, levels of estrogen (the "female hormone") start to rise and make the lining of the uterus (womb) grow and thicken. At the same time, an egg (ovum) in one of the ovaries starts to mature. At about day fourteen of a typical twenty-eight-day cycle, the egg leaves the ovary. This is called ovulation.

After the egg has left the ovary it travels through the fallopian tube to the uterus. Hormone levels rise and help prepare the uterine lining for pregnancy. A woman is most likely to get pregnant during the three days before ovulation or on the day of ovulation. Keep in mind, women with cycles that are shorter or longer than average may ovulate earlier or later than day fourteen.

If the egg is fertilized by a man's sperm cell and attaches to the uterine wall, the woman becomes pregnant. If the egg is not fertilized, it will break apart. If pregnancy does not occur, hormone levels drop, and the thickened lining of the uterus is shed during the menstrual period.

What is a typical menstrual period like?

During your period, the thickened uterine lining and extra blood are shed through the vaginal canal. Your period may not be the same every month and it may not be the same as other women's periods. Periods can be light, moderate, or heavy, and the length of the period also varies. While most periods last from three to five days, anywhere from two to seven days is normal. For the first few years after menstruation begins, longer cycles are common. A woman's cycle tends to shorten and become more regular with age. Most of the time, periods will be in the range of twenty-one to forty-five days apart.

What kinds of problems do women have with their periods?

Women can have a range of problems with their periods, including pain, heavy bleeding, and skipped periods.

Amenorrhea: The lack of a menstrual period. This term is used to describe the absence of a period in the following groups:

- Young women who haven't started menstruating by age fifteen
- Women who used to have regular periods, but haven't had one for ninety days
- Young women who haven't had a period for ninety days, even if they haven't been menstruating for long

Causes can include pregnancy, breastfeeding, and extreme weight loss caused by serious illness, eating disorders, excessive exercising, or stress. Hormonal problems, such as those caused by polycystic ovarian syndrome (PCOS) or problems with the reproductive organs, may be involved. It is important to talk to a doctor.

Dysmenorrhea: Painful periods, including severe cramps. When menstrual cramps occur in teens, the cause is too much of a chemical called prostaglandin. Most teens with dysmenorrhea do not have a serious disease even though the cramps can be severe. In older women, a disease or condition, such as uterine fibroids or endometriosis, sometimes causes the pain. For some women, using a heating pad or taking a warm bath helps ease their cramps. Some pain medicines available over the counter, such as ibuprofen (for instance, Advil®, Motrin®, Midol Cramp®), ketoprofen (for instance, Orudis KT®), or naproxen (for instance, Aleve®), can help with these symptoms. If pain is not relieved by these medicines or the pain interferes with work or school, you should see a doctor. Treatment depends on what is causing the problem and how severe it is.

Abnormal uterine bleeding: Vaginal bleeding that is different from normal menstrual periods. It includes very heavy bleeding or unusually long periods, periods too close together, and bleeding between periods. In both teens and women nearing menopause, hormonal changes can cause long periods along with irregular cycles. Even if the cause is hormonal changes, treatment is available. These changes can also go along with other serious medical problems such as uterine fibroids, polyps, or even cancer. You should see a doctor if these changes occur. Treatment for abnormal bleeding depends on the cause.

When does a girl usually get her first period?

In the United States, the average age is twelve. This does not mean that all girls start at the same age. A girl can start her period anytime between the ages of eight and fifteen. Usually, the first period starts about two years after breasts first start to grow. If a girl has not had her first period by age fifteen, or if it has been more than two to three years since breast growth started, she should see a doctor.

How long does a woman have periods?

Women usually have periods until menopause. Menopause occurs between the ages of forty-five and fifty-five, usually around age fifty. Menopause means that a woman is no longer ovulating (producing eggs) and can no longer get pregnant. Like menstruation, menopause can vary from woman to woman and these changes may take several years to occur. The time when your body begins its move into menopause is called the menopausal transition. This can last anywhere from two to eight years. Some women have early menopause because of surgery or other treatment, illness, or other reasons. If a woman doesn't have a period for ninety days, she should see her doctor to check for pregnancy, early menopause, or other medical problems that can cause periods to stop or become irregular.

When should I see a doctor about my period?

You should see your doctor if any of the following are true:

- You have not started menstruating by the age of fifteen, or by three years after breast growth began, or if breasts haven't started to grow by age thirteen.
- Your period suddenly stops for more than ninety days.
- Your periods become very irregular after having had regular, monthly cycles.
- Your period occurs more often than every twenty-one days or less often than every forty-five days.
- You are bleeding for more than seven days.
- You are bleeding more heavily than usual or using more than one pad or tampon every one to two hours.
- You bleed between periods.
- You have severe pain during your period.
- You suddenly get a fever and feel sick after using tampons.

How often should I change my pad/tampon?

Pads should be changed as often as needed, before the pad is soaked with blood. Each woman decides for herself what works best. Tampons should be changed at least every four to eight hours. Make sure that you use the lowest absorbency tampon needed for your flow. For example, use junior or regular absorbency on the lightest day of your period. If you use a super absorbency tampon on your lightest days, you may have a higher risk for toxic shock syndrome (TSS). TSS is a rare but sometimes deadly disease. Young women may be more likely to get TSS. Using any kind of tampon, at any absorbency, puts you at greater risk for TSS than using pads. The risk of TSS can be lessened or avoided by not using tampons, or by alternating between tampons and pads during your period.

The Food and Drug Administration (FDA) recommends the following tips to help avoid tampon problems:

- Follow package directions for insertion.

- Choose the lowest absorbency for your flow.
- Change your tampon at least every four to eight hours.
- Consider alternating pads with tampons.
- Know the warning signs of TSS (see below).
- Don't use tampons between periods.

If you have any of these symptoms of TSS while using tampons, take the tampon out and contact your doctor right away:

- Sudden high fever (over 102 degrees)
- Muscle aches
- Diarrhea
- Vomiting
- Dizziness or fainting
- Sunburn-like rash
- Sore throat
- Bloodshot eyes

Section 1.4

Puberty

Reprinted from "Puberty," National Institute of Child Health and Human Development, National Institutes of Health, January 22, 2007.

What is puberty?

Puberty is the time in life when a person becomes sexually mature. It is a physical change that usually happens between ages ten and fourteen for girls and ages twelve and sixteen for boys. Some African American girls start puberty earlier than white girls, making their age range for puberty nine to fourteen.

Puberty starts when a part of the brain called the hypothalamus begins releasing a hormone called gonadotropin releasing hormone (GnRH). GnRH then signals the pituitary gland to release two more hormones—luteinizing hormone (LH) and follicle-stimulating hormone (FSH)—to start sexual development.

A study funded in part by the National Institute of Child Health and Human Development (NICHD) has identified a gene that appears to be the crucial signal for the beginning of puberty. Without a functioning copy of the gene, known as GPR54, humans appear unable to enter puberty normally.

What are the signs of puberty?

Puberty affects boys and girls differently.

In females:

- The first sign of puberty is usually breast development.
- Other signs are the growth of hair in the pubic area and armpits, and acne.
- Menstruation (or a period) usually happens last.

In males:

- Puberty usually begins with the testicles and penis getting bigger.

- Then hair grows in the pubic area and armpits.
- Muscles grow, the voice deepens, and acne and facial hair develop as puberty continues.

Both boys and girls usually have a growth spurt (a rapid increase in height) that lasts for about two or three years along with the signs listed above. This brings them closer to their adult height, which they reach after puberty.

Does everyone go through puberty the same way?

Puberty can have different patterns, so everyone may not go through puberty in the same way. For example:

- Some children may begin puberty earlier than normal, a condition called precocious puberty. If signs of puberty occur early (before age seven or eight for girls and before age nine for boys), parents and caregivers should talk to their child's health care provider to see if treatment is needed.
- Other children may have delayed puberty, meaning the process begins later than normal. Sometimes there is a reason for puberty starting late; for example, many young girls who are gymnasts start puberty later than those who are not gymnasts. But in many cases, there is no known reason for the delay.

If development is later than normal, parents and caregivers should talk to a health care provider, who can make sure there is not a medical condition causing the delay. But most kids with delayed puberty need no treatment and begin puberty on their own body's time.

Section 1.5

Precocious Puberty

Reprinted from "Precocious Puberty," National Institute of Child Health and Human Development, National Institutes of Health, January 15, 2007.

What is precocious puberty?

Precocious puberty is puberty that begins before age eight years for girls and before age nine years for boys. The word "precocious" means developing unusually early.

What are the signs of precocious puberty?

The signs of precocious puberty are the same as those for regular puberty. The difference is that they start to occur at a younger age than normal.

For females, signs include development of breasts, pubic hair, and underarm hair; increased growth rate; and menstrual bleeding.

In boys, signs include growth of the penis and testicles, development of pubic and underarm hair, muscle growth, voice changes, and increased growth rate.

What causes precocious puberty?

Sometimes precocious puberty is the result of a structural problem in the brain that triggers puberty to begin too early. There are many conditions that may lead to precocious puberty, including the following:

- Congenital adrenal hyperplasia
- McCune-Albright syndrome
- Gonadal (testicles or ovaries) or adrenal gland disorders or tumors
- HCG-secreting tumors
- Hypothalamic hamartoma

But in many cases, there is no identifiable cause for the precocious puberty. Puberty just starts earlier than normal. If you think your child is beginning puberty early, talk to your child's health care provider.

What is the treatment for precocious puberty?

Treatment for precocious puberty can help stop puberty until the child is closer to the normal time for sexual development. One reason to consider treating precocious puberty is that rapid growth and bone maturation can prevent a child from reaching his or her full height potential.

Children grow rapidly in height during puberty and reach their final adult height after puberty. Children who go through puberty too early may not reach their full adult height potential because their growth stops too soon.

Another reason to consider treating precocious puberty is that a young child may not be psychologically ready for the physical and hormonal changes that occur in puberty.

If precocious puberty is caused by a specific medical problem, treating the underlying problem can often stop the puberty. In addition, precocious puberty can often be stopped by medical treatment to block the hormones that cause puberty.

Chapter 2

Nutrition and Wellness

Chapter Contents

Section 2.1

Tips for Healthy Eating

Excerpted from "Better Health and You: Tips for Adults," National Institute of Diabetes and Digestive and Kidney Diseases, National Institutes of Health, March 2008.

A balanced eating plan and regular physical activity are the building blocks of good health. Poor eating habits and physical inactivity may lead to overweight and related health problems. By eating right and being active, you may reach or maintain a healthy weight. You may also improve your physical health, improve your mental well-being, and set an example for others. Do it for yourself and your family!

Healthy Eating

What Is a Healthy Eating Plan?

A healthy eating plan includes the following components:

- Emphasizes fruits, vegetables, whole grains, and fat-free or low-fat milk and milk products
- Includes lean meats, poultry, fish, beans, eggs, and nuts
- Is low in saturated fats, trans fats, cholesterol, salt (sodium), and added sugars

Tips for Healthy Eating

Eat breakfast every day: People who eat breakfast are less likely to overeat later in the day. Breakfast also gives you energy and helps you get your day off to a healthy start. Choose whole grains more often. Try whole-wheat breads and pastas, oatmeal, brown rice, or bulgur.

Select a mix of colorful vegetables each day: Vegetables of different colors provide different nutrients. Choose dark leafy greens such as spinach, kale, collards, and mustard greens, and reds and oranges such as carrots, sweet potatoes, red peppers, and tomatoes.

Choose fresh, canned, or frozen fruit more often than fruit juice: Fruit juice has little or no fiber, and the calories may be high. Fresh, canned, or frozen fruit is often better for you. If you eat canned fruit, opt for fruit packed in water rather than syrup.

Use fats and oils sparingly: Olive, canola, and peanut oils, avocados, nuts and nut butters, olives, and fish provide heart-healthy fat as well as vitamins and minerals.

Eat sweets sparingly: Limit foods and beverages that are high in added sugars. Eat three meals every day. If you skip meals or replace a meal with a snack, you might overeat later on.

Have low-fat, low-sugar snacks on hand: Whether you are at home, at work, or on the go, healthy snacks may help to combat hunger and prevent overeating.

Quick Breakfast Ideas

- Low-fat yogurt sprinkled with low-fat granola
- Oatmeal with low-fat or fat-free milk, or soy-based beverage
- A slice of whole-wheat toast with a thin spread of peanut butter
- Fruit smoothie made with frozen fruit, low-fat yogurt, and juice
- High-fiber, low-sugar cereal with soy-based beverage or low-fat milk

Easy Snack Ideas

- Low-fat or fat-free yogurt
- Rice cakes
- Fresh or canned fruits
- Sliced vegetables or baby carrots
- Dried fruit and nut mix (no more than a small handful)
- Air-popped popcorn sprinkled with garlic powder or other spices
- High-fiber, low-sugar cereal

Healthy Weight

What Is a Healthy Weight?

Body mass index (BMI) is one way to tell whether you are at a healthy weight, overweight, or obese. It measures your weight in relation to your height.

A BMI of 18.5 to 24.9 is in the healthy range. A BMI of 25 to 29.9 is overweight, and a BMI of 30 or greater is considered obese.

In Figure 2.1, find your height in the left-hand column and move across the row to find your weight. If you are in the overweight or obese range on the chart, you may be at risk for certain health problems.

Another way to find out if you are at risk for health problems caused by overweight and obesity is to measure your waist. If you are a woman and your waist is more than thirty-five inches, or if you are a man and your waist is more than forty inches, your risk of disease is higher.

What Are the Health Risks of Being Overweight?

Extra weight may put you at higher risk for the following health conditions:

- Type 2 diabetes (high blood sugar)
- High blood pressure
- Coronary heart disease and stroke
- Some types of cancer
- Sleep apnea (when breathing stops for short periods during sleep)
- Osteoarthritis (wearing away of the joints)
- Gallbladder disease
- Irregular periods
- Problems with pregnancy, such as gestational diabetes (high blood sugar during pregnancy), high blood pressure, or increased risk for cesarean section (c-section)

Why Do People Become Overweight?

Many factors may play a part in why people gain weight.

Habits: Eating too many calories may become a habit. You may also develop a habit of doing sedentary activities like watching TV instead of being physically active. Over time, these habits can lead to weight gain.

Genes: Overweight and obesity tend to run in families. Although families often share diet and physical activity habits that can play a role in obesity, their shared genes increase the chance that family members will be overweight.

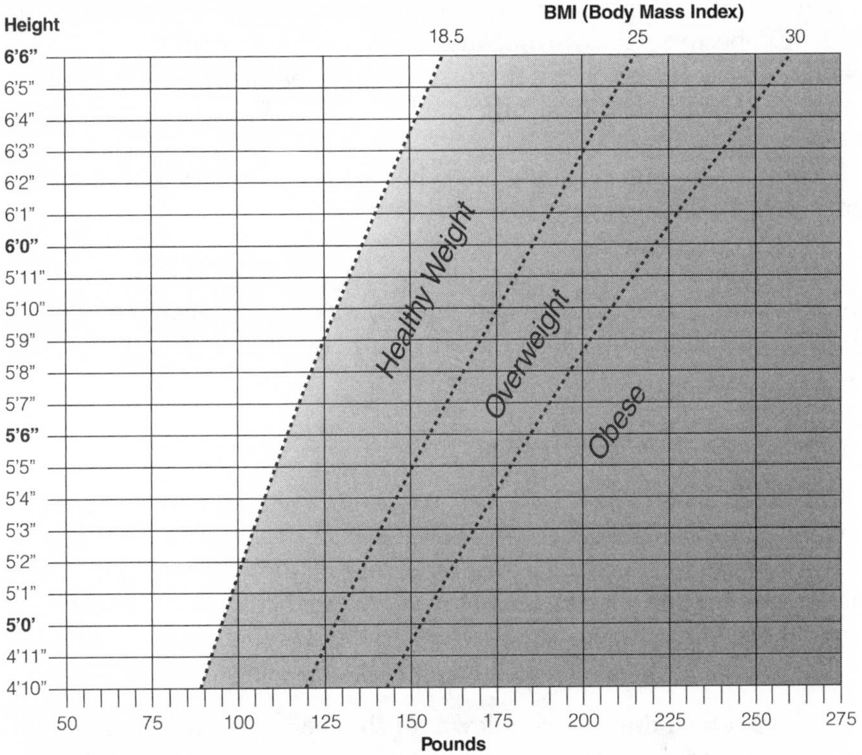

Find your weight on the bottom of the graph. Go straight up from that point until you come to the line that matches your height. Then look to find your weight group. The higher your BMI is over 25, the greater chance you may have of developing health problems.

Figure 2.1. *Body mass index chart (height is figured without shoes and weight is figured without clothes). Sources: George Bray, M.D., Pennington Biomedical Research Center, and National Heart, Lung, and Blood Institute's* Clinical Guidelines on the Identification, Evaluation, and Treatment of Overweight and Obesity in Adults: The Evidence Report.

Illness: Some diseases may lead to weight gain or obesity. These include hypothyroidism, Cushing syndrome, and depression. Talk to your health care provider if you think you have a health problem that could be causing you to gain weight.

Medicine: Some medicines may lead to weight gain. Ask your health care provider or pharmacist about the side effects of any medication you are taking.

The world around you: You can find food and messages about food at home, at work, at shopping centers, on TV, and at family and social events. People may eat too many foods high in fat, sugar, and salt just because they are always there. On top of that, our modern world—with its remote controls, drive-in banks, and escalators—makes it easy to be physically inactive.

Emotions: Many people eat when they are bored, sad, angry, or stressed, even when they are not hungry.

Although you may not be able to control all the factors that lead to overweight, you can change your eating and physical activity habits. And by changing those habits, you may be able to improve your weight and your health.

If You Need to Lose Weight

A weight loss of as little as 5 to 15 percent of your body weight over six months or longer has been shown to improve health. For example, if you weigh 200 pounds, losing 5 percent of your body weight means losing 10 pounds. Losing 15 percent of your body weight means losing 30 pounds. A safe rate of weight loss is 1/2 to 2 pounds per week.

Try some of these ideas to support your weight-loss efforts:

- Keep a food diary. Write down all the food you eat in a day. Also write down the time you eat and your feelings at the time. Writing down your feelings may help you identify your eating triggers. For example, you may notice that you sometimes overeat when you are in a big group, simply because everyone around you is eating. The next time you find yourself in this situation, be mindful of that eating trigger and try to limit your portion sizes.
- Shop from a list and shop when you are not hungry.

- Store foods out of sight, or do not keep many high-fat, high-sugar foods in your home.
- Dish up smaller servings. At restaurants, eat only half your meal and take the rest home.
- Eat at the table and turn off the TV.
- Be realistic about weight-loss goals. Aim for a slow, modest weight loss.
- Seek support from family and friends.
- Expect setbacks and forgive yourself if you regain a few pounds.
- Add moderate-to-vigorous-intensity physical activity to your weight-loss plan. Doing regular physical activity may help you control your weight.

Physical Activity

Getting Active

You do not have to be an athlete to benefit from regular physical activity. Even modest amounts of physical activity can improve your health. Start with small, specific goals, such as walking ten minutes a day, three days a week, and build up slowly from there. Keep an activity log to track your progress.

Try these activities to add more movement to your daily life:

- Take the stairs instead of the elevator. Make sure the stairs are well lit.
- Get off the bus one stop early if you are in an area safe for walking.
- Park the car farther away from entrances to stores, movie theaters, or your home.
- Take a short walk around the block with family, friends, or co-workers.
- In bad weather, walk around a mall.
- Rake the leaves or wash the car.
- Visit museums, the zoo, or an aquarium. You and your family can walk for hours and not realize it.
- Take a walk after dinner instead of watching TV.

Are You Ready to Be Even More Active?

As you become more fit, slowly increase your pace, the length of time you are active, and how often you are active. Before starting a vigorous physical activity program, check with your health care provider if you are a man over age forty or a woman over age fifty, or if you have chronic health problems.

For a well-rounded workout plan, combine aerobic activity, muscle-strengthening exercises, and stretching. Do at least thirty minutes a day of moderate-intensity physical activity on most or all days of the week. Add muscle-strengthening activities to your aerobic workout two to three times a week.

If you are trying to lose weight or maintain your weight loss, you may need to do more activity. Aim for sixty to ninety minutes on most days.

To reduce the risk of injury, do a slow aerobic warm-up, then stretch before aerobic or strengthening activities. Follow your workout with a few more minutes of stretching.

Aerobic activity is any activity that speeds up your heart and breathing while moving your body at a moderate or vigorous pace. (See below for examples.) If you have been inactive for a while, you may want to start with easier activities, such as walking at a gentle pace. This lets you build up to more intense activity without hurting your body.

Regular aerobic activity may help do the following:

- **Control weight:** Aerobic activity burns calories, which may help you manage your weight.
- **Prevent coronary heart disease and stroke:** Regular aerobic activity can strengthen your heart muscle and lower your blood pressure. It may also help lower "bad" cholesterol and raise "good" cholesterol.
- **Maintain strong bones:** Weight-bearing aerobic activities that involve lifting or pushing your own body weight, such as walking, jogging, or dancing, help to maintain strong bones.
- **Improve your outlook:** Aerobic exercise relieves tension and decreases stress. It may also help build your confidence and improve your self-image.

Choose aerobic activities that are fun. People are more likely to be active if they like what they are doing. It also helps to get support from a friend or a family member. Try one of these activities or others you enjoy:

- Brisk walking or jogging
- Bicycling
- Swimming
- Aerobic exercise classes
- Dancing (square dancing, salsa, African dance, swing)
- Playing basketball or soccer

Strengthening activities include lifting weights, using resistance bands, and doing push-ups or sit-ups. Besides building stronger muscles, strengthening activities may help you do the following:

- **Use more calories:** Not only do strengthening exercises burn calories, but having more muscle means you will burn slightly more calories throughout the day—even when you are sitting still.
- **Reduce injury:** Stronger muscles improve balance and support your joints, lowering the risk of injury.
- **Maintain strong bones:** Doing strengthening exercises regularly helps build bone and may prevent bone loss as you age.

Strengthening exercises should focus on working the major muscle groups of the body, such as the chest, back, abdominals, legs, and arms. Do exercises for each muscle group two or three times a week. Allow at least one day of rest for your muscles to recover and rebuild before another strengthening workout. (It is safe to do aerobic activity every day.)

Lifestyle activities are the day-to-day activities that you do. These activities can really add up and increase the number of calories you burn each day. They may also boost your energy and mood by getting your blood and muscles moving. Examples of lifestyle activities include the following:

- Taking the stairs instead of the elevator.
- Walking to your coworker's office instead of using the phone or e-mail.
- Gardening and doing household chores.

- Walking inside the bank rather than using the drive-through window.
- Parking farther from store entrances and walking the extra distance.
- Taking short breaks at work to get up, stretch, and walk.
- Playing with your children, nieces and nephews, and pets.

Be Good to Yourself

Many people feel stress in their daily lives. Stress can cause you to overeat, feel tired, and not want to do anything. Regular physical activity can give you more energy. Try some of these other ideas to help relieve stress and stay on track with your fitness and nutrition goals:

- Get plenty of sleep.
- Practice deep breathing while relaxing your muscles one at a time.
- Take a break and go for a walk.
- Take short stretch breaks throughout the day.
- Try taking a yoga or tai chi class to energize yourself and reduce stress.
- Try a new hobby, like a pottery class or any activity that sparks your interest.
- Surround yourself with people whose company you enjoy.

A balanced eating plan, regular physical activity, and stress relief can help you stay healthy for life.

Section 2.2

Nutrition for Women

"Facts about Women's Wellness—Nutrition," reprinted courtesy of the Illinois Department of Public Health (www.idph.state.il.us). The text of this document is available online at http://www.idph.state.il.us/about/womenshealth/factsheets/nut.htm; accessed May 12, 2008.

How do nutrition needs change for women throughout their lifespan?

During adolescence and early adulthood, women need to consume foods rich in calcium to build peak (maximum) bone mass. This will reduce the risk of developing osteoporosis, a progressive condition where there is a loss of bone that leaves those affected more susceptible to fractures. Women also need an adequate iron intake because they lose iron through menstruation. Women also need an adequate intake of calories to support energy and nutritional needs in order for the body to function properly. The amount of calories that an individual needs varies for each person and is based on age, gender, and activity level. As a general recommendation, women between twenty-three and fifty years of age generally need between 1,700 and 2,200 calories per day to maintain their current energy needs and body weight. Older women generally require fewer calories to support and sustain energy needs. Consuming fewer than 1,500 calories per day, even in attempts to lose weight, can put women at nutritional risk and can result in malnutrition and poor health.

What is a healthy diet?

A well-balanced diet, comprised of a variety of foods, adequately meets women's needs for vitamins, minerals, and energy. For good health, women need to pay special attention to calcium, iron, and folate (folic acid) intake. A healthy diet also should minimize the intake of fat and sugar. Diets high in saturated or trans fat can promote high levels of blood cholesterol and increase risk for heart disease. A diet that includes high sugar provides empty calories, or calories that do not provide any nutritional value and oftentimes replace more nutritious food selections.

Here are some more suggestions for healthy eating:

- Eat a variety of foods.
- Balance the food you eat with physical activity. Maintain a healthy body weight.
- Choose a diet with plenty of whole-grain products, vegetables, and fruits.
- Choose a diet low in fat, saturated fat, and cholesterol.
- Choose a diet moderate in sugars.
- Choose a diet moderate in salt and sodium.
- If you drink alcoholic beverages, do so in moderation.

How can I determine how much fat is ok to eat daily?

The total fat in your daily diet should average no more than 30 percent of your total calories consumed. And saturated fat should be no more than 10 percent of those 30 percent of calories. The amount of fat and saturated fat you eat depends on the foods you select and consume that have fat in them. Consider consulting with a nutrition professional to learn more about how to calculate your fat needs and to not exceed what are healthy amounts. There are many tools available to help you determine how much fat you should consume each day based on your current energy and nutrition needs. Reading food labels is one way to begin to identify where and how much fat is in particular food items.

Are dietary supplements such as vitamins and minerals important in a healthy diet?

It has not been scientifically established that large amounts of vitamins and minerals or dietary supplements help prevent or treat health problems or slow the aging process. Daily multivitamin tablets can be beneficial to some people who do not consume a balanced diet or a variety of foods. Generally, eating a well-balanced diet with a variety of foods provides the necessary nutrients your body needs. Eating whole foods is preferable to supplements because foods provide dietary fiber and other nutritional benefits that supplements do not. If you choose to take vitamin and mineral supplements, it is recommended to choose a multivitamin that does not exceed 100 percent of the recommended dietary intake (RDI).

How do you know which weight-loss programs are safe?

Many commercial weight-loss programs can work if they motivate you to decrease the amount of calories you eat or increase the amount of calories you burn each day. A responsible and safe weight-loss program should have the following features:

- The diet should include all of the recommended daily allowances for vitamins, minerals, and protein and be low-calorie, not low in essential foodstuffs.
- The program should direct an individual toward a slow, steady weight loss unless your doctor feels your particular health condition would benefit from more rapid weight loss. Expect to lose only about a pound a week after the first week or two.
- You should be evaluated and seen by your doctor before beginning any weight-loss program. Your physician also should be able to advise you on the need for weight loss, the appropriateness of the program you have in mind, and a sensible weight loss goal.
- The program should include plans for weight maintenance after the loss phase is over.
- The program should assist in encouraging healthy lifestyle behaviors such as changing your dietary habits and level of physical activity to enhance the likelihood of permanently adopting good health habits.
- A commercial weight-loss program should provide a detailed statement of fees and costs and of any additional items and should be recognized as safe by the FDA.

Why is calcium important?

All youth need calcium to build peak (maximum) bone mass during their early years of life. Low calcium intake is one important factor in the development of osteoporosis, a disease in which bone density decreases and leads to weak bones and future fractures. Women have a greater risk than men of developing osteoporosis. During adolescence and early adulthood, women should include good food sources of calcium in their diets This is when bone growth is occurring and calcium is being deposited into the bone. This occurs in women until they are thirty to thirty-five years of age. Women twenty-five to fifty years of age should have 1,000 mg of calcium each day, while women near or past menopause should have 1,200 mg of calcium daily if they are taking estrogen replacement therapy; otherwise, 1,500 mg per day is recommended. Women older than sixty-five years of age should have 1,500 mg per day.

What are goods sources of calcium?

Low-fat dairy products are excellent sources of calcium. Other good sources of calcium include salmon, tofu (soybean curd), certain vegetables (broccoli), legumes (peas and beans), calcium-enriched grain products, lime-processed tortillas, seeds and nuts. If you do not regularly consume adequate food sources of calcium, a calcium supplement can be considered to reach the recommended amount. The current recommendations for women for calcium are for a minimum of 1,200 mg per day.

Why is iron important for women?

Women need more of this mineral because they lose an average of 15 to 20 milligrams of iron each month during menstruation. Without enough iron, iron deficiency anemia can develop and cause symptoms that include fatigue and headaches. After menopause, body iron generally increases. Therefore, iron deficiency in women older than fifty years of age may indicate blood loss from another source and should be checked by a physician.

Animal products, such as meat, fish, and poultry are good and important sources of iron. Iron from plant sources is found in peas and beans, spinach and other green leafy vegetables, potatoes, and whole-grain and iron-fortified cereal products. The addition of even relatively small amounts of meat or foods containing vitamin C substantially increases the total amount of iron absorbed from the entire meal.

Section 2.3

Folic Acid: A Basic Requirement

Adapted from "Folic Acid—Easy to Read," National Women's Health Information Center, January 2005.

What is folic acid?

Folic acid is a B vitamin. Folic acid helps the body make healthy new cells.

Why should women take folic acid?

All women need folic acid. When a woman has enough folic acid before and during pregnancy, it can help prevent major birth defects of her baby's brain or spine.

Be sure to get enough folic acid every day. Start before you are pregnant. Folic acid is needed during the first few weeks, often before a woman knows she is pregnant. And half of all pregnancies in the United States are not planned. That is why it's so important to start taking folic acid each day, even when you are not planning to get pregnant.

Folic acid might also have other benefits for men and women of any age. Some studies show that folic acid might help prevent heart disease, stroke, some cancers, and possibly Alzheimer disease.

How can women get folic acid?

All women should aim to get at least 400 micrograms (400 mcg) of folic acid each day. There are a few easy ways she can do this:

- Take a daily vitamin that has folic acid in it. Most multivitamins sold in the United States have enough. Check the label on the vitamin to be sure. It should say "400 mcg" or "100%" next to folic acid. Some labels might use the word "folate" for folic acid. Or you can take a vitamin pill that only has folic acid in it. You can find both of these types at your local grocery, drug store, or discount store.

- Another way to get enough folic acid is to eat a serving of breakfast cereal that contains 100 percent of the daily value (DV) for folic acid each day. Check the label on the box to be sure it has enough.

Eat a healthy diet that contains lots of fruits and vegetables and other foods that have folic acid (or folate) in them or added to them. Broccoli, asparagus, bananas, oranges, peas, nuts, spaghetti, bread, cereal, and flour are some foods you can eat to get folic acid (or folate).

How can the food label help?

Look at the package and the food label to see if foods have folic acid in them. Find foods that say they have folic acid. The label will tell you how much folic acid is in it. Sometimes, the label will say folate instead of folic acid. It is the same thing.

How much folic acid should you take?

If you are able to get pregnant, you should take 400 micrograms (mcg) of folic acid every day. If you are pregnant, take 600 mcg of folic acid every day. If you are breastfeeding, take 500 mcg of folic acid every day. If you had a baby with spina bifida or anencephaly and want to get pregnant again, talk with your doctor and ask for a prescription for a higher dose of folic acid. You should take 4,000 mcg starting at least one to three months before getting pregnant and during the first three months of pregnancy. That's ten times the normal amount! But don't try to get the larger amount by taking more than one multivitamin or prenatal vitamin a day. You could get too much of another vitamin that could harm you or your baby. If you had a baby with spina bifida or anencephaly but you are not planning to have another baby, take 400 mcg of folic acid every day.

Section 2.4

Obesity and Weight Loss

Excerpted from "Obesity and Weight Loss," National Women's Health Information Center, February 2005.

How many people in the United States are overweight or obese?

Among U.S. women twenty years and older, over sixty-four million are overweight and over thirty-four million are obese.

How do I know if I'm overweight or obese?

Obesity is measured with a body mass index (BMI), a measure of body fat based on height and weight. Individuals with a BMI of 25 to 29.9 are considered overweight, while individuals with a BMI of 30 or more are considered obese.

What causes someone to become overweight or obese?

An unhealthy diet and physical inactivity are contributing factors to becoming overweight or obese. Overweight and obesity are problems that continue to get worse in the United States. Bigger portion sizes, little time to exercise or cook healthy meals, and relying on cars to get around are just a few reasons for this increase.

What are the health effects of being overweight or obese?

An unhealthy diet and physical inactivity can increase your chances of getting heart disease, cancer, stroke, type 2 diabetes, high blood pressure, breathing problems, arthritis, gallbladder disease, and osteoarthritis.

But body weight isn't the only problem. The places where you store your body fat also affect your health. Women with a "pear" shape tend to store fat in their hips and buttocks. Women with an "apple" shape store fat around their waists.

For most women, carrying extra weight around their waists (larger than 35 inches) raises health risks like heart disease, diabetes, or cancer more than carrying extra weight around the hips or thighs. Obesity can also affect medical care. Too much fat can obscure imaging tests, like x-rays, computed tomography (CT) scans, ultrasound, and magnetic resonance imaging (MRI). For example, in an ultrasound, the beam may not be able to get through layers of fat to get an image of a person's appendix, gallbladder, or kidneys. Too much body fat can make it harder for a doctor to make a medical diagnosis and treat a patient.

How do I find out what the best way is for me to lose weight?

Experts agree that the best way to lose weight is to follow a sensible eating plan and engage in regular physical activity. If you're interested in a weight-loss program, it should encourage healthy behaviors that help you lose weight that you can maintain over time. Before you start a weight-loss program, talk to your doctor.

Safe and effective weight-loss programs should include these components:

- Healthy eating plans that reduce calories but do not rule out specific foods or food groups
- Regular physical activity and/or exercise instruction
- Tips on healthy behavior changes that also consider your cultural needs
- Slow and steady weight loss of about 0.75 to 2 pounds per week and not more than 3 pounds per week (weight loss may be faster at the start of a program)
- Medical care if you are planning to lose weight by following a special formula diet, such as a very-low-calorie diet
- A plan to keep the weight off after you have lost it

What steps can I take to have a healthier diet?

Follow these tips on healthy eating.

Focus on fruits: Eat a variety of fruits—whether fresh, frozen, canned, or dried—rather than fruit juice for most of your fruit choices. For a 2,000-calorie diet, you will need two cups of fruit each day—like one small banana, one large orange, and one-quarter cup of dried apricots or peaches.

Vary your veggies: Eat more dark green veggies, such as broccoli, kale, and other dark leafy greens; orange veggies, such as carrots, sweet potatoes, pumpkin, and winter squash; and beans and peas, such as pinto beans, kidney beans, black beans, garbanzo beans, split peas, and lentils.

Get your calcium-rich foods: Get three cups of low-fat or fat-free milk—or an equivalent amount of low-fat yogurt and/or low-fat cheese (1.5 ounces of cheese equals 1 cup of milk)—every day. If you don't or can't consume milk, choose lactose-free milk products and/or calcium-fortified foods and drinks.

Make half your grains whole: Eat at least three ounces of whole-grain cereals, breads, crackers, rice, or pasta every day. One ounce is about one slice of bread, one cup of breakfast cereal, or one-half cup of cooked rice or pasta. Look to see that grains such as wheat, rice, oats, or corn are referred to as "whole" in the list of ingredients.

Go lean with protein: Choose lean meats and poultry. Bake it, broil it, or grill it. Vary your protein choices with more fish, beans, peas, nuts, and seeds.

Limit saturated fats: Get less than 10 percent of calories from saturated fatty acids. Most fats should come from sources of polyunsaturated and monounsaturated fatty acids, such as fish, nuts, and vegetable oils. When selecting and preparing meat, poultry, dry beans, and milk or milk products, make choices that are lean, low-fat, or fat-free.

Limit salt: Get less than 2,300 mg of sodium (approximately 1 teaspoon of salt) each day.

How can physical activity help?

An active lifestyle can help every woman. You don't have to be as fit as a professional athlete to benefit from physical activity. In fact, thirty minutes of moderate physical activity on most days of the week can greatly improve your health. Most people can get greater health benefits by engaging in physical activity of more vigorous intensity or longer duration. To help manage body weight and prevent gradual, unhealthy body weight gain, get about sixty minutes of moderate- to vigorous-intensity activity on most days of the week, while not exceeding caloric intake requirements. To keep weight loss off, get at least sixty to ninety minutes of daily moderate-intensity physical activity while not exceeding caloric intake requirements. Some people may need to consult with their doctor before participating in this level of activity. Achieve physical fitness by including cardiovascular conditioning, stretching exercises for flexibility, and resistance exercises or calisthenics for muscle strength and endurance. Physical activity has these benefits:

- Reduces your risk of dying from heart disease or stroke
- Lowers your risk of getting heart disease, stroke, high blood pressure, colon cancer, and diabetes
- Lowers high blood pressure
- Helps keep your bones, muscles, and joints healthy
- Reduces anxiety and depression and improves your mood
- Helps you handle stress and helps control your weight
- Protects against falling and bone fractures in older adults
- May help protect against breast cancer
- Helps control joint swelling and pain from arthritis
- Helps you feel more energetic and helps you sleep better

What drugs approved by the U.S. Department of Agriculture (USDA) are available for long-term treatment of obesity?

Sibutramine: Also called Meridia®, it is used together with a reduced-calorie diet to help you lose weight and keep the lost weight from returning. This medicine is approved for people whose initial body mass index (BMI) is at least 30. Patients with other risk factors, such as high blood pressure or diabetes, can be treated with the drug

Table 2.1. Increase your physical activity by taking small steps to change what you do everyday!

If you normally...	Then try this instead!
park as close as possible to the store	park farther away
let the dog out back	take the dog for a walk
take the elevator	take the stairs
have lunch delivered	walk to pick up lunch
relax while the kids play	get involved in their activity

if their BMI is 27 or higher. It can cause an increase in pulse and blood pressure. While you are taking sibutramine, your doctor will check your blood pressure and heart rate at regular visits. People with uncontrolled high blood pressure should not take sibutramine. Other side effects include dry mouth, headache, constipation, insomnia, anxiety, irritability or unusual impatience, nervousness, stuffy or runny nose, or trouble in sleeping.

Orlistat: Also called Xenical®, it prevents the body from absorbing some of the fat in food. It also prevents the body from absorbing some vitamins and beta carotene. Patients should take a vitamin supplement that contains fat-soluble (A, D, E, and K) vitamins and beta carotene. The most common side effects of orlistat are gas with discharge, fecal urgency, fatty/oily stools, and frequent bowel movements.

What surgical options are available for weight loss?

Vertical banded gastroplasty (VBG): Surgical staples are used to divide the stomach into two parts. The upper part is small, which limits space for food. Food empties from the upper pouch into the lower pouch through a small opening. A band is put around this opening so it doesn't stretch. Risks of VBG include wearing away of the band and breakdown of the staple line. In a small number of cases, stomach juices may leak into the abdomen or infection or death from complications may occur.

Laparoscopic gastric banding (Lap-Band): An inflatable band is placed around the upper stomach to create a small pouch and narrow passage into the remainder of the stomach. This limits food consumption and creates an earlier feeling of fullness. Once the band is in place, it is inflated with saline. The band is adjusted over time by increasing or decreasing the amount of salt solution to change the size of the passage. The band is intended for severely obese people—those at least one hundred pounds overweight or who are at least twice their ideal body weight—who have failed to lose weight by other methods such as a supervised diet and exercise. The band is intended to remain in place permanently, but it can be removed if necessary. People who get the band will need to diet and exercise in order to maintain their weight loss. Complications may include nausea and vomiting, heartburn, abdominal pain, band slippage, or pouch enlargement.

Roux-en-Y gastric bypass (RGB): The surgeon makes the stomach smaller by using surgical staples to create a small stomach pouch.

The pouch is attached to the middle part of the small intestine. Food bypasses the upper part of the small intestine and stomach and goes into the middle part of the small intestine through a small opening. Bypassing the stomach limits the amount of food a person can eat. By bypassing part of the intestine, the amount of calories and nutrients the body absorbs is reduced. The small opening slows down the rate food leaves the pouch. One risk for patients is "dumping syndrome." This happens when the stomach contents move too rapidly through the small intestine. Symptoms may include nausea, weakness, sweating, faintness, and diarrhea after eating. Side effects include infection, leaking, pulmonary embolism (sudden blockage in a lung artery), gallstones, and nutritional deficiency.

Biliopancreatic diversion (BPD): This procedure is not commonly used in the United States. A large part of the stomach is removed. The amount of food is restricted, in addition to stomach acid production. The small pouch that remains is connected directly to the final segment of the small intestine, completely bypassing other parts of the small intestine. A common channel remains in which bile and pancreatic digestive juices mix prior to entering the colon. Weight loss occurs since most of the calories and nutrients are routed into the colon, where they are not absorbed. This procedure is less frequently used than other types of surgery because of the high risk for nutritional deficiencies. A variation of BPD includes a "duodenal switch," which leaves a larger portion of the stomach intact, including the pyloric valve that regulates the release of stomach contents into the small intestine. It also keeps a small part of the duodenum.

Is liposuction a treatment for weight loss?

Liposuction is a procedure for shaping the body and is not recommended for weight loss. It is a surgical procedure in which fat is removed from under the skin with the use of a vacuum-suction cannula (a hollow pen-like instrument) or using an ultrasonic probe that breaks up the fat into small pieces and then removes it with suction. Persons with localized fat may decide to have liposuction to remove fat from that area. It doesn't guarantee permanent weight loss. To avoid weight gain after liposuction, people need to eat right and be physically active. Complications from liposuction may include infection, embolism (fat gets trapped in the blood vessels, gathers in the lungs, or travels to the brain), puncturing of organs, seroma, pain or numbness, swelling, burns, skin problems, and reactions to the anesthesia.

Chapter 3

Avoiding Risk Factors for Common Health Concerns

Chapter Contents

Section 3.1

Women and Cholesterol

Reprinted from "Cholesterol," U.S. Food and Drug Administration, 2005.

Did You Know . . . ?

- Women over age twenty should have their cholesterol checked by their doctor.
- Women over the age of fifty-five tend to have higher cholesterol levels than men.
- High cholesterol can increase your chance of having heart disease.

What Is Cholesterol?

Cholesterol is a fat-like material in your blood. Your body makes its own cholesterol. When you eat foods that have lots of fat or cholesterol, you can have too much cholesterol in your blood.

Cholesterol can build up on the inside of the blood vessels of your heart. If too much cholesterol builds up, then the blood cannot flow through to your heart. This can cause a heart attack.

Good vs. Bad Cholesterol

Not all cholesterol in your blood is bad for you. There are three kinds of blood cholesterol that you should know about: high-density lipoprotein (HDL, or good cholesterol), low-density lipoprotein (LDL, or bad cholesterol), and triglycerides.

What Can You Do?

There are things that you can do to lower your cholesterol:

- Cut back on foods with lots of fat such as fatty meats, fried foods, whole milk, fatty cheeses, butter, margarine, oils, lard, and creams.

- Cut back on food with lots of cholesterol, such as egg yolks and whole eggs.
- Eat more fruits and vegetables.
- Cut back on fatty snacks and desserts, such as candy, cookies, doughnuts, muffins, pastries, and pies.
- Exercise at least thirty minutes most days.
- If you are overweight, try to lose weight. Try to lose weight by cutting back on the amount that you eat. Even a small amount of weight loss can help lower your bad cholesterol, and you will also help your health in other ways.
- Ask your doctor if you need to take medicine to help lower your cholesterol. Triglycerides are another form of fat in your blood. They can also raise your risk for heart disease. Levels that are borderline high (150–99 mg/dL) or high (200 mg/dL or more) may need treatment.

What Are the Warning Signs of High Blood Cholesterol?

Most people do not have any signs. Sometimes cholesterol can build up in the blood vessels of your heart and cause chest pains.

How Do You Find Out If You Have High Cholesterol?

Go to the doctor and ask for a cholesterol test. The test will let you know how much good and bad cholesterol you have. The doctor will tell you the number for your total cholesterol level. Your total cholesterol number should be under 200.

Table 3.1. Good and Bad Cholesterol

Good Cholesterol	Bad Cholesterol
Good cholesterol is called HDL.	Bad cholesterol is called LDL.
Helps to keep the arteries from clogging up.	Causes buildup in your arteries and causes blockage of your arteries.
Protects against heart disease.	Causes heart disease.
Good level = 60 mg/dL or more.	Good level = under 100 mg/dL.

Section 3.2

Preventing and Controlling High Blood Pressure

Reprinted from "Preventing and Controlling High Blood Pressure," Centers for Disease Control and Prevention, August 22, 2007.

There are several things that you can do to keep your blood pressure healthy. These actions should become part of your regular lifestyle. You should discuss with your health care provider the best ways for you to address these issues.

Maintain a Healthy Weight

Being overweight or obese can raise your blood pressure, and losing weight can help you lower your blood pressure. Healthy weight status in adults is usually assessed by using weight and height to compute a number called the "body mass index" (BMI). BMI is used because it relates to the amount of body fat for most people. An adult who has a BMI of 30 or higher is considered to be obese. Overweight is a BMI between 25 and 29.9. Normal weight is a BMI of 18 to 24.9. Proper diet and regular physical activity can help to maintain a healthy weight. Other measures of excess body fat may include waist measurements or waist and hip measurements.

Be Active

Being physically inactive is related to high blood pressure, and physical activity can help to lower blood pressure. The Surgeon General recommends that adults should engage in moderate-level physical activities for at least thirty minutes on most days of the week.

Maintain a Healthy Diet

Along with healthy weight and regular physical activity, an overall healthy diet can help to maintain healthy blood pressure levels. This includes eating lots of fresh fruits and vegetables and lowering or cutting out salt or sodium and increasing potassium. High salt and sodium intake and a low potassium intake (due to not eating enough fruits and vegetables) can increase blood pressure. You need to watch the sodium that is already included in processed foods and to avoid adding sodium or salt in cooking or at the table. Low saturated fat and cholesterol are also part of an overall healthy diet. Recent studies such as the Dietary Approaches to Stop Hypertension (DASH) trial show that blood pressure can be significantly lowered through diet.

Moderate Alcohol Use

Excessive alcohol consumption is related to increased blood pressure. People who drink alcohol should do so in moderation. Based on current dietary guidelines, moderate drinking for women is defined as an average of one drink or less per day.

Prevent and Control Diabetes

People with diabetes have a higher risk of high blood pressure, but they can also work to reduce their risk. Recent studies suggest that all people can take steps to reduce their risk of diabetes. These include a healthy diet, weight loss, and regular physical activity.

No Tobacco

Smoking injures blood vessels and speeds up the process of hardening of the arteries. Further, smoking is a major risk for heart disease and stroke. If you don't smoke, don't start. Quitting smoking lowers one's risk of heart attack and stroke. Your doctor can suggest programs to help you quit smoking.

Medications

If you develop high blood pressure, your doctor may prescribe medications, in addition to lifestyle changes, to help bring it under control. Once your blood pressure is controlled, continuing your medication and doctor visits is critical to keep your blood pressure in check. The lifestyle changes noted above are just as important as taking your medicines as prescribed.

Genetic Factors

Genes can play a role in high blood pressure. It is also possible that an increased risk of high blood pressure within a family is due to factors such as a common sedentary lifestyle or poor eating habits. Therefore, lifestyle factors should be considered for preventing and controlling high blood pressure.

Section 3.3

Health Risks of Smoking and How to Quit

"Why It's Important to Quit" is reprinted from "Smoking and How to Quit: Why It's Important to Quit," and "How to Quit" is reprinted from "Smoking and How to Quit: How to Quit," National Women's Health Information Center, March 19, 2008.

Why It's Important to Quit

Women smoke for different reasons. Some women smoke to deal with stress or control weight. Younger women may start smoking to rebel, show independence, or be accepted by their peers. But there is never a good reason to smoke.

Health Reasons to Quit

Smoking causes serious health problems, including the following:

- Cancers of the lung, throat, mouth, larynx, esophagus, pancreas, kidney, bladder, cervix, and stomach
- Leukemia (a cancer of blood-forming tissues)
- Lung diseases
- Atherosclerosis, or hardening and narrowing of the arteries
- Heart attacks
- Stroke
- Gum disease
- Eye diseases that can lead to blindness

Smoking also has the following effects:

- Makes illnesses last longer
- Causes more wound infections after surgery
- Makes it harder to get pregnant
- Increases your risk of getting a hip fracture

Smoking during pregnancy is especially dangerous. Smoking while pregnant can cause the following:

- Placenta previa, where the placenta grows too close to the opening of the uterus or womb. As a result, the baby cannot be delivered through the vagina and must be delivered by cesarean section, or C-section.
- Placental abruption, where the placenta separates too early from the wall of the uterus. This can lead to early labor or infant death.
- Early rupture of membranes, or water breaking, before labor starts, so the baby is born too early.
- A baby with a low birth weight.
- Damage to an infant's lungs.

Other Benefits of Quitting

When you quit, you will never again have to leave your workplace, your home, or other places to smoke. Over time, you will see some of the other benefits of quitting:

- Your teeth will be cleaner.
- Your breath will smell better.
- The stain marks on your fingers will fade.
- Your skin will be less wrinkled.
- You will be able to smell and taste things better.

You will also feel stronger and be able to be more active.

How to Quit

Make the Decision to Quit and Feel Great!

If you have made the decision to quit smoking, congratulations! Not only will you improve your own health, you will also protect the health of your loved ones by no longer exposing them to secondhand smoke.

We know how hard it can be to quit smoking. Did you know that many people try to quit two or three times before they give up smoking for good? Nicotine is a very addictive drug—as addictive as heroin and cocaine. The good news is that millions of people have given up smoking for good. It's hard work to quit, but you can do it! Freeing yourself of an expensive habit that is dangerous to your health and the health of others will make you feel great!

Many women who smoke worry that they will gain weight if they quit. In fact, nearly 80 percent of people who quit smoking do gain weight, but the average weight gain is just five pounds. Keep in mind, however, that 56 percent of people who continue to smoke will gain weight too. The bottom line: The health benefits of quitting far exceed any risks from the weight gain that may follow quitting.

Tips to Help You Quit

Research has shown that the following five steps will help you to quit for good.

Pick a date to stop smoking: Before that day, get rid of all cigarettes, ashtrays, and lighters everywhere you smoke. Do not allow anyone to smoke in your home. Write down why you want to quit and keep this list as a reminder.

Get support from your family, friends, and coworkers: Studies have shown you will be more likely to quit if you have help. Let the people important to you know the date you will be quitting and ask them for their support. Ask them not to smoke around you or leave cigarettes out. Get more support ideas.

Find substitutes for smoking and vary your routine: When you get the urge to smoke, do something to take your mind off smoking. Talk to a friend, go for a walk, or go to the movies. Reduce stress with exercise, meditation, hot baths, or reading. Try sugar-free gum or candy to help handle your cravings. Drink lots of water and juices. You might want to try changing your daily routine as well. Try drinking tea instead of coffee, eating your breakfast in a different place, or taking a different route to work.

Talk to your doctor or nurse about medicines to help you quit: Some people have withdrawal symptoms when they quit smoking. These symptoms can include depression, trouble sleeping, feeling irritable or restless, and trouble thinking clearly. There are medicines to help relieve these symptoms. Most medicines help you quit smoking by giving you small, steady doses of nicotine, the drug in cigarettes that causes addiction.

Talk to your doctor or nurse to see if one of these medicines may be right for you:

- *Nicotine patch:* Worn on the skin and supplies a steady amount of nicotine to the body through the skin
- *Nicotine gum or lozenge:* Releases nicotine into the bloodstream through the lining in your mouth
- *Nicotine nasal spray:* Inhaled through your nose and passes into your bloodstream
- *Nicotine inhaler:* Inhaled through the mouth and absorbed in the mouth and throat
- *Bupropion:* An antidepressant medicine that reduces nicotine withdrawal symptoms and the urge to smoke
- *Varenicline (Chantix®):* A medicine that reduces nicotine withdrawal symptoms and the pleasurable effects of smoking

Be prepared for relapse: Most people relapse, or start smoking again, within the first three months after quitting. Don't get discouraged if you relapse. Remember, many people try to quit several times before quitting for good. Think of what helped and didn't help the last time you tried to quit. Figuring these out before you try to quit again will increase your chances for success. Certain situations can increase your chances of smoking. These include drinking alcohol, being around other smokers, gaining weight, stress, or becoming depressed. Talk to your doctor or nurse for ways to cope with these situations.

Where to Get Help

Get more help if you need it. Join a quit-smoking program or support group to help you quit. These programs can help you handle withdrawal and stress and teach you skills to resist the urge to smoke. Contact your local hospital, health center, or health department for information about quit-smoking programs and support groups in your area.

Section 3.4

Alcohol: A Women's Health Issue

Excerpted from "Alcohol: A Women's Health Issue," National Institute on Alcohol Abuse and Alcoholism, National Institutes of Health, NIH Publication No. 04-4956, March 2005.

Women and Drinking

Exercise, diet, hormones, and stress: keeping up with all the health issues facing women is a challenge.

Alcohol presents yet another health challenge for women. Even in small amounts, alcohol affects women differently than men. In some ways, heavy drinking is much more risky for women than it is for men.

With any health issue, accurate information is key. There are times and ways to drink that are safer than others. Every woman is different. No amount of drinking is 100 percent safe, 100 percent of the time, for every woman. With this in mind, it's important to know how alcohol can affect a woman's health and safety.

How Much Is Too Much?

Sixty percent of U.S. women have at least one drink a year. Among women who drink, 13 percent have more than seven drinks per week.

For women, this level of drinking is above the recommended limits published in the *Dietary Guidelines for Americans*, which are issued jointly by the U.S. Department of Agriculture and the U.S. Department of Health and Human Services.

The *Dietary Guidelines* define moderate drinking as no more than one drink a day for women and no more than two drinks a day for men.

The *Dietary Guidelines* point out that drinking more than one drink per day for women can increase the risk for motor vehicle crashes, other injuries, high blood pressure, stroke, violence, suicide, and certain types of cancer.

Some people should not drink at all:

- Anyone under age 21

- People of any age who are unable to restrict their drinking to moderate levels
- Women who may become pregnant or who are pregnant
- People who plan to drive, operate machinery, or take part in other activities that require attention, skill, or coordination
- People taking prescription or over-the-counter medications that can interact with alcohol

Why are lower levels of drinking recommended for women than for men? Because women are at greater risk than men for developing alcohol-related problems. Alcohol passes through the digestive tract and is dispersed in the water in the body. The more water available, the more diluted the alcohol. As a rule, men weigh more than women, and, pound for pound, women have less water in their bodies than men. Therefore, a woman's brain and other organs are exposed to more alcohol and to more of the toxic byproducts that result when the body breaks down and eliminates alcohol.

What Is a Drink?

A standard drink is as follows:

- One 12-ounce bottle of beer or wine cooler
- One 5-ounce glass of wine
- 1.5 ounces of 80-proof distilled spirits

Keep in mind that the alcohol content of different types of beer, wine, and distilled spirits can vary quite substantially.

Moderate Drinking: Benefits and Risks

Moderate drinking can have short- and long-term health effects, both positive and negative.

Among the benefits are the following:

- **Heart disease:** Once thought of as a threat mainly to men, heart disease also is the leading killer of women in the United States. Drinking moderately may lower the risk for coronary heart disease, mainly among women over age fifty-five. However, there are other factors that reduce the risk of heart disease, including a healthy diet, exercise, not smoking, and keeping a healthy weight. Moderate drinking provides little, if any, net health benefit for younger people. (Heavy drinking can actually damage the heart.)

Risks are as follows:

- **Drinking and driving:** It doesn't take much alcohol to impair a person's ability to drive. The chances of being killed in a single-vehicle crash are increased at a blood alcohol level that a 140-pound woman would reach after having one drink on an empty stomach.
- **Medication interactions:** Alcohol can interact with a wide variety of medicines, both prescription and over-the-counter. Alcohol can reduce the effectiveness of some medications, and it can combine with other medications to cause or increase side effects. Alcohol can interact with medicines used to treat conditions as varied as heart and blood vessel disease, digestive problems, and diabetes. In particular, alcohol can increase the sedative effects of any medication that causes drowsiness, including cough and cold medicines and drugs for anxiety and depression. When taking any medication, read package labels and warnings carefully.
- **Breast cancer:** Research suggests that as little as one drink per day can slightly raise the risk of breast cancer in some women, especially those who have a family history of breast cancer. It is not possible, however, to predict how alcohol will affect the risk for breast cancer in any one woman.
- **Fetal alcohol syndrome:** Drinking by a pregnant woman can harm her unborn baby, and may result in a set of birth defects called fetal alcohol syndrome (FAS).

Another risk of drinking is that a woman may at some point abuse alcohol or become alcoholic (alcohol dependent). Drinking more than seven drinks per week increases a woman's chances of abusing or becoming dependent on alcohol. Even women who drink fewer than seven drinks a week are at increased risk of developing alcohol abuse or dependence if they occasionally have four or more drinks on any given day.

Heavy Drinking

An estimated 5.3 million women in the United States drink in a way that threatens their health, safety, and general well-being. A strong case can be made that heavy drinking is more risky for women than men:

- Heavy drinking increases a woman's risk of becoming a victim of violence and sexual assault.
- Drinking over the long term is more likely to damage a woman's health than a man's, even if the woman has been drinking less alcohol or for a shorter length of time than the man.

The health effects of alcohol abuse and alcoholism are serious. Some specific health problems include the following:

- **Alcoholic liver disease:** Women are more likely than men to develop alcoholic hepatitis (liver inflammation) and to die from cirrhosis.
- **Brain disease:** Most alcoholics have some loss of mental function, reduced brain size, and changes in the function of brain cells. Research suggests that women are more vulnerable than men to alcohol-induced brain damage.
- **Cancer:** Many studies report that heavy drinking increases the risk of breast cancer. Alcohol also is linked to cancers of the digestive tract and of the head and neck (the risk is especially high in smokers who also drink heavily).
- **Heart disease:** Chronic heavy drinking is a leading cause of cardiovascular disease. Among heavy drinkers, men and women have similar rates of alcohol-related heart disease, even though women drink less alcohol over a lifetime than men.

Finally, many alcoholics smoke; smoking in itself can cause serious long-term health consequences.

Women and Problem Drinking

Fewer women than men drink. However, among the heaviest drinkers, women equal or surpass men in the number of problems that result from their drinking. For example, female alcoholics have death rates 50 to 100 percent higher than those of male alcoholics, including deaths from suicides, alcohol-related accidents, heart disease and stroke, and liver cirrhosis.

An Individual Decision

A woman's genetic makeup shapes how quickly she feels the effects of alcohol, how pleasant drinking is for her, and how drinking alcohol over the long term will affect her health, even the chances that she could have problems with alcohol. A family history of alcohol problems, a woman's risk of illnesses like heart disease and breast cancer, medications she is taking, and age are among the factors for each woman to weigh in deciding when, how much, and how often to drink.

What Are Alcohol Abuse and Alcoholism?

Alcohol abuse is a pattern of drinking that is harmful to the drinker or others. The following situations, occurring repeatedly in a twelve-month period, would be indicators of alcohol abuse:

- Missing work or skipping child care responsibilities because of drinking
- Drinking in situations that are dangerous, such as before or while driving
- Being arrested for driving under the influence of alcohol or for hurting someone while drunk
- Continuing to drink even though there are ongoing alcohol-related tensions with friends and family

Alcoholism or alcohol dependence is a disease. It is chronic, or lifelong, and it can be both progressive and life threatening. Alcoholism is based in the brain. Alcohol's short-term effects on the brain are what cause someone to feel high, relaxed, or sleepy after drinking.

In some people, alcohol's long-term effects can change the way the brain reacts to alcohol, so that the urge to drink can be as compelling as the hunger for food. Both a person's genetic makeup and his or her environment contribute to the risk for alcoholism. The following are some of the typical characteristics of alcoholism:

- **Craving:** A strong need, or compulsion, to drink
- **Loss of control:** the inability to stop drinking once a person has begun
- **Physical dependence:** withdrawal symptoms, such as nausea, sweating, shakiness, and anxiety, when alcohol use is stopped after a period of heavy drinking
- **Tolerance:** the need for increasing amounts of alcohol to get "high."

Know the Risks

Research suggests that a woman is more likely to drink excessively if she has any of the following:

- Parents and siblings (or other blood relatives) with alcohol problems
- A partner who drinks heavily
- The ability to "hold her liquor" more than others
- A history of depression
- A history of childhood physical or sexual abuse

The presence of any of these factors is a good reason to be especially careful with drinking.

How Do You Know If You Have a Problem?

Answering the following four questions can help you find out if you or someone close to you has a drinking problem:

- Have you ever felt you should cut down on your drinking?
- Have people annoyed you by criticizing your drinking?
- Have you ever felt bad or guilty about your drinking?
- Have you ever had a drink first thing in the morning to steady your nerves or to get rid of a hangover?

One "yes" answer suggests a possible alcohol problem. If you responded "yes" to more than one question, it is very likely that you have a problem with alcohol. In either case, it is important that you see your health care provider right away to discuss your responses to these questions.

Even if you answered "no" to all of the above questions, if you are having drinking-related problems with your job, relationships, health, or with the law, you should still seek help.

Treatment for Alcohol Problems

Treatment for an alcohol problem depends on its severity. Women who have alcohol problems but who are not yet alcohol dependent may be able to stop or reduce their drinking with minimal help. Routine doctor visits are an ideal time to discuss alcohol use and its potential problems. Health care providers can help a woman take a good hard look at what effect alcohol is having on her life and can give advice on ways to stop drinking or to cut down.

Section 3.5

Dangers of Tanning and Ultraviolet Rays

"Protect Yourself from the Sun" is excerpted from a document by the same title produced by the Centers for Disease Control and Prevention, May 17, 2007. Text under the title "The Truth about Indoor Tanning" is reprinted from www.osteopathic.org, © 2003–2008, American Osteopathic Association. Reprinted with the consent of the American Osteopathic Association. This document is available online at http://www.osteopathic.org/index.cfm?PageID=you_indoortan; accessed May 12, 2008.

Protect Yourself from the Sun

Summer is a great time to have fun outdoors. It's also a time to take precautions to avoid sunburns, which can increase your risk of skin cancer.

Skin cancer is the most common form of cancer in the United States. Exposure to the sun's ultraviolet (UV) rays appears to be the most important environmental factor involved with developing skin cancer. During the summer months, UV radiation tends to be greater.

To help prevent skin cancer while still having fun outdoors, regularly use sun protective practices such as the following:

- Seek shade, especially during midday hours (10:00 a.m. to 4:00 p.m.), when UV rays are strongest and do the most damage.
- Cover up with clothing to protect exposed skin.
- Get a hat with a wide brim to shade the face, head, ears, and neck.
- Grab shades that wrap around and block as close to 100 percent of both ultraviolet A (UVA) and ultraviolet B (UVB) rays as possible.
- Rub on sunscreen with sun protective factor (SPF) 15 or higher, and both UVA and UVB protection.

It's always wise to choose more than one way to cover up when you're in the sun. Use sunscreen, and put on a T-shirt. Seek shade, and grab your sunglasses. Wear a hat, but rub on sunscreen too. Combining these sun protective actions helps protect your skin from the sun's damaging UV rays.

UV rays reach you on cloudy and hazy days, as well as bright and sunny days. UV rays will also reflect off any surface like water, cement, sand, and snow. Additionally, UV rays from artificial sources of light, like tanning beds, cause skin cancer and should be avoided.

Most forms of skin cancer can be cured. However, the best way to avoid skin cancer is to protect your skin from the sun.

Remember, when in the sun, seek shade, cover up, get a hat, wear sunglasses, and use sunscreen!

The Truth about Indoor Tanning

As the temperatures rise and shorts replace pants, pale winter skin may sway some to consider the speedy effects of indoor tanning to achieve a bronze summer glow. However, indoor tanning is even more dangerous than outdoor sun exposure.

"The myth of health associated with a suntan is simply that—a myth," explains Craig Wax, D.O., an osteopathic family physician practicing in Mullica Hill, New Jersey. "Some people expose themselves to the sun for the vitamin D. The amount of vitamin D made available is minimal compared with the risk of skin cancer with prolonged exposure."

He further explains that tanning is the body's way of protecting itself against ultraviolet (UV) ray exposure. The brown pigment melanin produced by skin is spread throughout the exposed areas. This pigment only minimally protects the skin against further damage from UV radiation.

Despite this information, the use of indoor tanning devices which emit ultraviolet light, both in tanning salons and at home, has never been more popular. The industry serves twenty-eight million people; generates $5 billion a year; and is represented by 30,000 tanning facilities across the country, according to the Skin Cancer Foundation.

"Many patients consider indoor tanning to be a safer alternative to sun tanning," he explains. "But it is just the opposite; tanning beds emit up to twice as much skin damaging radiation."

Dr. Wax explains that overexposure to UV rays can cause eye injury, premature wrinkling and aging of the skin, light-induced skin rashes, and increased chances of developing skin cancer.

"Young women are prone to use tanning salons," explains Dr. Wax, "because while the aging effects and skin cancer might take years to surface, the perceived social value of a tan is immediate." He warns that the dangers of tanning are serious and increase the potential for skin cancer, including:

- **Malignant melanoma:** The deadliest form of skin cancer, often surfacing as a flat or slightly raised discolored patch that has irregular borders. This is the result of intense exposure in childhood, resulting in multiple sunburns.
- **Basal cell carcinoma (BCC):** The most common form of skin cancer, BCC can be identified by an open sore, a red patch of skin, a shiny bump, a pink growth or scar-like area. This type of skin cancer follows a similar pattern to melanoma and is best identified by a physician.

Dr. Wax further explains that the health risks associated with UV radiation are even more likely with smoking, the use of birth control pills, anti-depressants, acne medication, ingredients found in antidandruff shampoos, lime oil, and some cosmetics.

"If you or someone you know is using an indoor tanning device, it is important to educate them on the hazards of tanning," explains Dr. Wax.

Further, he explains that if skin shows signs of possible cancer, it is important to consult a physician immediately.

Section 3.6

Preventing Allergic Reactions to Cosmetics

Reprinted from "Cosmetics," U.S. Food and Drug Administration, 2006.

People use cosmetics to look and smell good. These products can range from eye shadow to deodorants. They can have many different ingredients. The U.S. Food and Drug Administration (FDA) does not test cosmetics before they are put in stores. The law says they must be safe if used in the usual way, or the way the label says to use them.

How do allergies start?

Some people may react to something in a product, For example, they may have itching, redness, rash, sneezing, or wheezing. Allergies may happen the first time you use a product or after you have used it more than once.

Are "testers" at makeup counters safe?

Lots of people use the testers at makeup counters. Testers can have lots of germs because so many people use them. Do you want to test a product at the counter anyway? If so, use a new sponge or cotton swab.

Are labels important?

Yes! Always read them carefully. The law says a label must tell you the following things:

- What the product is
- If there are things to know about how to use the product safely
- How much of the product the package contains
- What company makes the product or distributes it

Also, if it is sold at retail to consumers, there must be a list telling what's in the product. Usually this is on the label. In any case, it should be in a place where you can see it when you buy it.

How do I know if it's a cosmetic or a drug?

If a product is meant to keep you from getting sick, make you well, or change the way your body works, it is a drug. For example, products to treat dandruff and pimples are drugs. The law treats them differently from cosmetics. For example, they have different rules for how ingredients are listed. Some products are both cosmetics and drugs. For example, a shampoo that is just for washing your hair is a cosmetic. A product for stopping dandruff is a drug. A shampoo that is used for washing your hair and stopping dandruff is both a cosmetic and a drug. It must follow the rules for both cosmetics and drugs.

I have seen the term AHA. What does it mean?

AHA is the short term for alpha hydroxy acid. Cosmetic makers claim that AHAs lessen wrinkles. They say that they soften other signs of aging, too.

Many people have had skin problems after using AHAs. They have sent complaints to the FDA about the following:

- Redness
- Swelling
- Burning
- Blisters
- Bleeding
- Rash
- Itching
- Changes in skin color

Can I use AHA products safely?

Protect your skin from the sun while you are using the product and for a week after you stop using it. Buy only products that contain 10 percent AHAs or less. Buy only products with pH of 3.5 or more. Do a test first on a small patch of skin. Stop using the product if you have itching, burning, swelling, or other problems. See your skin doctor (called a dermatologist) if you have problems.

What should I do if I have a bad reaction to a cosmetic?

First, call your doctor to find out how to take care of the problem. You also can report a problem to FDA.

Safety Tips for Beauty

- Follow directions on the label carefully, including all "Cautions" and "Warnings."
- Keep makeup closed tight when not in use.
- Wash your hands before you put on makeup.
- Do not put on makeup while you are driving.
- Do not share makeup with anyone else.
- Do not add liquid to makeup.
- Stop using a product if you get a rash or other problem where you are using it.
- Throw away makeup if the color changes.
- Throw away makeup if it gets an odor.
- Be extra careful not to keep mascara too long. Some companies say three months is long enough.
- Do not use eye makeup if you have an eye infection. Throw away eye makeup you were using when you got the infection.
- Keep makeup out of the sun.
- Do not use spray cans while you are smoking or near a source of heat. It could also cause a fire.

Chapter 4

Recommended Screenings and Checkups for Women

Chapter Contents

Section 4.1

Preventive Health Care for Women

Excerpted from "Women: Stay Healthy at Any Age—Your Checklist for Health," Agency for Healthcare Research and Quality, AHRQ Publication No. 07-IP005-A, February 2007.

What can you do to stay healthy and prevent disease? You can get certain screening tests, take preventive medicine if you need it, and practice healthy behaviors.

Top health experts from the U.S. Preventive Services Task Force suggest that when you go for your next checkup, you should talk to your doctor or nurse about how you can stay healthy, no matter what your age.

Screening Tests for Women: What You Need and When

The most important things you can do to stay healthy are as follows:

- Get recommended screening tests.
- Be tobacco free.
- Be physically active.
- Eat a healthy diet.
- Stay at a healthy weight.
- Take preventive medicines if you need them.

Screening tests can find diseases early, when they are easier to treat. Health experts from the U.S. Preventive Services Task Force have made recommendations, based on scientific evidence, about testing for the conditions below. Talk to your doctor about which ones apply to you and when and how often you should be tested.

- **Obesity:** Have your body mass index (BMI) calculated to screen for obesity. (BMI is a measure of body fat based on height and weight.)

- **Breast cancer:** Have a mammogram every one to two years starting at age forty.
- **Cervical cancer:** Have a Pap smear every one to three years if you have ever been sexually active and are between the ages of twenty-one and sixty-five.
- **High cholesterol:** Have your cholesterol checked regularly starting at age forty-five. If you are younger than forty-five, talk to your doctor about whether to have your cholesterol checked if you have diabetes, you have high blood pressure, heart disease runs in your family, or you smoke.
- **High blood pressure:** Have your blood pressure checked at least every two years. High blood pressure is 140/90 or higher.
- **Colorectal cancer:** Have a test for colorectal cancer starting at age fifty. Your doctor can help you decide which test is right for you. If you have a family history of colorectal cancer, you may need to be screened earlier.
- **Diabetes:** Have a test for diabetes if you have high blood pressure or high cholesterol.
- **Depression:** Your emotional health is as important as your physical health. If you have felt "down," sad, or hopeless over the last two weeks or have felt little interest or pleasure in doing things, you may be depressed. Talk to your doctor about being screened for depression.
- **Osteoporosis (thinning of the bones):** Have a bone density test beginning at age sixty-five to screen for osteoporosis. If you are between the ages of sixty and sixty-four and weigh 154 pounds or less, talk to your doctor about being tested.
- **Chlamydia and other sexually transmitted infections:** Have a test for chlamydia if you are twenty-five or younger and sexually active. If you are older, talk to your doctor about being tested. Also ask whether you should be tested for other sexually transmitted diseases.
- **Human immunodeficiency virus (HIV):** Have a test to screen for HIV infection if you have had unprotected sex with multiple partners; are pregnant; have used or now use injection drugs; exchange sex for money or drugs or have sex partners who do; have past or present sex partners who are HIV-infected, are bisexual, or use injection drugs; are being treated for sexually

transmitted diseases; or had a blood transfusion between 1978 and 1985.

Daily Steps to Health

Don't smoke: If you do smoke, talk to your doctor about quitting. If you are pregnant and smoke, quitting now will help you and your baby. Your doctor or nurse can help you. And, you can also help yourself.

Be physically active: Walking briskly, mowing the lawn, dancing, swimming, and bicycling are just a few examples of moderate physical activity. If you are not already physically active, start small and work up to thirty minutes or more of moderate physical activity most days of the week.

Eat a healthy diet: Emphasize fruits, vegetables, whole grains, and fat-free or low-fat milk and milk products; include lean meats, poultry, fish, beans, eggs, and nuts; and eat foods low in saturated fats, trans fats, cholesterol, salt (sodium), and added sugars.

Stay at a healthy weight: Balance calories from foods and beverages with calories you burn off by your activities. To prevent gradual weight gain over time, make small decreases in food and beverage calories and increase physical activity.

Drink alcohol only in moderation: If you drink alcohol, have no more than one drink a day. (A standard drink is one 12-ounce bottle of beer or wine cooler, one 5-ounce glass of wine, or 1.5 ounces of 80-proof distilled spirits.) If you are pregnant, avoid alcohol.

Should You Take Medicines to Prevent Disease?

- **Hormones:** Do not take hormones to prevent disease. Talk to your doctor if you need relief from the symptoms of menopause.
- **Breast cancer drugs:** If your mother, sister, or daughter has had breast cancer, talk to your doctor about the risks and benefits of taking medicines to prevent breast cancer.
- **Aspirin:** Ask your doctor about taking aspirin to prevent heart disease if you are older than forty-five, or younger than forty-five and have high blood pressure, have high cholesterol, have diabetes, or smoke.

- **Immunizations:** Stay up-to-date with your immunizations. Have a flu shot every year starting at age fifty. If you are younger than fifty, ask your doctor whether you need a flu shot. Have a pneumonia shot once after you turn sixty-five. If you are younger, ask your doctor whether you need a pneumonia shot.

Section 4.2

Breast Cancer Screening: Mammograms

Reprinted from "Mammograms," National Women's Health Information Center, April 2006.

What is the best method of detecting breast cancer?

A mammogram, or x-ray of the breast, along with a clinical breast exam (an exam done by your doctor) is the most effective way to detect breast cancer early. Mammograms have both benefits and limitations. For example, some cancers can't be detected by a mammogram, but may be detectable by breast exam.

Checking your own breasts for lumps or other changes is called a breast self-exam (BSE). Studies so far have not shown that BSE alone reduces the numbers of deaths from breast cancer. BSE should not take the place of clinical breast exam and a mammogram.

What is a mammogram?

A mammogram is a safe test used to look for any problems with a woman's breasts. The test uses a special, low-dose x-ray machine to take pictures of both breasts. The results are recorded on x-ray film or directly onto a computer for a radiologist to examine.

Mammograms allow the doctor to have a closer look for breast lumps and changes in breast tissue. They can show small lumps or growths that a doctor or woman may not be able to feel when doing a clinical breast exam. Mammography is the best screening tool that doctors have for finding breast cancer.

If a lump is found, your doctor may order other tests, such as ultrasound or a biopsy—a test where a small amount of tissue is taken from the lump and area around the lump. The tissue is sent to a lab to look for cancer or changes that may mean cancer is likely to develop. Breast lumps or growths can be benign (not cancer) or malignant (cancer). Finding breast cancer early means that a woman has a better chance of surviving the disease. There are also more choices for treatment when breast cancer is found early.

Are there different types of mammograms?

- Screening mammograms are done for women who have no symptoms of breast cancer. When you reach age forty, you should have a mammogram every one to two years.
- Diagnostic mammograms are done when a woman has symptoms of breast cancer or a breast lump. This mammogram takes longer than screening mammograms because more pictures of the breast are taken.
- Digital mammograms take an electronic image of the breast and store it directly in a computer. Current research has not shown that digital images are better at finding cancer than x-ray film images.

How is a mammogram done?

You stand in front of a special x-ray machine. The person who takes the x-rays, called a radiologic technologist, places your breasts (one at a time) between two plastic plates. The plates press your breast to make it flat. You will feel pressure on your breast for a few seconds. It may cause you some discomfort; and you might feel squeezed or pinched. But, the flatter your breast, the better the picture. Most often, two pictures are taken of each breast—one from the side and one from above. A screening mammogram takes about fifteen minutes from start to finish.

What if I have breast implants?

If you have breast implants, be sure to tell your mammography facility that you have them when you make your appointment. You will need an x-ray radiologic technologist who is trained in x-raying patients with implants. This is important because breast implants can hide some breast tissue, which could make if difficult for the radiologist to see breast cancer when looking at your mammograms. For this reason, to take a mammogram of a breast with an implant, the x-ray technician might gently lift the breast tissue slightly away from the implant.

How often should I get a mammogram?

Women forty years and older should get a mammogram every one to two years. Women who have had breast cancer or other breast problems or who have a family history of breast cancer might need to start getting mammograms before age forty, or they might need to get them more often. Talk to your doctor about when to start and how often you should have a mammogram.

Where can I get a mammogram?

Be sure to get a mammogram from a facility certified by the U.S. Food and Drug Administration (FDA). These places must meet high standards for their x-ray machines and staff. Some of these facilities also offer digital mammograms.

Your doctor, local medical clinic, or local or state health department can tell you where to get no-cost or low-cost mammograms.

How do I get ready for my mammogram?

First, check with the place you are having the mammogram for any special instructions you may need to follow before you go. Here are some general guidelines to follow:

- Make your mammogram appointment for one week after your period. Your breasts hurt less after your period.
- If you have breast implants, be sure to tell your mammography facility that you have them when you make your appointment.
- Wear a shirt with shorts, pants, or a skirt. This way, you can undress from the waist up and leave your shorts, pants, or skirt on when you get your mammogram.
- Don't wear any deodorant, perfume, lotion, or powder under your arms or on your breasts on the day of your mammogram appointment. These things can make shadows show up on your mammogram.

Are there any problems with mammograms?

As with any medical test, mammograms have limits. These limits include the following:

- They are only part of a complete breast exam. Your doctor also should do a clinical breast exam. If your mammogram finds something abnormal, your doctor will order other tests.
- "False negatives" can happen. This means everything may look normal, but cancer is actually present. False negatives don't happen often. Younger women are more likely to have a false negative mammogram than are older women. This is because the breast tissue is denser, making cancer harder to spot.
- "False positives" can happen. This is when the mammogram results look like cancer is present, even though it is not. False positives are more common in younger women than older women.

Section 4.3

Screening for Cervical Cancer: Pap Tests

Reprinted from "Pap Test," National Women's Health Information Center, March 2006.

What is a Pap test?

The Pap test, also called a Pap smear, checks for changes in the cells of your cervix. The cervix is the lower part of the uterus (womb) that opens into the vagina (birth canal). The Pap test can tell if you have an infection, abnormal (unhealthy) cervical cells, or cervical cancer.

Why do I need a Pap test?

A Pap test can save your life. It can find the earliest signs of cervical cancer—a common cancer in women. If caught early, the chance of curing cervical cancer is very high. Pap tests also can find infections and abnormal cervical cells that can turn into cancer cells. Treatment can prevent most cases of cervical cancer from developing.

Getting regular Pap tests is the best thing you can do to prevent cervical cancer. About 13,000 women in America will find out they have cervical cancer this year. And in 2004, 3,500 women died from cervical cancer in the United States.

Do all women need Pap tests?

It is important for all women to have pap tests, along with pelvic exams, as part of their routine health care. You need a Pap test if you are twenty-one years or older or under twenty-one years old and have been sexually active for three years or more.

There is no age limit for the Pap test. Even women who have gone through menopause (when a woman's periods stop) need regular Pap tests.

How often do I need to get a Pap test?

It depends on your age and health history. Talk with your doctor about what is best for you. The American College of Obstetricians and Gynecologists recommends the following:

- If you are younger than thirty years old, you should get a Pap test every year.
- If you are age thirty or older and have had normal Pap tests for three years in a row, talk to your doctor about spacing out Pap tests to every two or three years.
- If you are ages sixty-five to seventy and have had at least three normal Pap tests and no abnormal Pap tests in the last ten years, ask your doctor if you can stop having Pap tests.

You should have a Pap test every year no matter how old you are if any of the following are true:

- You have a weakened immune system because of organ transplant, chemotherapy, or steroid use.
- Your mother was exposed to diethylstilbestrol (DES) while pregnant.
- You are human immunodeficiency virus (HIV)-positive.

Women who are living with HIV, the virus that causes acquired immunodeficiency syndrome (AIDS), are at a higher risk of cervical cancer and other cervical diseases. The U.S. Centers for Disease Control and Prevention recommends that all HIV-positive women get an initial Pap test, and get re-tested six months later. If both Pap tests are normal, then these women can get yearly Pap tests in the future.

Who does not need regular Pap tests?

The only women who do not need regular Pap tests are the following:

- Women over age sixty-five who have had a number of normal Pap tests and have been told by their doctors that they don't need to be tested anymore.
- Women who do not have a cervix and are at low risk for cervical cancer. These women should speak to their doctor before stopping regular Pap tests.

I had a hysterectomy. Do I still need Pap tests?

It depends on the type of hysterectomy (surgery to remove the uterus) you had and your health history. Women who have had a hysterectomy should talk with their doctor about whether they need routine Pap tests.

Usually during a hysterectomy, the cervix is removed with the uterus. This is called a total hysterectomy. Women who have had a total hysterectomy for reasons other than cancer may not need regular Pap tests. Women who have had a total hysterectomy because of abnormal cells or cancer should be tested yearly for vaginal cancer until they have three normal test results. Women who have had only their uterus removed but still have a cervix need regular Pap tests. Even women who have had hysterectomies should see their doctors yearly for pelvic exams.

How can I reduce my chances of getting cervical cancer?

Aside from getting Pap tests, the best way to avoid cervical cancer is by steering clear of the human papilloma virus (HPV). HPV is a major cause of cervical cancer. HPV infection is also one of the most common sexually transmitted diseases (STDs). So, a woman boosts her chances of getting cervical cancer if she has the following risk factors:

- Starts having sex before age eighteen
- Has many sex partners
- Has sex partners who have other sex partners
- Has or has had a sexually transmitted disease (STD)

What should I know about human papilloma viruses (HPV)?

Human papilloma viruses are a group of more than one hundred different viruses. About forty types of HPV are spread during sex. Some types of HPVs can cause cervical cancer when not treated. HPV infection is one of the most common sexually transmitted diseases. About 75 percent of sexually active people will get HPV sometime in their life. Most women with untreated HPV do *not* get cervical cancer. Some HPVs cause genital warts but these HPVs do not cause cervical cancer. Since HPV rarely causes symptoms, most people don't know they have the infection.

How would I know if I had human papilloma virus (HPV)?

Most women never know they have HPV. It usually stays hidden and doesn't cause symptoms like warts. When HPV doesn't go away on its own, it can cause changes in the cells of the cervix. Pap tests usually find these changes.

How do I prepare for a Pap test?

Many things can cause wrong test results by washing away or hiding abnormal cells of the cervix. So, doctors suggest that for two days before the test you avoid the following:

- Douching
- Using tampons
- Using vaginal creams, suppositories, and medicines
- Using vaginal deodorant sprays or powders
- Having sex

Should I get a Pap test when I have my period?

No. Doctors suggest you schedule a Pap test when you do not have your period. The best time to be tested is ten to twenty days after the first day of your last period.

How is a Pap test done?

Your doctor can do a Pap test during a pelvic exam. It is a simple and quick test. While you lie on an exam table, the doctor puts an instrument called a speculum into your vagina, opening it to see the cervix. He or she will then use a special stick or brush to take a few cells from inside and around the cervix. The cells are placed on a glass slide and sent to a lab for examination. While usually painless, a Pap test is uncomfortable for some women.

When will I get the results of my Pap test?

Usually it takes three weeks to get Pap test results. Most of the time, test results are normal. If the test shows that something might be wrong, your doctor will contact you to schedule more tests. There are many reasons for abnormal Pap test results. It usually does not mean you have cancer.

What do abnormal Pap test results mean?

It is scary to hear that your Pap test results are "abnormal." But abnormal Pap test results usually do not mean you have cancer. Most often there is a small problem with the cervix.

Some abnormal cells will turn into cancer. But most of the time, these unhealthy cells will go away on their own. By treating these unhealthy cells, almost all cases of cervical cancer can be prevented. If you have abnormal results, to talk with your doctor about what they mean.

My Pap test was "abnormal," what happens now?

There are many reasons for "abnormal" Pap test results. If results of the Pap test are unclear or show a small change in the cells of the cervix, your doctor will probably repeat the Pap test.

If the test finds more serious changes in the cells of the cervix, the doctor will suggest more powerful tests. Results of these tests will help your doctor decide on the best treatment. These include the following:

- **Colposcopy:** The doctor uses a tool called a colposcope to see the cells of the vagina and cervix in detail.
- **Endocervical curettage:** The doctor takes a sample of cells from the endocervical canal with a small spoon-shaped tool called a curette.
- **Biopsy:** The doctor removes a small sample of cervical tissue. The sample is sent to a lab to be studied under a microscope.

The U.S. Food and Drug Administration (FDA) recently approved the LUMA Cervical Imaging System. The doctor uses this device right after a colposcopy. This system can help doctors see areas on the cervix that are likely to contain precancerous cells. This device shines a light on the cervix and looks at how different areas of the cervix respond to this light. It gives a score to tiny areas of the cervix. It then makes a color map that helps the doctor decide where to further test the tissue with a biopsy. The colors and patterns on the map help the doctor tell the difference between healthy tissue and tissue that might be diseased.

My Pap test result was a "false positive." What does this mean?

Pap tests are not always 100 percent correct. False positive and false negative results can happen. This can be upsetting and confusing. A false positive Pap test is when a woman is told she has abnormal cervical cells, but the cells are really normal. If your doctor says your Pap results were a false positive, there is no problem.

A false negative Pap test is when a woman is told her cells are normal, but in fact, there is a problem with the cervical cells that was missed. False negatives delay the discovery and treatment of unhealthy cells of the cervix. But having regular Pap tests boosts your chances of finding any problems. If abnormal cells are missed at one time, they will probably be found on your next Pap test.

I don't have health insurance. How can I get a free or low-cost Pap test?

Programs funded by the National Breast and Cervical Cancer Early Detection Program (NBCCEDP) offer free or low-cost Pap tests to women in need. These and other programs are available throughout the United States. Also, your state or local health department can direct you to places that offer free or low-cost Pap tests.

Section 4.4

Colorectal Cancer Screening

Reprinted from "Colorectal Cancer: Basic Facts on Screening," Centers for Disease Control and Prevention, January 2006.

What Is Colorectal Cancer?

Colorectal cancer is cancer that occurs in the colon or rectum. Sometimes it is called colon cancer, for short. The colon is the large intestine or large bowel. The rectum is the passageway that connects the colon to the anus.

It's the Second Leading Cancer Killer

Colorectal cancer is the second leading cancer killer in the United States, but it doesn't have to be. If everybody age fifty or older had regular screening tests, at least one-third of deaths from this cancer could be avoided. So if you are fifty or older, start screening now.

Who Gets Colorectal Cancer?

- Both men and women can get colorectal cancer.
- Colorectal cancer is most often found in people fifty and older.
- The risk for getting colorectal cancer increases with age.

Are You at High Risk?

Your risk for colorectal cancer may be higher than average if any of the following are true:

- You or a close relative have had colorectal polyps or colorectal cancer.
- You have inflammatory bowel disease.

People at high risk for colorectal cancer may need earlier or more frequent tests than other people. Talk to your doctor about when you should begin screening and how often you should be tested.

Screening Saves Lives

If you're 50 or older, getting a screening test for colorectal cancer could save your life. Here's how:

- Colorectal cancer usually starts from polyps in the colon or rectum. A polyp is a growth that shouldn't be there.
- Over time, some polyps can turn into cancer.
- Screening tests can find polyps, so they can be removed before they turn into cancer.
- Screening tests can also find colorectal cancer early. When it is found early, the chance of being cured is good.

Colorectal Cancer Can Start With No Symptoms

People who have polyps or colorectal cancer sometimes don't have symptoms, especially at first. This means that someone could have polyps or colorectal cancer and not know it. That is why having a screening test is so important.

What Are the Symptoms?

Some people with colorectal polyps or colorectal cancer do have symptoms. They may include the following:

- Blood in or on your stool (bowel movement).
- Pain, aches, or cramps in your stomach that happen a lot and you don't know why.
- A change in bowel habits, such as having stools that are narrower than usual.
- Losing weight and you don't know why.

If you have any of these symptoms, talk to your doctor. These symptoms may also be caused by something other than cancer. However, the only way to know what is causing them is to see your doctor.

Types of Screening Tests

There are several different screening tests that can be used to find polyps or colorectal cancer. Each one can be used alone. Sometimes they are used in combination with each other. Talk to your doctor about which test or tests are right for you and how often you should be tested.

Fecal occult blood test or stool test: For this test, you receive a test kit from your doctor or health care provider. At home, you put a small piece of stool on a test card. You do this for three bowel movements in a row. Then you return the test cards to the doctor or a lab. The stool samples are checked for blood. This test should be done every year.

Flexible sigmoidoscopy: For this test, the doctor puts a short, thin, flexible, lighted tube into your rectum. The doctor checks for polyps or cancer inside the rectum and lower third of the colon. This test should be done every five years.

Fecal occult blood test plus flexible sigmoidoscopy: Your doctor may ask you to have both tests. Some experts believe that by using both tests, there is a better chance of finding polyps or colorectal cancer.

Colonoscopy: This test is similar to flexible sigmoidoscopy, except the doctor uses a longer, thin, flexible, lighted tube to check for polyps or cancer inside the rectum and the entire colon. During the test, the doctor can find and remove most polyps and some cancers. This test should be done every ten years.

Colonoscopy may also be used as a follow-up test if anything unusual is found during one of the other screening tests.

Double contrast barium enema: This test is an x-ray of your colon. You are given an enema with a liquid called barium. Then the doctor takes an x-ray. The barium makes it easy for the doctor to see the outline of your colon on the x-ray to check for polyps or other abnormalities. This test should be done every five years.

Will Insurance or Medicare Pay for Screening Tests?

Many insurance plans and Medicare help pay for colorectal cancer screening tests. Check with your plan to find out which tests are covered for you.

The Bottom Line

If you're fifty or older, talk with your doctor about getting screened.

Section 4.5

Screening for Osteoporosis

Reprinted from "Osteoporosis: The Diagnosis," National Institute of Arthritis and Musculoskeletal and Skin Diseases, National Institutes of Health, November 2005.

Osteoporosis is a condition of low bone density that can progress silently over a long period of time. If diagnosed early, the fractures associated with the disease can often be prevented. Unfortunately, osteoporosis frequently remains undiagnosed until a fracture occurs.

An examination to diagnose osteoporosis can involve several steps that predict your chances of future fracture, diagnose osteoporosis, or both. It might include the following:

- An initial physical exam
- Various x-rays that detect skeletal problems
- Laboratory tests that reveal important information about the metabolic process of bone breakdown and formation
- A bone density test to detect low bone density

Before performing any tests, your doctor will record information about your medical history and lifestyle and will ask questions related to the following:

- Risk factors, including information about any fractures you have had
- Your family history of disease, including osteoporosis
- Medication history
- General intake of calcium and vitamin D
- Exercise pattern
- For women, menstrual history

In addition, the doctor will note medical problems and medications you may be taking that can contribute to bone loss (including glucocorticoids, such as cortisone). He or she will also check your height for changes and your posture to note any curvature of the spine from vertebral fractures, which is known as kyphosis.

Risk Factors

Risk factors for osteoporotic fracture include the following:

- Personal history of fracture as an adult
- History of fracture in a first-degree relative
- Caucasian or Asian race, although African Americans and Hispanic Americans are at significant risk as well
- Advanced age
- Being female
- Dementia
- Poor health, frailty, or both
- Current cigarette smoking
- Low body weight
- Anorexia nervosa
- Estrogen deficiency: Past menopause, menopause before age forty-five, having both ovaries removed, or the absence of menstrual periods for a year or more prior to menopause (women lose bone rapidly in the first four to eight years following menopause, making them more susceptible to osteoporosis)
- Use of certain medications such as corticosteroids and anticonvulsants
- Lifelong low calcium intake
- Excessive alcohol intake
- Impaired eyesight despite adequate correction
- Recurrent falls
- Inadequate physical activity

X-Ray Tests

If you have back pain, your doctor may order an x-ray of your spine to determine whether you have had a fracture. An x-ray also may be appropriate if you have experienced a loss of height or a change in posture. However, since an x-ray can detect bone loss only after 30 percent of the skeleton has been depleted, the presence of osteoporosis may be missed.

Bone Mineral Density Tests

A bone mineral density (BMD) test is the best way to determine your bone health. BMD tests can identify osteoporosis, determine your risk for fractures (broken bones), and measure your response to osteoporosis treatment. The most widely recognized bone mineral density test is called a dual-energy x-ray absorptiometry or DXA test. It is painless: a bit like having an x-ray, but with much less exposure to radiation. It can measure bone density at your hip and spine.

During a BMD test, an extremely low energy source is passed over part or all of the body. The information is evaluated by a computer program that allows the doctor to see how much bone mass you have. Since bone mass serves as an approximate measure of bone strength, this information also helps the doctor accurately detect low bone mass, make a definitive diagnosis of osteoporosis, and determine your risk of future fractures.

BMD tests provide doctors with a measurement called a T-score, a number value that results from comparing your bone density to optimal bone density. When a T-score appears as a negative number such as -1, -2, or -2.5, it indicates low bone mass. The more negative the number, the greater the risk of fracture.

Although no bone density test is 100 percent accurate, this type of test is the single most important predictor of whether a person will fracture in the future.

Bone Scans

For some people, a bone scan may be ordered. A bone scan is different from the BMD test just described, although the term "bone scan" often is used incorrectly to describe a bone density test. A bone scan can tell the doctor whether there are changes that may indicate cancer, bone lesions, inflammation, or new fractures. In a bone scan, the person being tested is injected with a dye that allows a scanner to identify differences in the conditions of various areas of bone tissue.

Laboratory Tests

A number of laboratory tests may be performed on blood and urine samples. The results of these tests can help your doctor identify conditions that may be contributing to your bone loss.

The most common blood tests evaluate the following:

- Blood calcium levels
- Blood vitamin D levels
- Thyroid function
- Parathyroid hormone levels
- Estradiol levels to measure estrogen (in women)
- Follicle stimulating hormone (FSH) test to establish menopause status
- Testosterone levels (in men)
- Osteocalcin levels to measure bone formation

The most common urine tests are as follows:

- Twenty-four-hour urine collection to measure calcium metabolism
- Tests to measure the rate at which a person is breaking down or resorbing bone

Treatment

In addition to diagnosing osteoporosis, results from BMD tests assist the doctor in deciding whether to begin a prevention or treatment program. Once you and your doctor have definitive information based on your history, physical examination, and diagnostic tests, a specific treatment program can be developed for you.

Recommendations for optimizing bone health include a comprehensive program that consists of a well-balanced diet rich in calcium and vitamin D, physical activity, and a healthy lifestyle (including not smoking, avoiding excessive alcohol use, and recognizing that some prescription medications and chronic diseases can cause bone loss). If you already have experienced a fracture, your doctor may refer you to a specialist in physical therapy or rehabilitation medicine to help you with daily activities, safe movement, and exercises to improve your strength and balance.

Chapter 5

Recommended Vaccinations for Women

Chapter Contents

Section 5.1

Vaccination Schedule for Adults

"Vaccinations for Adults," April 2008. Reprinted with permission from the Immunization Action Coalition, www.immunize.org, © 2008.

Getting immunized is a lifelong, life-protecting job. Don't leave your healthcare provider's office without making sure you've had all the vaccinations you need.

Influenza Vaccine

If you are between nineteen and forty-nine years of age, you need a dose yearly if you have a chronic health problem, are a healthcare worker, have close contact with certain individuals (consult your healthcare provider to determine your level of risk for infection and your need for this vaccine), or you simply want to avoid getting influenza or spreading it to others.

If you are aged fifty or older, you need a does every fall or winter.

Pneumococcal Vaccine

Between the ages of nineteen and sixty-four, you need one to two doses of this vaccine if you have certain chronic medical conditions (consult your healthcare provider to determine your level of risk for infection and your need for this vaccine). You need one dose at age sixty-five (or older) if you've never been vaccinated. You may also need a second dose.

Tetanus, Diphtheria, Pertussis (Td, Tdap) Vaccine

If you haven't had at least three tetanus-and-diphtheria-containing shots sometime in your life, you need to get them now. Start with dose number one, followed by dose number two in one month, and dose number three in six months. All adults need Td booster doses every ten years. If you're younger than age sixty-five and haven't had pertussis-containing vaccine as an adult, one of the doses that you receive should have pertussis (whooping cough) vaccine in it—known as Tdap. Be sure to consult your healthcare provider if you have a deep or dirty wound.

Hepatitis B (HepB) Vaccine

You need this vaccine if you have a specific risk factor for hepatitis B virus infection (consult your healthcare provider to determine your level of risk for infection and your need for this vaccine) or you simply wish to be protected from this disease. The vaccine is given as a three-dose series (dose number one now, followed by dose number two in one month, and with dose number three usually given five months later).

Hepatitis A (HepA) Vaccine

You need this vaccine if you have a specific risk factor for hepatitis A virus infection (consult your healthcare provider to determine your level of risk for infection and your need for this vaccine) or you simply wish to be protected from this disease. The vaccine is usually given as two doses, six to eighteen months apart.

Human Papillomavirus (HPV) Vaccine

You need this vaccine if you are a woman who is age twenty-six or younger. The vaccine is given in three doses over six months.

Measles, Mumps, Rubella (MMR) Vaccine

You need at least one dose of MMR if you were born in 1957 or later. You may also need a second dose. Consult your healthcare provider to determine your level of risk for infection and your need for this vaccine.

Varicella (Chickenpox) Vaccine

If you've never had chickenpox or you were vaccinated but received only one dose, talk to your healthcare provider about whether you need this vaccine.

Meningococcal Vaccine

If you are a young adult going to college and plan to live in a dormitory, you need to get vaccinated against meningococcal disease.

People with certain medical conditions should also receive this vaccine (consult your healthcare provider to determine your level of risk for infection and your need for this vaccine).

Zoster (Shingles) Vaccine

If you are age sixty or older, you should get this vaccine now.

Vaccines for Travelers

Do you travel outside the United States? If so, you may need additional vaccines. The Centers for Disease Control and Prevention (CDC) operates an international traveler's health information line. You may also consult a travel clinic or your healthcare provider.

Section 5.2

Human Papillomavirus Vaccine

Reprinted from "HPV (Human Papillomavirus) Vaccine: What You Need to Know," Centers for Disease Control and Prevention, February 2, 2007.

What Is Human Papillomavirus?

Genital human papillomavirus (HPV) is the most common sexually transmitted virus in the United States.

There are about forty types of HPV. About 20 million people in the United States are infected, and about 6.2 million more get infected each year. HPV is spread through sexual contact.

Most HPV infections don't cause any symptoms, and go away on their own. But HPV is important mainly because it can cause cervical cancer in women. Every year in the United States about 10,000 women get cervical cancer and 3,700 die from it. It is the second leading cause of cancer deaths among women around the world.

HPV is also associated with several less common types of cancer in both men and women. It can also cause genital warts and warts in the upper respiratory tract.

More than 50 percent of sexually active men and women are infected with HPV at some time in their lives.

There is no treatment for HPV infection, but the conditions it causes can be treated.

HPV Vaccine: Why Get Vaccinated?

HPV vaccine is an inactivated (not live) vaccine which protects against four major types of HPV.

These include two types that cause about 70 percent of cervical cancer and two types that cause about 90 percent of genital warts. HPV vaccine can prevent most genital warts and most cases of cervical cancer.

Protection from HPV vaccine is expected to be long-lasting. But vaccinated women still need cervical cancer screening because the vaccine does not protect against all HPV types that cause cervical cancer.

Who Should Get HPV Vaccine and When?

Routine Vaccination

HPV vaccine is routinely recommended for girls eleven to twelve years of age. Doctors may give it to girls as young as nine.

Why is HPV vaccine given to girls at this age? It is important for girls to get HPV vaccine before their first sexual contact—because they have not been exposed to HPV. For these girls, the vaccine can prevent almost 100 percent of disease caused by the four types of HPV targeted by the vaccine.

However, if a girl or woman is already infected with a type of HPV, the vaccine will not prevent disease from that type.

Catch-Up Vaccination

The vaccine is also recommended for girls and women thirteen to twenty-six years of age who did not receive it when they were younger.

HPV vaccine is given as a three-dose series: the first dose now, the second dose two months after dose one, and the third dose six months after dose one. Additional (booster) doses are not recommended.

HPV vaccine may be given at the same time as other vaccines.

Who Should Not Get the Vaccine?

Some girls or women should not get HPV vaccine or should wait.

Anyone who has ever had a life-threatening allergic reaction to yeast, to any other component of HPV vaccine, or to a previous dose of HPV vaccine should not get the vaccine. Tell your doctor if the person getting the vaccine has any severe allergies.

Pregnant women should not get the vaccine. The vaccine appears to be safe for both the mother and the unborn baby, but it is still being studied. Receiving HPV vaccine when pregnant is not a reason to consider terminating the pregnancy. Women who are breast feeding may safely get the vaccine.

People who are mildly ill when the shot is scheduled can still get HPV vaccine. People with moderate or severe illnesses should wait until they recover.

What Are the Risks from HPV Vaccine?

HPV vaccine does not appear to cause any serious side effects.

However, a vaccine, like any medicine, could possibly cause serious problems, such as severe allergic reactions. The risk of any vaccine causing serious harm, or death, is extremely small.

Several mild problems may occur with HPV vaccine:

- Pain at the injection site (about eight people in ten)
- Redness or swelling at the injection site (about one person in four)
- Mild fever (100°F) (about one person in ten)
- Itching at the injection site (about one person in thirty)
- Moderate fever (102°F) (about one person in sixty-five)

These symptoms do not last long and go away on their own.

Life-threatening allergic reactions from vaccines are very rare. If they do occur, it would be within a few minutes to a few hours after the vaccination.

Like all vaccines, HPV vaccine will continue to be monitored for unusual or severe problems.

What If There Is a Severe Reaction?

Look for any unusual condition, such as a high fever or behavior changes. Signs of a serious allergic reaction can include difficulty breathing, hoarseness or wheezing, hives, paleness, weakness, a fast heart beat or dizziness.

If a severe reaction occurs, take the following steps:

- Call a doctor, or get the person to a doctor right away.
- Tell your doctor what happened, the date and time it happened, and when the vaccination was given.
- Ask your doctor, nurse, or health department to report the reaction by filing a Vaccine Adverse Event Reporting System (VAERS) form.

How Can I Learn More?

- Ask your doctor or nurse. They can show you the vaccine package insert or suggest other sources of information.
- Call your local or state health department.
- Contact the Centers for Disease Control and Prevention.

Chapter 6

Women's Health: A Statistical Overview

Life Expectancy

A baby girl born in the United States in 2004 could expect to live 80.4 years, 5.2 years longer than her male counterpart, whose life expectancy would be 75.2 years. The life expectancy at birth for white females was 80.8 years; for black females, the life expectancy at birth was 76.3 years.

Between 1970 and 2004, white females' life expectancy increased from 75.6 to 80.8 years (6.9 percent). Black females' life expectancy increased from 68.3 to 76.3 years (11.7 percent) during the same period.

Physical Activity

Regular physical activity promotes health, psychological well-being, and a healthy body weight. To reduce the risk of chronic disease, the *Dietary Guidelines for Americans, 2005* recommends engaging in at least thirty minutes of moderate-intensity physical activity on most days of the week for adults. To prevent weight gain over time, the *Guidelines* recommend about sixty minutes of moderate to vigorous physical activity on most days while not exceeding caloric intake requirements.[1]

Excerpted from "Women's Health USA 2007," U.S. Department of Health and Human Services, Health Resources and Services Administration, 2007.

In 2005, only 50.9 percent of women reported engaging in at least ten minutes of moderate leisure-time physical activity per week, and 32.0 percent reported at least ten minutes of vigorous activity.

Nutrition

The *Dietary Guidelines for Americans, 2005* recommends eating a variety of nutrient-dense foods while not exceeding caloric needs. For most people, this means eating a daily assortment of fruits and vegetables, whole grains, lean meats and beans, and low-fat or fat-free milk products, while limiting added sugar, sodium, saturated and trans fats, and cholesterol.[1]

Some fats, mostly those that come from sources of polyunsaturated or monounsaturated fatty acids, such as fish, nuts, and vegetable oils, are an important part of a healthy diet. However, high intake of saturated fats, trans fats, and cholesterol may increase the risk of coronary heart disease. Most Americans should consume fewer than 10 percent of calories from saturated fats, less than 300 mg/day of cholesterol, and keep trans fatty acid consumption to a minimum. In 2003–04, 63.5 percent of women exceeded the recommended maximum daily intake of saturated fat—most commonly non-Hispanic white women and non-Hispanic black women (65.9 and 64.4 percent, respectively). Salt, or sodium chloride, also plays an important role in heart health, as high salt intake can contribute to high blood pressure. Almost 70 percent of women exceed the recommended intake of less than 2,300 mg/day of sodium (about 1 teaspoon of salt).

Cigarette Smoking

According to the U.S. Surgeon General, smoking damages every organ in the human body. Cigarette smoke contains toxic ingredients that prevent red blood cells from carrying a full load of oxygen, impairs genes that control the growth of cells, and binds to the airways of smokers. This contributes to numerous chronic illnesses, including several types of cancers, chronic obstructive pulmonary disease (COPD), cardiovascular disease, reduced bone density and fertility, and premature death.[2]

In 2005, over sixty million people in the United States aged twelve and older smoked cigarettes within the past month. Smoking was less common among females aged twelve and older (22.5 percent) than among males of the same age group (27.4 percent). The rate has declined over the past several decades among both sexes. In 1985, the rate among males was 43.4, percent while the rate among females was 34.5 percent.

Quitting smoking has major and immediate health benefits, including reducing the risk of diseases caused by smoking and improving overall health.[2] In 2005, over 42 percent of smokers reported trying to quit at least once in the past year. Females were more likely than males to try to quit smoking (44.8 versus 40.7 percent). Among both males and females, non-Hispanic blacks were the most likely to attempt to quit (48.4 and 49.6 percent, respectively).

Smoking during pregnancy can have a negative impact on the health of infants and children by increasing the risk of complications during pregnancy, premature delivery, and low birth weight—a leading cause of infant mortality.[2]

According to the National Survey on Drug Use and Health, 16.6 percent of pregnant women aged fifteen to forty-four smoked in 2004–05; however, this varied by race and ethnicity. Non-Hispanic white women (21.5 percent) were more likely to smoke during pregnancy than women of other races. Hispanic women were least likely to smoke during pregnancy (7.2 percent), while 15 percent of non-Hispanic black women did so.

Alcohol Use

In 2005, 51.8 percent of the total U.S. population aged twelve and older reported using alcohol in the past month; among those aged eighteen and older, the rate was 55.9 percent. According to the Centers for Disease Control and Prevention, alcohol is a central nervous system depressant that, in small amounts, can have a relaxing effect. Although there is some debate over the health benefits of small amounts of alcohol consumed regularly, the negative health effects of excessive alcohol use and abuse are well established. Short-term effects can include increased risk of motor vehicle injuries, falls, domestic violence, and child abuse. Long-term effects can include pancreatitis, high blood pressure, liver cirrhosis, various cancers, and psychological disorders, including dependency.

Overall, males are more likely to drink alcohol than females, with past-month alcohol use reported by 58.1 percent of males and 45.9 percent of females aged twelve years and older. This is true across all age groups with the exception of twelve- to seventeen-year-olds; in that group, 17.2 percent of females and 15.9 percent of males reported past-month use. Males are also more likely than females to engage in binge drinking, which is defined as drinking five or more drinks on the same occasion at least once in the past month (30.5 versus 15.2 percent), and heavy drinking, which is defined as five or more drinks on the same occasion at least five times in the past month (10.3 versus 3.1 percent).

Alcohol use during pregnancy can be a special concern for women of childbearing age. Drinking alcohol during pregnancy can contribute to fetal alcohol syndrome (FAS), low birth weight in infants, and developmental delays. In 2004–05, 12.1 percent of pregnant women reported drinking alcohol in the past month. This was most common in the fifteen to seventeen and twenty-six to forty-four year age groups (13.9 and 13.5 percent, respectively) and least common among those in the eighteen to twenty-five year age group (9.7 percent).

Illicit Drug Use

Illicit drugs are associated with serious health and social consequences, such as addiction. Illicit drugs include marijuana/hashish, cocaine, inhalants, hallucinogens, crack, and prescription-type psychotherapeutic drugs used for non-medical purposes. In 2005, nearly 12.7 million women aged eighteen years and older reported using an illicit drug within the past year; this represents 11.2 percent of women. The past-year illicit drug use rate was significantly higher among women aged eighteen to twenty-five years than among women twenty-six years and older (30.1 percent versus 8.1 percent). Among adolescent females aged twelve to seventeen years, 20.0 percent reported using illicit drugs in the past year.

According to the National Survey on Drug Use and Health's 2004–05 estimates, 3.9 percent of pregnant women reported using illicit drugs in the past month. Among pregnant fifteen- to seventeen-year-olds, 12.3 percent, or 1 in 8, reported past month illicit drug use. Women eighteen and older were less likely to report illicit drug use during pregnancy: the rate was 7.0 percent among eighteen- to twenty-five-year-olds, and 1.6 percent among those aged twenty-six to forty-four years.

HIV/AIDS

Acquired immunodeficiency syndrome (AIDS) is the final stage of the human immunodeficiency virus (HIV), which destroys or disables the cells that are responsible for fighting infection. AIDS is diagnosed when HIV has weakened the immune system enough that the body has a difficult time fighting infections.[3] In 2005, there were an estimated 10,774 new AIDS cases among adolescent and adult females, compared to 29,766 new cases among males of the same age group.

Men have been disproportionately affected by AIDS, but the rate among women is increasing at a faster pace; since 2001, new AIDS cases have increased by 7.2 percent among females compared to a 6.7 percent increase among males.

Arthritis

Arthritis, the leading cause of disability among Americans over fifteen years of age, comprises more than one hundred different diseases that affect areas in or around the joints.[4] The most common type is osteoarthritis, which is a degenerative joint disease that causes pain and loss of movement due to deterioration in the cartilage covering the ends of bones in the joints. Other types of arthritis include rheumatoid arthritis, lupus arthritis, gout, and fibromyalgia.

In 2005, over 21 percent of adults in the United States reported that they had ever been diagnosed with arthritis. Arthritis was more common in women than men (25.5 versus 17.4 percent), and rates of arthritis increased dramatically with age for both sexes. Fewer than 10 percent of women in the eighteen to forty-four year age group had been diagnosed with arthritis, compared to 52.7 percent among women aged sixty-five to seventy-four years, and almost 60 percent of women seventy-five years and older.

In 2005, the rate of arthritis among women varied by race and ethnicity. It was most common among non-Hispanic white women (282.1 per 1,000 women), followed by non-Hispanic black women (243.3 per 1,000). The lowest rates of arthritis were among Asian and Hispanic women (124.4 and 144.2 per 1,000, respectively).

Asthma

Asthma is a chronic inflammatory disorder of the airway characterized by episodes of wheezing, chest tightness, shortness of breath, and coughing. This disorder may be aggravated by allergens, tobacco smoke, and other irritants; exercise; and infections of the respiratory tract. However, by taking certain precautions, persons with asthma may be able to effectively manage this disorder and participate in daily activities.

In 2005, women had higher rates of asthma than men (91.9 per 1,000 women versus 51.1 per 1,000 men); this was true in every racial and ethnic group. Among women, non-Hispanic black women had the highest asthma rate (108.4 per 1,000 women), followed by non-Hispanic white women (93.8 per 1,000); Asian women had the lowest asthma rate (55.6 per 1,000).

Autoimmune Diseases

Autoimmune diseases comprise more than eighty serious, chronic illnesses that can involve almost every human organ system. The common thread among these diseases is that the body's own immune system attacks itself. For largely unknown reasons, about 75 percent of autoimmune diseases occur in women, most frequently in women of childbearing age.

The most common autoimmune diseases include thyroid disease and systemic lupus erythematosus. Hashimoto disease, or hypothyroiditis, is a disease in which the immune system destroys the thyroid, and it occurs in ten women for every one man. Graves disease, in which excessive amounts of thyroid hormone are produced, is another thyroid disease that occurs more frequently in women than men.

Lupus is an inflammation of the connective tissues that can affect multiple organ systems; it occurs in nine women for every one man. In addition to lupus, connective tissue diseases include rheumatoid arthritis, a disorder in which the membranes around joints become inflamed; Sjögren syndrome, in which patients slowly lose the ability to secrete saliva and tears; and scleroderma, which activates immune cells to produce scar tissue in the skin, internal organs, and small blood vessels.

Multiple sclerosis, twice as common in women as in men, is a disease of the central nervous system characterized by numbness, weakness, tingling, or paralysis of the limbs, impaired vision, and/or lack of coordination. Myasthenia gravis also results in gradual muscle weakness. Antiphospholipid syndrome occurs when antibodies attack body tissues and organs and results in the formation of blood clots in arteries or veins. Autoimmune thrombocytopenic purpura is characterized by the failure of blood to clot as it should. Autoimmune hepatitis and primary biliary cirrhosis both cause the liver to become inflamed, which can lead to cirrhosis, or scarring, of the liver and liver failure.

Autoimmune diseases are poorly understood and little comprehensive data exist. However, the LUMINA (Lupus in Minority Populations: Nature vs. Nurture) study has provided new data about the relationship between ethnicity and outcomes among patients with lupus. The study found that black and Hispanic lupus patients have more active disease and more organ system involvement than white patients. Data also showed that black patients may accrue more renal damage than white patients and more skin damage than either Hispanic or white patients.[5]

Diabetes

Diabetes is a chronic condition and a leading cause of death and disability in the United States. Complications of diabetes are serious and may include blindness, kidney damage, heart disease, stroke, and nervous system disease.

In 2005, women and men reported similar rates of having ever been told they had diabetes, though women under the age of forty-five were slightly more likely than men of the same age group. The rate of diabetes increased with age for both sexes; however, older men were more likely to have diabetes than their female counterparts. The rate of diabetes among women under the age of forty-five was 25.1 per 1,000 women, compared to 22.9 per 1,000 men of the same age. The rates among women and men seventy-five years and older were 146.4 and 170.1 per 1,000, respectively.

Non-Hispanic black women were more likely than women of other racial and ethnic groups to have diabetes: the rate of diabetes among this group was 106.8 per 1,000 in 2005, compared to a rate of 77.1 per 1,000 Hispanic women, 71.6 per 1,000 American Indian/Alaska natives and women of multiple races, and 69.1 per 1,000 non-Hispanic white women. Asian women had the lowest rate of diabetes (49.7 per 1,000). Most women with diabetes of all racial and ethnic groups do not take insulin, which may indicate that they have Type 2 diabetes. Non-Hispanic white and Hispanic women with diabetes were less likely than non-Hispanic black women to take insulin in 2005.

Cancer

Lung and bronchus cancer is the leading cause of cancer death among females, accounting for 26 percent of cancer deaths, followed by breast cancer, which is responsible for 15 percent of deaths. Colon and rectal cancer, pancreatic cancer, and ovarian cancer are also significant causes of cancer deaths among females. Due to the varying survival rates for different types of cancer, the most common causes of cancer death are not always the most common types of cancer. For instance, although lung and bronchus cancers cause the greatest number of deaths, breast cancer is the most common type of cancer among women. Other types of cancer that are common among females but are not among the top ten causes of cancer deaths include melanoma, thyroid cancer, and cancer of the kidney and renal pelvis. In addition, other types of cancer, such as some skin cancers, are common but may not lead to death.

Gynecological and Reproductive Disorders

Gynecological disorders affect the internal and external organs in a woman's pelvic and abdominal areas and may affect a woman's fertility. These disorders include vulvodynia—unexplained chronic discomfort or pain of the vulva—and chronic pelvic pain, which is a consistent and severe pain occurring mostly in the lower abdomen for at least six months. While the causes of vulvodynia are unknown, recent evidence suggests that it may occur in up to 16 percent of women, usually beginning before age twenty-five, and that Hispanic women are at greater risk for this disorder.[6] Chronic pelvic pain may be symptomatic of an infection or indicate a problem with one of the organs in the pelvic area.[7]

Reproductive disorders may affect a woman's ability to get pregnant. Examples of these disorders include polycystic ovary syndrome (PCOS), endometriosis, and uterine fibroids. PCOS occurs when immature follicles in the ovaries form together to create a large cyst, preventing mature eggs from being released. In most cases, the failure of the follicles to release the eggs results in a woman's inability to become pregnant. An estimated 5 to 10 percent of women in the United States are affected by PCOS. Endometriosis, in which tissue resembling that of the uterine lining grows outside of the uterus, is estimated to affect nearly 5.5 million women in North America. Uterine fibroids are noncancerous tumors that grow underneath the lining, between the muscles, or on the outside of the uterus. A hysterectomy—abdominal surgery to remove the uterus—is one option to treat certain conditions including chronic pelvic pain, uterine fibroids, PCOS, and endometriosis when symptoms are severe.[7]

In 2004, 8.1 percent of women aged twenty to fifty-four years had endometriosis and 15.6 percent had uterine fibroids, but the prevalence of both disorders varied with age. Of women aged twenty to fifty-four years, endometriosis was most common among the thirty-five- to forty-four-year-old age group (12.4 percent), while uterine fibroids were most common among forty-five- to fifty-four-year-olds (27.6 percent). Women aged twenty to thirty-four years were least likely to have either disorder (4.1 and 2.1 percent, respectively).

Heart Disease and Stroke

In 2004, heart disease was the leading cause of death among women. Heart disease describes any disorder that prevents the heart from functioning normally.

In 2005, adult women under forty-five years had a higher rate of heart disease than men of the same age (50.9 versus 35.2 per 1,000 adults, respectively). However, men had a slightly higher overall rate of heart disease than women. Heart disease rates among both sexes increased with age.

In 2005, the highest rate of heart disease was among non-Hispanic white women (128.7 per 1,000), followed by non-Hispanic black women (107.1 per 1,000); Asian women had the lowest rate (51.1 per 1,000). Although non-Hispanic white women experience the highest rates of heart disease, deaths from heart disease are highest among non-Hispanic black women.

Hypertension

Hypertension, also known as high blood pressure, is a risk factor for a number of conditions, including heart disease and stroke. It is defined as a systolic pressure (during heartbeats) of 140 or higher, and/or a diastolic pressure (between heartbeats) of 90 or higher. In 2005, women had higher overall rates of hypertension than men (265.9 versus 249.9 per 1,000 population); however, these rates varied by race and ethnicity. For instance, non-Hispanic black and Hispanic women had higher rates of hypertension than their male counterparts, while non-Hispanic white and Asian women had rates similar to men. Among women, non-Hispanic blacks had the highest rate of hypertension (353.8 per 1,000 women), followed by non-Hispanic whites (264.5 per 1,000); Asian women had the lowest rate (190.4 per 1,000).

Rates of hypertension increase substantially with age and are highest among those seventy-five years and older, which demonstrates the chronic nature of the disease. The rate among women aged eighteen to forty-four years was 90.7 per 1,000 women in 2005, compared to a rate of 345.8 per 1,000 women aged forty-five to sixty-four years, 570.6 per 1,000 women aged sixty-five to seventy-four years, and 633.0 per 1,000 women aged seventy-five years and older. This means that almost two-thirds of those in the oldest age group have ever been diagnosed with hypertension.

Leading Causes of Death

In 2004, there were 1,215,947 female deaths in the United States. Of these deaths, nearly half were attributable to heart disease and malignant neoplasms (cancer), responsible for 330,513 and 267,058 deaths, respectively. The next two leading causes of death were cerebrovascular diseases (stroke), which accounted for 7.5 percent of deaths, followed by chronic lower respiratory disease, which accounted for 5.2 percent.

Heart disease was the leading cause of death for women in almost every racial and ethnic group; the exception was Asian/Pacific Islander females, for whom the leading cause of death was cancer. One of the most noticeable differences in leading causes of death by race and ethnicity is that chronic lower respiratory disease was the fourth leading cause of death among non-Hispanic white females while it was the seventh leading cause of death among other racial and ethnic groups. Similarly, diabetes mellitus was the eighth leading cause of death among non-Hispanic white females, while it was the fourth among other racial and ethnic groups. Among Hispanic females, death in the perinatal period was the ninth leading cause of death, and hypertension was the tenth leading cause among Asian/Pacific Islander females. Also noteworthy is that Native American/Alaska Native females experienced a higher proportion of deaths due to unintentional injury (8.5 percent) and liver disease (4.2 percent) than females of other racial and ethnic groups.

Mental Illness and Suicide

Mental illness affects both sexes, although many types of mental disorders are more prevalent among women. Among adults interviewed in 2001–03, 23.0 percent of women had experienced any anxiety disorder in the past year, compared to 13.8 percent of men.

Other common mental disorders include social phobia, generalized anxiety disorder, and major depressive disorder, all of which are more common among women than men.

Among women, mental disorders are most common among those aged eighteen to twenty-five years. Serious psychological distress occurs among almost 23 percent of women in this age group, compared to nearly 16 percent of women aged twenty-six to forty-nine years and 9.0 percent of women aged fifty years and older. Major depressive disorder displays a similar pattern, occurring most frequently among those women eighteen to twenty-five years (12.9 percent), compared to twenty-six- to forty-nine-year-olds and those aged fifty years and older (10.5 and 6.6 percent, respectively).

Although most people who suffer from mental illness do not commit suicide, mental illness is a major risk factor. Women attempt suicide three times as often as men, but men are much more likely to die of suicide injury than women.[8] In 2004, the female suicide death rate among those aged fifteen years and older was 5.7 per 100,000 females,

Table 6.1. Ten Leading Causes of Death Among Females (All Ages), by Race/Ethnicity, 2004

Rank	Cause	Total %	Non-Hispanic White %	Non-Hispanic Black %	Hispanic %	Asian/ Pacific Islander %	American Indian/ Alaska Native %
1	Heart Disease	27.2	27.5	26.9	23.8	23.7	19.4
2	Malignant Neoplasms (cancer)	22.0	22.0	21.3	21.4	26.9	19.2
3	Cerebrovascular Diseases (stroke)	7.5	7.5	7.4	6.6	9.8	5.6
4	Chronic Lower Respiratory Disease	5.2	5.8	2.4	2.7	2.3	4.2
5	Alzheimer Disease	3.9	4.2	2.2	2.4	1.8	N/A
6	Unintentional Injury	3.3	3.2	2.9	4.8	4.0	8.5
7	Influenza and Pneumonia	3.1	2.8	2.1	2.8	3.4	2.5
8	Diabetes Mellitus	2.7	2.6	5.1	5.8	4.0	6.4
9	Nephritis (kidney inflammation)	1.8	1.6	3.0	2.0	1.7	2.3
10	Septicemia (blood poisoning)	1.5	1.4	2.3	N/A	N/A	1.6

Source: Centers for Disease Control and Prevention, National Center for Injury Prevention and Control

Note: N/A = not in the top ten leading causes of death for this racial/ethnic group.

compared to a rate of 22.4 per 100,000 males. Although mental disorders affect women in younger age groups more often than women in older age groups, women aged forty-five to fifty-four years have the highest suicide death rate among females (8.6 per 100,000). Among males, the highest suicide death rate occurs in the sixty-five to eighty-four age group (27.2 per 100,000).

There are also disparities in suicide rates among racial and ethnic groups. Among females aged fifteen years and older, American Indian/Alaska natives have the highest suicide rate (8.0 per 100,000 females), followed by non-Hispanic whites (6.8 per 100,000). Non-Hispanic black females have the lowest suicide rates among all racial and ethnic groups (2.3 per 100,000), closely followed by Hispanic females (2.5 per 100,000).

Osteoporosis

Osteoporosis is the most common underlying cause of fractures in the elderly, but it is not frequently diagnosed or treated, even among individuals who have already suffered a fracture. An estimated ten million Americans now have osteoporosis, while another thirty-four million have low bone mass and are at risk for developing osteoporosis; 80 percent of them are women. By 2020, an estimated 1 in 2 Americans over age fifty will be at risk for osteoporosis and low bone mass. Each year more than 1.5 million people suffer a bone fracture related to osteoporosis, with the most common breaks in the wrist, spine, and hip. Fractures can have devastating consequences. For example, hip fractures are associated with an increased risk of mortality, and nearly 1 in 5 hip fracture patients ends up in a nursing home within a year. Direct care for osteoporotic fractures costs $18 billion yearly.[9]

In 2003–04, women aged eighteen years and older were more likely than men to report having been told by a health professional that they have osteoporosis (10.0 versus 1.7 percent, respectively.) In addition, 72.4 percent of women with osteoporosis received treatment, compared to 52.1 percent of men. The rate of osteoporosis among women varied significantly with age. While only 5.3 percent aged eighteen to sixty-four years had osteoporosis in 2003–04, 33.8 percent of women aged seventy-five to eighty-four years and 32.9 percent of those aged eighty-five years and older reported having osteoporosis.

Overweight and Obesity

Being overweight or obese increases the risk for numerous ailments, including high blood pressure, diabetes, heart disease, stroke, arthritis, cancer, and poor reproductive health.[10] According to the Centers for Disease Control and Prevention, 61.5 percent of women were overweight or obese in 2003–04.

Since 1960, rates of overweight and obesity among women have increased dramatically. In 1960–62, 24.5 percent of women were overweight and 15.7 percent were obese, compared to 27.4 and 34.0 percent, respectively, in 2001–04. This marks an 11.8 percent increase in female overweight and a 116.6 percent increase in female obesity over the past four decades.

Rates of overweight and obesity among women vary by race and ethnicity. In 2003–04, Hispanic women (32.1 percent) were more likely than non-Hispanic white and non-Hispanic black women to be overweight (28.4 and 26.9 percent, respectively). Non-Hispanic black women were most likely to be obese (53.0 percent), while non-Hispanic white women were least likely to be obese (30.3 percent).

Sexually Transmitted Infections

Reported rates of sexually transmitted infections (STIs) among females vary by a number of factors, including age and race/ethnicity. Rates are highest among adolescents and young adults, and non-Hispanic blacks and American Indian/Alaska natives. In 2005, there were 1,729 cases of chlamydia and 590 cases of gonorrhea per 100,000 non-Hispanic black females, compared to 237 and 43 cases, respectively, per 100,000 non-Hispanic white females. American Indian/Alaska native females also have high rates of STIs with 1,778 and 170 cases of chlamydia and gonorrhea, respectively, per 100,000 females.

Although these STIs are treatable with antibiotics, they can have serious health consequences. Active infections can increase the odds of contracting another STI, such as HIV, and untreated STIs can lead to pelvic inflammatory disease, infertility, and adverse pregnancy outcomes.

Another STI, genital human papillomavirus (HPV), has been estimated to affect at least 50 percent of the sexually active population. The first study to examine the prevalence of HPV in the United States was recently released, based on data from the National Health and Nutrition Examination Survey. Overall, 26.8 percent of females aged fourteen to fifty-nine years were found to have HPV, with the highest rates occurring among the twenty- to twenty-four-year-old age group (44.8 percent). There are many different types of HPV, and some, which are referred to as "high-risk," can cause cancer. In 2006, the Food and Drug Administration approved a vaccine that protects women from four strains of HPV that can be the source of cervical cancer, precancerous lesions, and genital warts.[11]

Sleep Disorders

Sleep is a necessity of life; however, in a 2007 poll by the National Sleep Foundation, almost one-third of women reported getting "a good night's sleep" (as defined by respondents) only a few nights a month or less. In the same poll, 39 percent of women reported getting a good night's sleep every night or almost every night, while another 32 percent report getting a good night's sleep a few nights a week. Pregnant and postpartum women were more likely than women overall to report rarely or never getting a good night's sleep (30 and 42 percent versus 15 percent, respectively).

Overall, about two-thirds of women reported experiencing a sleep problem at least a few nights a week within the past month, with 46 percent reporting that this occurred every night or almost every night. The most common sleep problem was waking up feeling unrefreshed, which was reported to occur at least a few nights a week by half of all women. Almost half of women (49 percent) reported being awake a lot during the night at least a few nights a week, 37 percent reported difficulty falling asleep a few nights a week, and just over one-third of women reported waking up too early and not being able to fall back asleep.

References

1. U.S. Department of Health and Human Services; U.S. Department of Agriculture. *Dietary Guidelines for Americans 2005*. Washington, DC: U.S. Government Printing Office, January 2005.

2. U.S. Department of Health and Human Services. *The health consequences of smoking: a report of the Surgeon General. 2004.*

3. Centers for Disease Control and Prevention. HIV/AIDS Basic Information. Available from: http://www.cdc.gov/hiv/topics/basic/index.htm. Viewed 8/15/07.

4. Arthritis Foundation. The facts about arthritis. 2004. http://www.arthritis.org. Viewed 4/18/07.

5. Alarcon, GS, K Brooks, J Reveille, JR Lisse. Do Patients of Hispanic and African-American Ethnicity with Lupus Experience

Worse Outcomes than Patients with Lupus from Other Populations? The LUMINA Study. *SLE in Clinical Practice*. 1999; 2(3).

6. Harlow et al A Population-Based Assessment of Chronic Unexplained Vulvar Pain: Have we underestimated the prevalence of vulvodynia? *JAMWA*. 2003; 58: 82–88.

7. National Institutes of Health, National Institute of Child Health and Human Development. www.nichd.nih.gov. Viewed 4/16/07.

8. Centers for Disease Control and Prevention, National Center for Injury Prevention and Control. Suicide: Fact Sheet. www.cdc.gov/ncipc. Viewed 4/18/07.

9. U.S. Department of Health and Human Services. *Bone Health and Osteoporosis: A Report of the Surgeon General*. Rockville, MD: Office of the Surgeon General; 2004.

10. Centers for Disease Control and Prevention, National Center for Chronic Disease Prevention and Health Promotion. Overweight and obesity. June 2004. www.cdc.gov/nccdphp/dnpa/obesity. Viewed 4/16/07.

11. *FDA News*. FDA Licenses New Vaccine for Prevention of Cervical Cancer and Other Diseases in Females Caused by Human Papillomavirus. June 8, 2006.

Chapter 7

Health Disparities Affecting Minority Women

Health Disparities Affecting Minorities: African Americans

According to the 2000 U.S. census, African Americans account for 13 percent of the U.S. population, or 36.4 million individuals.

Major health disparities for African Americans are as follows:

- **Human immunodeficiency virus/acquired immunodeficiency syndrome (HIV/AIDS):** In 2001, African Americans accounted for more than 50 percent of all new HIV/AIDS diagnoses.
- **Heart disease and stroke:** In 2001, the African American age-adjusted death rate for heart disease (316.9 per 100,000) was 30.1 percent higher than that of white Americans (243.5) and 41.2 percent higher than that of white Americans for stroke (78.8 per 100,000 vs. 55.8).
- **Cancer:** The age-adjusted death rate for cancer was 25.4 percent higher for African Americans (243.1 per 100,000) than for white Americans (193.9) in 2001.

Excerpted from "Health Disparities Affecting Minorities: African Americans," "Health Disparities Affecting Minorities: American Indian/Alaska Natives," "Health Disparities Affecting Minorities: Asian Americans," "Health Disparities Affecting Minorities: Native Hawaiian and Other Pacific Islanders," and "Health Disparities Affecting Minorities: Hispanic/Latino Americans," Centers for Disease Control and Prevention, October 2005.

- **Adult immunization:** Influenza vaccination coverage among adults sixty-five years of age and older was 70.2 percent for whites and 52.0 percent for African Americans in 2001. The gap for pneumococcal vaccination coverage among older adults was even wider, with 60.6 percent for whites and 36.1 percent for African Americans.
- **Diabetes:** The age-adjusted death rate for African Americans in 2001 was more than twice that for white Americans (49.2 per 100,000 vs. 23.0).

Health Disparities Affecting Minorities: American Indian/Alaska Natives

According to the 2000 U.S. census, American Indians and Alaska natives (AI/AN) comprise 0.9 to 1.5 percent of the U.S. population and have the highest poverty rates of all Americans.

Major health disparities for American Indian/Alaska Natives include the following:

- **Chronic diseases:** The 2002 age-adjusted prevalence rate of diabetes was over twice that for all U.S. adults, and the AI/AN mortality rate from chronic liver disease was nearly three times higher.
- **Infant mortality:** AI/AN rates were 1.6 times higher than non-Hispanic white rates. The AI/AN sudden infant death syndrome (SIDS) rate was the highest of any population group, more than double that of whites in 1999.
- **Sexually transmitted diseases (STDs):** The syphilis rate among AI/AN was six times higher than the syphilis rate among the non-Hispanic white population, the chlamydia rate was 5.5 times higher, the gonorrhea rate was four times higher, and the AIDS rate was 1.5 times higher in 2001.
- **Injuries:** In 2001 AI/AN death rates for unintentional injuries and motor vehicle crashes were 1.7 to 2.0 times higher than the rates for all racial/ethnic populations, while suicide rates for AI/AN youth were three times greater than rates for whites of similar age.

Health Disparities Affecting Minorities: Asian Americans

According to the 2000 U.S. census, Asian Americans represent 4.2 percent of the U.S. population, or 11.9 million individuals.

Major health disparities for Asian Americans are as follows:

- **Cancer:** During 1988–92, the highest age-adjusted incidence rate of cervical cancer occurred among Vietnamese American women (43 per 100,000), almost five times higher than the rate among non-Hispanic white women (7.5).
- **Tuberculosis:** Asian Americans and Pacific Islanders had the highest tuberculosis (TB) case rates (33 per 100,000) of any racial and ethnic population in 2001 (14 per 100,000 for non-Hispanic blacks, 12 per 100,000 for Hispanics/Latinos, 11 per 100,000 for American Indians/Alaska natives, and 2 per 100,000 for non-Hispanic whites).
- **Hepatitis B virus (HBV):** The rate of acute hepatitis B (HBV) among Asian Americans and Pacific Islanders has been decreasing, but the reported rate in 2001 was more than twice as high among Asian Americans and Pacific Islanders (2.95 per 100,000) than among white Americans (1.31).

Health Disparities Affecting Minorities: Native Hawaiian and Other Pacific Islanders

According to the 2000 U.S. census, Native Hawaiian and other Pacific Islanders represent 0.3 percent of the U.S. population, or 874,000 individuals.

Major health disparities for Native Hawaiians and other Pacific Islanders are as follows:

- **Diabetes:** During 1996–2000, Native Hawaiians were 2.5 times more likely to be diagnosed with diabetes than non-Hispanic white residents of Hawaii of similar age.
- **Infant mortality:** In 2000, infant mortality among Native Hawaiians was 9.1 per 1,000, almost 60 percent higher than among whites (5.7).
- **Hepatitis B virus (HBV):** The rate if acute hepatitis B (HBV) among Asian Americans and Pacific Islanders has been decreasing, but the reported rate in 2001 was more than twice as high among Asian Americans and Pacific Islanders (2.95 per 100,000) than among white Americans (1.31).
- **Asthma:** Native Hawaiians in Hawaii have an asthma rate of 139.5 per 1,000 in 2000, almost twice the rate for all other races in Hawaii (71.5).

Health Disparities Affecting Minorities: Hispanic/Latino Americans

According to the 2000 U.S. census, Hispanics/Latinos represent 13.3 percent of the U.S. population, or 38.8 million individuals.

Major health disparities for Hispanics/Latinos are as follows:

- **HIV/AIDS:** The age-adjusted death rate for HIV in 1999 was 32.7 per 100,000 for Puerto Ricans living on the mainland U.S., higher than any other racial or ethnic groups, more than six times the national average (5.4), and more than thirteen times the rate for non-Hispanic whites (2.4).
- **Diabetes:** The diabetes death rate in 2000 was highest among Puerto Ricans (172 per 100,000), Mexican Americans (122), and Cuban Americans (47) for Hispanics/Latinos.
- **Adult immunization:** Influenza vaccination coverage among adults sixty-five years of age and older is 70.2 percent for whites and 46.7 percent for Hispanics/Latinos. The gap for pneumococcal vaccination coverage among older adults is even wider, with 60.6 percent for whites and 23.8 percent for Hispanics/Latinos in 2002.
- **Asthma:** In the northeast United States, from 1993–95, Hispanics/Latinos had an asthma death rate of 34 per million, more than twice the rate for white Americans (15.1).

What You Can Do to Eliminate Health Disparities

Healthcare providers can take these steps:

- Advise and encourage clients to reduce their risk for chronic and infectious illnesses
- Ensure that standing orders are in place for screening tests
- Advise seniors and medically compromised clients to get pneumococcal and influenza vaccinations
- Provide culturally competent and linguistically appropriate care

Individuals can do the following:

- Think prevention—see a healthcare provider annually, even if you feel healthy

- Eat more fruits and vegetables and less fat and sugar
- Get at least thirty minutes of physical activity daily—taking the stairs burns five times more calories than taking the elevator
- Take loved ones to a healthcare provider
- Stop smoking

Communities can participate in these ways:

- Join with others to promote community-wide health activities and campaigns
- Form coalitions with civic, professional, religious, and educational organizations to advocate health policies, programs, and services
- Support policies that promote healthcare access for all

Chapter 8

Lesbian Health Concerns

What challenges do lesbian women face in the health care system?

Lesbians face unique challenges within the health care system that can cause poorer mental and physical health. Many doctors, nurses, and other health care providers have not had sufficient training to understand the specific health experiences of lesbians, or that women who are lesbians, like heterosexual women, can be healthy normal females. There can be barriers to optimal health for lesbians, such as the following:

- Fear of negative reactions from their doctors if they disclose their sexual orientation
- Doctors' lack of understanding of lesbians' disease risks, and issues that may be important to lesbians
- Lack of health insurance because of no domestic partner benefits
- Low perceived risk of getting sexually transmitted diseases and some types of cancer

For the above reasons, lesbians often avoid routine health exams and even delay seeking medical care when health problems occur.

Reprinted from "Lesbian Health," National Women's Health Information Center, January 2005.

What are important health issues for lesbians to discuss with their doctors or nurses?

Heart disease: Heart disease is the number one killer of all women. Factors that raise women's risk for heart disease—such as obesity, smoking, and stress—are high among lesbians. The more risk factors (or things that increase risk) a woman has, the greater the chance that she will develop heart disease. There are some factors that you can't control, such as getting older, family health history, and race. But you can do something about some of the biggest risk factors for heart and cardiovascular disease—smoking, high blood pressure, lack of exercise, diabetes, and high blood cholesterol.

Exercise: Studies have shown that physical inactivity adds to a person's risk for getting heart and cardiovascular disease, as well as some cancers. People who are not active are twice as likely to develop heart and cardiovascular disease compared to those who are more active. The more overweight you are, the higher your risk for heart disease. More research with lesbians in this area is needed.

Obesity: Being obese can make you more likely to get heart disease, and cancers of the uterus, ovary, breast, and colon. Many studies have found that lesbians have a higher body mass than heterosexual women. Studies suggest that lesbians may store fat more in the abdomen and have a greater waist circumference, which places them at higher risk for heart disease and other obesity-related issues such as premature death. Additionally, some suggest that lesbians are less concerned about weight issues than heterosexual women.

At this time, more research is needed in these areas: physical activity in lesbians; possible dietary differences between lesbians and heterosexual women; if a higher body mass index (BMI) is a reflection of lean tissue and not excess fat; and if there's a different cultural norm among lesbians about thinness. In addition, other important factors for researchers to consider are race/ethnic background, age, health status, education, cohabitation with a female relationship partner, and having a disability. Studies have reported that among lesbian and bisexual women, African American or Latina ethnicity, older age, poorer health status, lower educational attainment, lower exercise frequency, and cohabiting with a female relationship partner increases a lesbian woman's likelihood of having a higher BMI.

Nutrition: Research supports that lesbian and bisexual women are less likely to eat fruits and vegetables every day. More research on food consumption and dietary differences in relation to health and lesbians and bisexuals is needed.

Smoking: Smoking can lead to heart disease and multiple cancers, including cancers of the lung, throat, stomach, colon, and cervix. Lesbians are more likely to smoke, compared to heterosexual women. Researchers think that high rates of smoking in this population are a consequence of several things, like social factors, such as low self-esteem, stress resulting from discrimination, concealing one's sexual orientation, and tobacco advertising targeted toward gays and lesbians. Studies have also found that smoking rates are higher among gay and lesbian adolescents compared to the general population. Smoking as a teen increases the risk of becoming an adult smoker. We know that about 90 percent of adult smokers started smoking as teens.

Depression and anxiety: Many factors cause depression and anxiety among all women. Studies show that lesbian and bisexual women report higher rates of depression and anxiety than heterosexual women do. This may result from the fact that lesbian women may also face social stigma, rejection by family members, abuse and violence, being treated unfairly in the legal system, hiding some or all aspects of one's life, and lacking health insurance.

Lesbians often feel they have to conceal their lesbian status to family, friends, and employers. Lesbians can also be recipients of hate crimes and violence. Despite strides in our larger society, discrimination against lesbians does exist, and discrimination for any reason may lead to depression and anxiety.

Alcohol and drug abuse: Substance abuse is as serious a public health problem for the lesbians, gay men, bisexuals, and transgendered people (LGBT) as it is for the general U.S. population. Overall, recent data suggest that substance use among lesbians—particularly alcohol use—has declined over the past two decades. Reasons for this decline may include greater awareness and concern about health; more moderate drinking among women in the general population; some lessening of the social stigma and oppression of lesbians; and changing norms associated with drinking in some lesbian communities. However, both heavy drinking and use of drugs other than alcohol appear to be prevalent among young lesbians and among some older groups of lesbians.

Cancers: Lesbian women may be at a higher risk for uterine, breast, cervical, endometrial, and ovarian cancers because of the health profiles listed above. However, more research is needed.

In addition, there are several other reasons that may contribute to this risk:

- Lesbians have traditionally been less likely to bear children. Hormones released during pregnancy and breastfeeding are believed to protect women against breast, endometrial, and ovarian cancers.
- Lesbians have higher rates of alcohol use, poor nutrition, and obesity. These factors may increase the risk of breast, endometrial, and ovarian cancers, and other cancers.
- Lesbians are less likely to visit a doctor or nurse for routine screenings, such as a Pap, which can prevent or detect cervical cancer. The viruses that cause most cervical cancer can be sexually transmitted between women. Lesbians have similar rates of mammography testing (for breast cancer) as heterosexual women.

Domestic violence: Also called intimate partner violence, this is when one person purposely causes either physical or mental harm to another. Domestic violence can occur in lesbian relationships as it does in heterosexual relationships, though there is some evidence that it occurs less often. But for many reasons, lesbian victims are more likely to stay silent about the violence. Some reasons include fewer services available to help them; fear of discrimination; threats from the batterer to "out" the victim; or fear of losing custody of children.

Polycystic ovarian syndrome (PCOS): This is the most common hormonal reproductive problem in women of childbearing age. PCOS is a health problem that can affect a woman's menstrual cycle, fertility, hormones, insulin production, heart, blood vessels, and appearance.

Women with PCOS have these characteristics:

- High levels of male hormones, also called androgens
- An irregular or no menstrual cycle
- May or may not have many small cysts (fluid-filled sacs) in their ovaries

An estimated 5 to 10 percent of women of childbearing age have PCOS (ages twenty to forty). There is evidence that lesbians may have a higher rate of PCOS than heterosexual women.

Osteoporosis: Millions of women already have or are at risk for osteoporosis. Osteoporosis means that your bones get weak, and you're more likely to break a bone. Osteoporosis in lesbian women has not yet been well studied.

Sexual health: Lesbian women are at risk for many of the same sexually transmitted diseases (STDs) as heterosexual women. Lesbian women can transmit STDs to each other through skin-to-skin contact, mucosa contact, vaginal fluids, and menstrual blood. Sharing sex toys is another method of transmitting STDs.

These are common STDs that can be passed between women:

- *Bacterial vaginosis (BV):* Although we don't know for sure that BV is caused by a sexually transmitted agent, BV occurs more commonly among women who have recently acquired other STDs, or who have recently had unprotected sex. For reasons that are unclear, BV is more common in lesbian and bisexual women than heterosexual women, and frequently occurs in both members of lesbian couples. BV happens when the normal bacteria in the vagina get out of balance. Sometimes, BV causes no symptoms, but over half of affected women have a vaginal discharge with a fishy odor or vaginal itching. If left untreated, BV can increase a woman's chances of getting other STDs such as human immunodeficiency virus (HIV), chlamydia, gonorrhea, and pelvic inflammatory disease.
- *Human papillomavirus (HPV):* HPV can cause genital warts and abnormal changes on the cervix that can lead to cancer, if it is not treated. Most people with HPV or genital warts don't know they are infected until they have had a Pap test because they may not have symptoms, but the virus can still be spread by contact. Lesbians can transmit HPV through direct genital skin-to-skin contact or by the virus traveling on hands or sex toys. Some women and their doctors wrongly assume that lesbian women do not need a regular Pap test. However, the virus can be spread by lesbian sexual activity, and many lesbians have been sexual with men so it is recommended that lesbian women have a Pap test. This simple test is an effective method of detecting abnormal cells on the cervix that can lead to cancer. Begin getting Pap tests no later than age twenty-one or sooner if

you're sexually active. These recommendations apply equally to lesbians who've never had sex with men, as cervical cancer caused by HPV has been seen in this group of women.

- *Trichomoniasis ("Trich"):* It is caused by a parasite that can be passed from one person to another during sexual contact. It can also be picked up from contact with damp, moist objects such as towels or wet clothing. Trich is spread through sexual contact with an infected person. Signs include yellow, green, or gray vaginal discharge (often foamy) with a strong odor; discomfort during sex and when urinating; irritation and itching of the genital area; and lower abdominal pain in rare cases. To tell if you have trich, your doctor or nurse will do a pelvic exam and lab test. A pelvic exam can show small red sores, or ulcerations, on the wall of the vagina or on the cervix. Trich is treated with antibiotics.
- *Herpes:* Herpes is a virus that can produce sores (also called lesions) in and around the vaginal area, on the penis, around the anal opening, and on the buttocks or thighs. Occasionally, sores also appear on other parts of the body where the virus has entered through broken skin. Most people get genital herpes by having sex with someone who is shedding the herpes virus during periods when an outbreak is not visible. The most common cause of recurrent genital herpes is HSV-2, which is transmitted through direct genital contact. HSV-1 is another herpes virus that usually infects the mouth and causes oral cold sores, but can also be transmitted to the genital area through oral sex. Lesbians can transmit this virus to each other if they have intimate contact with someone with a lesion or touch infected skin even when an outbreak is not visible.
- *Syphilis:* Syphilis is an STD caused by bacteria. Syphilis is passed through direct contact with a syphilis sore during vaginal, anal, or oral sex. If untreated, syphilis can infect other parts of the body. Syphilis remains uncommon in the general population, but has been increasing in men who have sex with men. It is extremely rare among lesbians. However, lesbians should talk to their doctor if they have any nonhealing ulcers.

What other STDs can lesbian women get?

Chlamydia: Most women have no symptoms. Women with symptoms may have abnormal vaginal discharge, burning when urinating, or bleeding between menstrual periods.

Infections that are not treated, even if there are no symptoms, can lead to lower abdominal pain, low back pain, nausea, fever, pain during sex, or bleeding between periods.

Gonorrhea: Symptoms are often mild, but most women have no symptoms. Even when women have symptoms, they can sometimes be mistaken for a bladder or other vaginal infection. Symptoms include pain or burning when urinating, yellowish and sometimes bloody vaginal discharge, and bleeding between menstrual periods.

Hepatitis B: Some women have no symptoms. Women with symptoms may have mild fever, headache and muscle aches, tiredness, loss of appetite, nausea or vomiting, diarrhea, dark-colored urine and pale bowel movements, stomach pain, and skin and whites of eyes turning yellow.

Human immunodeficiency virus (HIV)/acquired immunodeficiency syndrome (AIDS): Some women may have no symptoms for ten years or more. Women with symptoms may have extreme fatigue, rapid weight loss, frequent low-grade fevers and night sweats, frequent yeast infections (in the mouth), vaginal yeast infections and other STDs, pelvic inflammatory disease (PID), menstrual cycle changes, and red, brown, or purplish blotches on or under the skin or inside the mouth, nose, or eyelids.

Pubic lice: Symptoms include itching and finding lice.

What can lesbian women do to protect their health?

Find a doctor who is sensitive to your needs to help you get regular check ups: The Gay and Lesbian Medical Association provides online health care referrals.

Get a Pap test: The Pap test finds changes in your cervix early, so you can be treated before the problem becomes serious. Begin getting Pap tests no later than age twenty-one or within three years of first having sexual intercourse. After two to three yearly Pap tests have been normal, talk to your doctor or nurse about getting a Pap test at least once every three years.

Talk to your doctor or nurse about an HPV test if your Pap test is abnormal: In combination with a Pap test, an HPV test helps prevent cervical cancer. It can detect the types of HPV that cause cervical cancer. The Food and Drug Administration (FDA) has approved an HPV DNA test for women as a follow-up to a Pap test with results that are abnormal or in combination with a Pap test in women aged thirty and older.

Practice safer sex: Get tested for STDs like chlamydia or herpes before beginning a relationship. If you're unsure about a partner's status, practice methods to reduce the likelihood of sharing vaginal fluid or blood, including condoms on sex toys.

Have a balanced, healthy diet: Eat a variety of whole grains, fruits, and vegetables. These foods give you energy, plus vitamins, minerals, and fiber. Besides, they taste good! Try foods like brown rice or whole-wheat bread. Bananas, strawberries, and melons are some great-tasting fruits. Try vegetables raw, on a sandwich, or in a salad. Be sure to pick a variety of colors and kinds of fruits and vegetables. You can vary the form—try fresh, frozen, canned, or dried.

Drink moderately: If you drink alcohol, don't have more than one drink per day. Too much alcohol raises blood pressure and can raise your risk for stroke, heart disease, osteoporosis, many cancers, and other problems.

Get moving: An active lifestyle can help every woman. Thirty minutes of moderate physical activity on most days of the week can greatly improve your health and decrease your risk of heart disease and some cancers!

Don't smoke: If you do smoke, try to quit. Avoid secondhand smoke as much as you can.

Try different strategies to deal with your stress: Stress from discrimination is a tough challenge in the life of every lesbian. Relax using deep breathing, yoga, meditation, and massage therapy. You can also take a few minutes to sit and listen to soothing music, or read a book. Talk to your friends or get help from a professional if you need it.

Talk to your doctor or nurse about screening tests you may need: Regular preventive screenings are critical to staying healthy. All the tests that heterosexual women need, lesbian women need too.

Get help for domestic violence: Call the police or leave if you or your children are in danger! Call a crisis hotline or the National Domestic Violence Hotline at 800-799-SAFE or TDD 800-787-3224, which is available 24 hours a day, 365 days a year, in English, Spanish, and other languages. The Helpline can give you the phone numbers of local hotlines and other resources.

Build strong bones: Exercise. Get a bone density test. Make sure you get enough calcium and vitamin D each day. Reduce your chances of falling by making your home safer. For example, use a rubber bathmat in the shower or tub. Keep your floors free from clutter. Lastly, talk to your doctor or nurse about taking medicines to prevent or treat bone loss.

Know the signs of a heart attack: Women are less likely than men to believe they are having a heart attack and more likely to delay in seeking treatment. For women, chest pain may not be the first sign your heart is in trouble. Before a heart attack, women have said that they have unusual tiredness, trouble sleeping, problems breathing, indigestion, and anxiety. These symptoms can happen a month or so before the heart attack. During a heart attack, women often have pain or discomfort in the center of the chest; pain or discomfort in other areas of the upper body, including the arms, back, neck, jaw, or stomach; or other symptoms, such as shortness of breath, breaking out in a cold sweat, nausea, or light-headedness.

Know the signs of a stroke: The signs of a stroke happen suddenly and are different from the signs of a heart attack. Signs you should look for are weakness or numbness on one side of your body, dizziness, loss of balance, confusion, trouble talking or understanding speech, headache, nausea, or trouble walking or seeing. Remember: Even if you have a "mini-stroke," you may have some of these signs.

Chapter 9

Violence Against Women and Ways to Prevent It

What Is Abuse?

Sometimes it is hard and confusing to admit that you are in an abusive relationship, or to find a way out. There are clear signs to help you know if you are being abused. If the person you love or live with does any of these things to you, it's time to get help:

- Monitors what you're doing all the time
- Criticizes you for little things
- Constantly accuses you of being unfaithful
- Prevents or discourages you from seeing friends or family, or going to work or school
- Gets angry when drinking alcohol or using drugs
- Controls how you spend your money
- Controls your use of needed medicines
- Humiliates you in front of others
- Destroys your property or things that you care about

Excerpted from "Violence Against Women: What Is Abuse?" "Violence Against Women: Safety Planning List," "Violence Against Women: Dating Violence," "Violence Against Women: Domestic and Intimate Partner Violence," "Violence Against Women: Emotional and Verbal Abuse," "Violence Against Women: Sexual Assault and Abuse," and "Violence Against Women: Ways to Prevent and End Violence," National Women's Health Information Center, September 2007.

- Threatens to hurt you, the children, or pets, or does hurt you (by hitting, beating, pushing, shoving, punching, slapping, kicking, or biting)
- Uses or threatens to use a weapon against you
- Forces you to have sex against your will
- Blames you for his or her violent outbursts

Safety Planning List

Here are some helpful items to get together when you are planning on leaving an abusive situation. Keep these items in a safe place until you are ready to leave, or if you need to leave suddenly. If you have children, take them. And take your pets, too (if you can):

- Identification for yourself and your children
    - Birth certificates
    - Social security cards (or numbers written on paper if you can't find the cards)
    - Driver's license
    - Photo identification or passports
    - Welfare identification
    - Green card
- Important personal papers
    - Marriage certificate
    - Divorce papers
    - Custody orders
    - Legal protection or restraining orders
    - Health insurance papers and medical cards
    - Medical records for all family members
    - Children's school records
    - Investment papers/records and account numbers
    - Work permits
    - Immigration papers
    - Rental agreement/lease or house deed
    - Car title, registration, and insurance information

- Funds
    - Cash
    - Credit cards
    - Automatic teller machine (ATM) card
    - Checkbook and bankbook (with deposit slips)
- Keys
    - House
    - Car
    - Safety deposit box or post office box
- A way to communicate
    - Phone calling card
    - Cell phone
    - Address book
- Medications
    - At least one month's supply for all medicines you and your children are taking, as well as a copy of the prescriptions
- A way to get by
    - Jewelry or small objects you can sell if you run out of money or stop having access to your accounts
- Things to help you cope
    - Pictures
    - Keepsakes
    - Children's small toys or books

Dating Violence

Dating violence is when one person purposely causes physical or psychological harm to another person they are dating, including sexual assault, physical abuse, and psychological/emotional abuse. It is a serious crime that occurs in both casual and serious relationships, and in both heterosexual and same-sex relationships. Sometimes, a victim might unknowingly be given alcohol or "date rape" drugs like Rohypnol. Date rape drugs are often slipped into a victim's drink while a person is in a social setting such as a club or party. These drugs, as well as alcohol, can make a person unable to resist assault, and cause a type of amnesia so she is uncertain about what happened. The victim is then left to deal with the trauma of the sexual assault and the uncertainty surrounding the specifics of the crime. Unfortunately, most cases of dating violence are not reported to the police.

Violence against women by anyone is always wrong, whether the abuser is someone you date; a current or past spouse, boyfriend, or girlfriend; a family member; an acquaintance; or a stranger. You are not at fault. You did not cause the abuse to occur, and you are not responsible for the violent behavior of someone else.

If you or someone you know has been the victim of dating violence, seek help from other family members and friends or community organizations. Reach out for support or counseling. Talk with a health care provider, especially if you have been physically hurt. Learn how to minimize your risk of becoming a victim of dating violence before you find yourself in an uncomfortable or threatening situation.

Domestic and Intimate Partner Violence

What Is It?

Domestic violence and abuse, also called intimate partner violence, is when one person purposely causes either physical or mental harm to another, including the following:

- Physical abuse
- Psychological or emotional abuse
- Sexual assault
- Isolation
- Controlling all of the victim's money, shelter, time, food, etc.

Often, the violent person is a husband, former husband, boyfriend, or ex-boyfriend, but sometimes the abuser is female. Domestic violence and abuse are common and must be taken very seriously.

One in four women report that they have been physically assaulted or raped by an intimate partner. These crimes occur in both heterosexual and same-sex relationships. Physical and emotional trauma can lead to increased stress, depression, lowered self-esteem, and post-traumatic stress disorder (an emotional state of discomfort and stress connected to the memories of a disturbing event).

Violence against women by anyone is always wrong, whether the abuser is a current or past spouse, boyfriend, or girlfriend; someone you date; a family member; an acquaintance; or a stranger. You are not at fault. You did not cause the abuse to happen, and you are not responsible for the violent behavior of someone else.

If you or someone you know has been a victim of intimate partner violence, seek help from family members, friends, or community organizations. An important part of getting help is knowing if you are in an abusive relationship. It can be hard to admit you're in an abusive relationship. But, there are clear signs to help you know if you are being abused.

Get Help for Domestic Abuse

If you are being abused or have a loved one who is being abused, get help. Don't ignore it. It won't go away. Keep in mind, you're not alone. Many women are victims of domestic abuse.

Here are things you can do:

- Make a plan in case you need to leave. Set aside some money and find a place to go. Put important papers and items in a place where you can get them quickly. Review a full checklist of items you'll need, such as marriage license, birth certificates, and checkbook.
- If you're in danger, call the police or leave.
- If you're hurt, go to a local hospital emergency room.
- Call the National Domestic Violence Hotline at 800-799-SAFE or TDD 800-787-3224, which is available 24 hours a day, 365 days a year, in English, Spanish, and other languages. The Helpline can give you the phone numbers of local domestic violence shelters and other resources.
- Look up state resources for a list of local places to get help.
- Reach out to someone you trust—a family member, friend, coworker, or spiritual leader.
- Contact your family court (or domestic violence court, if offered by your state) for information about getting a court order of protection.

Domestic Violence Shelters

Domestic violence shelters offer victims of domestic violence and their children temporary housing as well as counseling and assistance. Services may include the following:

- Individual counseling
- Family counseling
- Support groups
- Job training
- Legal help

Transitional Housing

Transitional housing focuses on giving families a safe space and time to recover from domestic violence. Families live independently, in separate apartments, while they also receive needed services. Services can include the following:

- Individual counseling
- Family counseling
- Support groups
- Job training
- Help finding affordable, permanent housing
- Legal help

Visitation Centers

Families dealing with divorce, domestic violence, or custody issues often have a hard time finding a comfortable, neutral place for children to visit with a parent. A visitation center is a safe place where children from families dealing with these issues can visit with a parent.

Impact of Domestic Violence on Children

Violence in the home doesn't just affect the person being abused; it affects everyone in the home, including children.

Children may witness abuse in a number of different ways:

- They may be in the room and see their mother being abused.
- They may hear their parents fighting.
- They may see the aftermath of the abuse when they see their mother's bruises.

Studies have shown that children who grow up in violent homes are more likely to withdraw and have behavioral problems. As they get older, these children often blame themselves for not stopping the abuse. This can lead to further withdrawal, depression, and substance abuse.

Children who grow up in abusive homes are more likely to become abusers or be abused themselves. A boy who grows up with a father who beats his mother tends to see women as weak and submissive and repeat the cycle of abuse in his own relationships. A girl who sees the abuse of her mother is likely to think that abuse is part of a normal relationship and become involved with an abuser herself.

If you're being abused, it's important to get help for yourself, but also for your children.

Human Immunodeficiency Virus (HIV) and Domestic Violence

Domestic violence and HIV are connected in two ways:

- If you've been abused in the past or are currently in an abusive relationship, you are more likely to get HIV. If you were physically or sexually abused as a child, you're more likely to have a higher number of partners and less likely to use condoms each time, putting you at greater risk for HIV. If you're currently in an abusive relationship, you may be forced to have sex and you probably can't insist that your partner use a condom, putting you at risk for HIV.
- Women with HIV who disclose their HIV status to their partners also are at risk of physical abuse. If you're planning to tell your partner you have HIV, take these steps to lower the risk that your partner will react violently:
  - Tell your partner that you are HIV positive **before** you get sexually involved.
  - Tell your partner that you are HIV positive in a semi-public place. A public park is a good place, because it gives you some privacy, but there are others around in case you need help.
  - If you feel at all threatened by your partner's reaction, keep meetings public for a while.

Why Women Don't Leave

Most people who have never been in an abusive relationship wonder, "Why doesn't she just leave?" There are many reasons why a woman may not leave an abusive relationship. She may have little or no money and have no way to support herself and her children. She may reach out for help only to find that all the local domestic violence shelters are full. She may not be able to contact friends and family who could help her. Or she may worry about the safety of herself and her children if she leaves.

Emotional and Verbal Abuse

"You're so stupid. You never do anything right!" If this sounds familiar, you may be a victim of emotional abuse.

Emotional and verbal abuse—attempts to isolate, threaten, or intimidate—can harm you, even if you are not being abused physically. Moreover, emotional and verbal abuse often are a sign that physical abuse will follow.

Some examples of emotional and verbal abuse include the following:

- Yelling
- Criticizing
- Name-calling
- Blaming you for everything
- Playing mind games or manipulating you
- Ordering you around
- Keeping you from spending time with friends and family
- Threatening to hurt you

No one deserves to be abused, physically or verbally.

Sexual Assault and Abuse

Sexual assault and abuse is any type of sexual activity that you do not agree to, including the following:

- Inappropriate touching
- Vaginal, anal, or oral penetration
- Child molestation

Sexual assault can be verbal, visual, or anything that forces a person to join in unwanted sexual contact or attention. Examples of this are voyeurism, exhibitionism, incest, and sexual harassment.

Rape is forced sexual intercourse, including vaginal, anal, or oral penetration. It is a common form of sexual assault and can be committed in many situations—on a date, by a friend or an acquaintance, or when you think you are alone. Educate yourself on "date rape" drugs. They can be slipped into a drink when a victim is not looking. Never leave your drink unattended—no matter where you are. Try to always be aware of your surroundings. Date rape drugs make a person unable to resist assault and have a type of memory loss so the victim doesn't know what happened.

Violence against women by anyone is always wrong, whether the abuser is someone you date; a current or past spouse, boyfriend, or girlfriend; a family member; an acquaintance; or a stranger. You are not at fault. You did not cause the abuse to occur, and you are not responsible for the violent behavior of someone else. If you or someone you know has been sexually assaulted, seek help from other family members and friends or community organizations. Reach out for support or counseling. Talk with a health care provider, especially if you have been physically hurt. Learn how to minimize your risk of becoming a victim of sexual assault or sexual abuse before you find yourself in an uncomfortable or threatening situation. And, learn about how to get help for sexual assault and abuse. Another important part of getting help is knowing if you are in an abusive relationship. There are clear signs to help you know if you are being abused.

Get Help for Sexual Assault

Take steps right away if you've been sexually assaulted:

- Get away from the attacker to a safe place as fast as you can. Then call 911 or the police.
- Call a friend or family member you trust. You also can call a crisis center or a hotline to talk with a counselor. Feelings of shame, guilt, fear, and shock are normal. It is important to get counseling from a trusted professional.
- Do not wash, comb, or clean any part of your body. Do not change clothes if possible, so the hospital staff can collect evidence. Do not touch or change anything at the scene of the assault.
- Go to your nearest hospital emergency room as soon as possible. You need to be examined and treated for any injuries you may have. Ask to be screened for sexually transmitted diseases (STDs) and for emergency contraception to help prevent pregnancy. The

doctor will collect evidence using a rape kit to find fibers, hairs, saliva, semen, or clothing that the attacker may have left behind.

- You or the hospital staff can call the police from the emergency room to file a report.
- Ask the hospital staff about possible support groups you can attend right away.

You can help someone who is abused or who has been assaulted by listening and offering comfort. Go with her or him to the police, the hospital, or to counseling. Reinforce the message that she or he is not at fault, and that it is natural to feel angry and ashamed.

Ways to Prevent and End Violence

There are some ways you can help prevent and end violence:

- Call the police if you see or hear evidence of domestic violence.
- Support a friend or family member who may be in an abusive relationship.
- Volunteer at a local domestic violence shelter or another organization helping survivors or working to prevent violence.
- Raise your children to respect others. Teach your children to respect others and to treat others as they would like to be treated. Lead by example.
- Protect yourself. Take a self-defense class.
- Become an activist. Participate in a Take Back the Night march, a yearly march held in most major cities to raise awareness about violence against women. Or tell your congressional representatives that you expect their support for the funding of domestic violence survivor services and prevention programs.

If you're a victim of abuse or violence at the hands of someone you know or love, or you are recovering from an assault by a stranger, you are not alone.

To get immediate help and support, call the National Domestic Violence Hotline at 800-799-SAFE (7233) or the National Sexual Assault Hotline at 800-656-4673.

Part Two

Breast and Gynecological Concerns

Chapter 10

Nonmalignant Breast Conditions

Chapter Contents

Section 10.1

Understanding Breast Changes

Excerpted from "Knowing Your Breasts and Common Breast Conditions," National Women's Health Information Center, 2007.

Conditions in the Breast

General breast lumpiness (fibrocystic changes): This lumpiness happens around the nipple and areola and in the upper-outer part of the breast. Your breast may feel rubbery, firm, or hard to the touch. Changes or infection could cause your breasts to feel painful or full and lumpy. Some women can feel these lumps before and during their periods. The lumps usually go away by the end of their periods. During pregnancy, the milk-producing glands become swollen, and the breasts may feel lumpier than usual. Your breasts also can feel very painful or feel lumpy when you're breastfeeding. You may feel lumpiness in your breasts more as you approach middle age, and the milk-producing tissue of your breasts turns into soft, fatty tissue. Unless you are taking hormone therapy, this type of lumpiness generally goes away after menopause.

Cyst or "fluid-filled lump": A cyst is a sac or capsule in your breast that is filled with fluid. It can get larger right before your period. If it gets large enough, it feels like a lump, moves around when you touch it, and may be painful. Cysts may go away on their own, or your doctor can drain the fluid. They are usually not cancer.

Fibroadenoma: These breast tumors are not cancerous. They are round masses that can be small or large. You may feel them as a moveable, painless, firm, or rubbery lump. They may get bigger during pregnancy and smaller after menopause. Sometimes, they stop growing or shrink on their own. They can also be removed by surgery.

Intraductal papilloma: These growths usually occur in the milk ducts near the nipple. The growths cause bleeding from the nipple. They may also cause pain and breast enlargement. Sometimes, you can feel the lump. It is treated by taking out the growth and the part of the duct where it has grown.

Mastitis: This breast infection causes soreness or a lump in the breast. It can happen when you are breastfeeding or if you get a crack in the skin around the nipple. It causes a fever and flu-like symptoms, such as feeling run down or very achy. Some women also have nausea and vomiting. It can cause yellowish discharge from the nipple. Your breasts may feel warm or hot to the touch. You also can have redness and swelling on the skin of your breast over the area that is infected. It usually occurs only in one breast. Mastitis is treated with self-care (such as applying warm compresses, getting plenty of rest and fluids) and antibiotics.

Duct ectasia: This condition happens to women nearing menopause. The ducts under the nipple become inflamed and clogged. Symptoms are a thick, green or black, sticky discharge; pain; or a hard lump. This problem can go away on its own, or you may be treated with warm compresses, antibiotics, or surgery.

Abscess: Severe infections in the breast, like mastitis, can lead to an abscess. An abscess is a build-up of pus. The breast may be tender and swollen in that area. The abscess can be drained and treated with antibiotics.

Fat necrosis: When the breast is hurt from an injury, scar tissue can form and cause a lump. The lump may or may not be painful, depending on how long ago you were injured. The skin may be red, bruised, or look dimpled. The lump may go away on its own or may be removed by surgery.

Section 10.2

Breast Infection

Breast infections are classified as breast abscesses or as mastitis.

Abscesses

Abscesses are well-defined collections of infected material or pus that generally require some form of drainage for management. Symptoms will typically include redness or warmth in the area of the abscess and breast pain. Infections including fever or chills may be present.

Breast abscesses that occur directly behind the nipple are often caused by a condition known as periductal mastitis or duct ectasia. These types of breast abscesses are notorious for their ability to recur even after satisfactory drainage and antibiotic therapy. Multiple recurrences of abscesses behind the nipple may eventually lead to the recommendation to have the diseased ducts surgically removed.

Abscesses that occur further away from the nipple in other quadrants of the breast can be seen in the immediate postpartum period. These abscesses may respond to drainage using a needle-guided approach but occasionally will require surgical drainage in addition to antibiotic therapy.

Breast abscesses in postmenopausal women that occur outside of the nipple area require special consideration. Without an underlying cause such as lactation or periductal mastitis, it is uncommon for postmenopausal women to develop abscesses. It is important to perform a thorough imaging evaluation including mammogram and ultrasound to exclude an underlying breast cancer. Drainage of an abscess in this age group always requires close follow-up to make sure there is not an underlying breast tumor.

Mastitis

Mastitis refers to an infection in the soft tissue of the breast, but no well-defined collection that requires drainage. This is most commonly seen in women who are lactating and breastfeeding. Most cases of mastitis will respond to antibiotic therapy. Severe cases may require intravenous antibiotics and when symptoms begin to improve, oral antibiotics can be utilized. Women who are beyond childbearing age who develop symptoms of diffuse redness in one breast should be evaluated for inflammatory carcinoma.

Section 10.3

Fibrocystic Breast Disease

Reprinted from "Fibrocystic Breast Disease,"

Alternative Names

Mammary dysplasia; benign breast disease

Definition

Fibrocystic breast disease is described as common, benign (noncancerous) changes in the tissues of the breast. The term "disease" in this case is misleading, and many providers prefer the term "change."

The condition is so commonly found in breasts, it is believed to be a variation of normal. Other related terms include "mammary dysplasia," "benign breast disease," and "diffuse cystic mastopathy."

Causes

The cause is not completely understood, but the changes are believed to be associated with ovarian hormones since the condition usually subsides with menopause, and may vary in consistency during the menstrual cycle.

The incidence of it is estimated to be over 60 percent of all women. It is common in women between the ages of thirty and fifty, and rare in postmenopausal women. The incidence is lower in women taking birth control pills. The risk factors may include family history and diet (such as excessive dietary fat, and caffeine intake), although these are controversial.

Symptoms

- A dense, irregular and bumpy "cobblestone" consistency in the breast tissue
- Usually more marked in the outer upper quadrants
- Breast discomfort that is persistent, or that occurs off and on (intermittent)
- Breast(s) feel full
- Dull, heavy pain and tenderness
- Premenstrual tenderness and swelling
- Breast discomfort improves after each menstrual period
- Nipple sensation changes, itching

Note: Symptoms may range from mild to severe. Symptoms typically peak just before each menstrual period, and improve immediately after the menstrual period.

Exams and Tests

Physical examination reveals the presence of mobile (non-anchored) breast "masses." These masses are usually rounded, with smooth borders, and either rubbery or slightly changeable in shape. Dense tissue may make the breast examination more difficult to interpret:

- Mammography may be difficult to interpret due to dense tissue.
- A biopsy of the breast may be necessary to rule out other disorders.
- Aspiration of the breast with a fine needle can often diagnose and treat larger cysts.

Treatment

Self care may include restricting dietary fat to approximately 25 percent of the total daily calorie intake, and eliminating caffeine.

Performing a breast self-examination monthly, and wearing a well-fitting bra to provide good breast support are important.

The effectiveness of vitamin E, vitamin B_6, and herbal preparations, such as evening primrose oil, are somewhat controversial. Discuss their use with your health care provider.

Oral contraceptives may be prescribed because they often decrease the symptoms. A synthetic androgen may be prescribed by a doctor in severe cases, when the potential benefit is thought to outweigh the potential adverse effects.

Outlook (Prognosis)

If dietary changes decrease the symptoms, and are maintained, the benefit most likely will persist. A combination of treatment and use of medications may be necessary to obtain relief for severe cases.

Possible Complications

Because fibrocystic changes may make breast examination and mammography more difficult to interpret, early cancerous lesions may occasionally be overlooked.

When to Contact a Medical Professional

Call your health care provider if you feel a new, unusual, or "dominant" lump during a breast self-examination.

Call for an appointment with your health care provider if you are a woman, aged twenty or older, who has never been taught, or does not currently know how, to perform breast self-examination. Also call if you are a woman, aged forty or older, who has not had a screening mammogram.

Prevention

Reduction of dietary fat and caffeine if you have fibrocystic breast changes has been suggested, although recent studies have questioned the role of caffeine and fat in fibrocystic disease.

Chapter 11

Premenstrual Syndrome and Premenstrual Dysphoric Disorder

What is premenstrual syndrome (PMS)?

Premenstrual syndrome (PMS) is a group of symptoms linked to the menstrual cycle. PMS symptoms occur in the week or two weeks before your period (menstruation or monthly bleeding). The symptoms usually go away after your period starts. PMS can affect menstruating women of any age. It is also different for each woman. PMS may be just a monthly bother or it may be so severe that it makes it hard to even get through the day. Monthly periods stop during menopause, bringing an end to PMS.

What causes PMS?

The causes of PMS are not clear. It is linked to the changing hormones during the menstrual cycle. Some women may be affected more than others by changing hormone levels during the menstrual cycle. Stress and emotional problems do not seem to cause PMS, but they may make it worse.

Diagnosis of PMS is usually based on your symptoms, when they occur, and how much they affect your life.

What are the symptoms of PMS?

PMS often includes both physical and emotional symptoms. Common symptoms are as follows:

Reprinted from "Premenstrual Syndrome," National Women's Health Information Center, January 2007.

- Acne
- Breast swelling and tenderness
- Feeling tired
- Having trouble sleeping
- Upset stomach, bloating, constipation, or diarrhea
- Headache or backache
- Appetite changes or food cravings
- Joint or muscle pain
- Trouble concentrating or remembering
- Tension, irritability, mood swings, or crying spells
- Anxiety or depression

Symptoms vary from one woman to another. If you think you have PMS, keep track of which symptoms you have and how severe they are for a few months. You can use a calendar to write down the symptoms you have each day or you can use a form to track your symptoms. If you go to the doctor for your PMS, take this form with you.

How common is PMS?

Estimates of the percentage of women affected by PMS vary widely. According to the American College of Obstetricians and Gynecologists, at least 85 percent of menstruating women have at least one PMS symptom as part of their monthly cycle. Most of these women have symptoms that are fairly mild and do not need treatment. Some women (about 3 to 8 percent of menstruating women) have a more severe form of PMS, called premenstrual dysphoric disorder (PMDD). This will be discussed further below.

PMS occurs more often in women who have the following characteristics:

- Are between their late twenties and early forties
- Have at least one child
- Have a family history of depression
- Have a past medical history of either postpartum depression or a mood disorder

What is the treatment for PMS?

Many things have been tried to ease the symptoms of PMS. No treatment works for every woman, so you may need to try different ones to see what works. If your PMS is not so bad that you need to see a doctor, some lifestyle changes may help you feel better. Below are some lifestyle changes that may help ease your symptoms:

- Take a multivitamin every day that includes 400 micrograms of folic acid. A calcium supplement with vitamin D can help keep bones strong and may help ease some PMS symptoms.
- Exercise regularly.
- Eat healthy foods, including fruits, vegetables, and whole grains.
- Avoid salt, sugary foods, caffeine, and alcohol, especially when you are having PMS symptoms.
- Get enough sleep. Try to get eight hours of sleep each night.
- Find healthy ways to cope with stress. Talk to your friends, exercise, or write in a journal.
- Don't smoke.

Over-the-counter pain relievers such as ibuprofen, aspirin, or naproxen may help ease cramps, headaches, backaches, and breast tenderness.

In more severe cases of PMS, prescription medicines may be used to ease symptoms. One approach has been to use drugs such as birth control pills to stop ovulation from occurring. Women on the pill report fewer PMS symptoms, such as cramps and headaches, as well as lighter periods.

Table 11.1. Amounts of Calcium You Need Each Day

Ages	Milligrams per day
9–18	1300
19–50	1000
51 and older	1200

Note: Pregnant or nursing women need the same amount of calcium as other women of the same age.

What is premenstrual dysphoric disorder (PMDD)?

There is evidence that a brain chemical called serotonin plays a role in a severe form of PMS, called premenstrual dysphoric disorder (PMDD). The main symptoms, which can be disabling, include the following:

- Feelings of sadness or despair, or possibly suicidal thoughts
- Feelings of tension or anxiety
- Panic attacks
- Mood swings, crying
- Lasting irritability or anger that affects other people
- Disinterest in daily activities and relationships
- Trouble thinking or focusing
- Tiredness or low energy
- Food cravings or binge eating
- Having trouble sleeping
- Feeling out of control
- Physical symptoms, such as bloating, breast tenderness, headaches, and joint or muscle pain

You must have five or more of these symptoms to be diagnosed with PMDD. Symptoms occur during the week before your period and go away after bleeding starts.

Making some lifestyle changes may help ease PMDD symptoms. See the question, "What is the treatment for PMS?" above for more information.

Antidepressants called selective serotonin reuptake inhibitors (SSRIs) that change serotonin levels in the brain have also been shown to help some women with PMDD. The Food and Drug Administration (FDA) has approved three medications for the treatment of PMDD:

- Sertraline (Zoloft®)
- Fluoxetine (Sarafem®)
- Paroxetine HCI (Paxil CR®)

Individual counseling, group counseling, and stress management may also help relieve symptoms.

Chapter 12

Menstrual Irregularities

Chapter Contents

Section 12.1

Dysfunctional Uterine Bleeding

Reprinted from "Dysfunctional Uterine Bleeding (DUB)," © 2008 A.D.A.M., Inc. Reprinted with permission. Updated February 5, 2008.

Alternative Names

Anovulatory bleeding; Bleeding—dysfunctional uterine; DUB; Abnormal uterine bleeding

Definition

Dysfunctional uterine bleeding (DUB) is abnormal bleeding from the vagina that is not due to a physical (anatomical) cause.

Causes

DUB may be caused by an imbalance of hormones—estrogen or progesterone.

Risk factors include:

- emotional stress;
- excessive exercise;
- obesity.

DUB occurs in women during their reproductive years (they have started their period but have not reached menopause). About 20 percent of DUB cases occur in adolescents and 40 percent occur in women over forty.

Symptoms

- Abnormal menstrual periods
- Bleeding from the vagina between periods
- Changing menstrual cycles (usually less than twenty-eight days between menstrual periods)

- Changing menstrual flow ranging from very little to a lot
- Excessive growth of body hair in a male pattern (hirsutism)
- Hot flashes
- Infertility
- Mood swings
- Tenderness of the vagina

Exams and Tests

Dysfunctional uterine bleeding (DUB) is diagnosed after all other causes of abnormal uterine bleeding are ruled out. This includes:

- disease;
- early pregnancy disorders;
- infection;
- structure problems;
- tumors.

The health care provider will do a pelvic examination. Tests usually include:

- complete blood count (CBC);
- blood clotting profile;
- hormone tests;
- follicle stimulating hormone (FSH);
- luteinizing hormone (LH);
- male hormone (androgen) levels;
- prolactin;
- progesterone;
- serum human chorionic gonadotropin (HCG)—to rule out pregnancy;
- thyroid function tests.

The following procedures may be done:

- dilatation and curettage (D and C);
- endometrial biopsy;

- hysteroscopy;
- pelvic ultrasound.

Treatment

Young women within a few years of their first period are not treated unless symptoms are very severe, such as heavy blood loss causing anemia.

In other women, the goal of treatment is to control the menstrual cycle. Oral birth control pills or progestogen therapy are often used for this purpose. Women with anemia may get iron supplements.

If you want to get pregnant, you may be given medication to stimulate ovulation.

Women whose symptoms are severe and resistant to medical therapy may need surgical treatments including:

- burning or removing the lining of the uterus (endometrial ablation);
- hysterectomy.

Older women who may be getting close to menopause may receive hormones or surgery to relieve symptoms.

Outlook (Prognosis)

Hormone therapy usually relieves symptoms.

Possible Complications

- Infertility from lack of ovulation
- Severe anemia from prolonged or heavy menstrual bleeding
- Buildup of the uterine lining without enough menstrual bleeding (a possible factor in the development of endometrial cancer)

When to Contact a Medical Professional

Call your health care provider if you have unusual vaginal bleeding.

References

Rakel P, ed. *Conn's Current Therapy 2005*. 57th ed. Philadelphia, Pa: WB Saunders; 2005:1286–88.

Stenchever A. *Comprehensive Gynecology*. 4th ed. St. Louis, Mo: Mosby; 2001:1082–84.

Katz VL, Lentz GM, Lobo RA, Gershenson DM. Katz: *Comprehensive Gynecology*. 5th ed. Philadelphia, Pa: Mosby; 2007.

Section 12.2

Amenorrhea

Reprinted from "Amenorrhea," National Institute of Child Health and Human Development, National Institutes of Health, May 14, 2007.

What is amenorrhea?

Amenorrhea is the absence of a menstrual period:

- Primary amenorrhea is when a young woman has not yet had a period by age sixteen.
- Secondary amenorrhea describes someone who used to have a regular period but then it stopped for at least three months (this can include pregnancy).

What are the signs of amenorrhea?

The main sign of amenorrhea is missing a menstrual period.

Regular periods are a sign of overall good health. Missing a period may mean that you are pregnant or that something is going wrong. It's important to tell your health care provider if you miss a period so he or she can begin to find out what is happening in your body.

Amenorrhea itself is not a disease, but is usually a symptom of another condition. Depending on that condition, a woman might experience other symptoms, such as headache, vision changes, hair loss, or excess facial hair.

What are the causes of amenorrhea?

Amenorrhea is a symptom of a variety of conditions, ranging from not serious to serious.

With primary amenorrhea:

- Chromosomal or genetic abnormalities can cause the eggs and follicles involved in menstruation to deplete too early in life.
- Hypothalamic or pituitary diseases and physical problems, such as problems with reproductive organs, can prevent periods from starting.
- Moderate or excessive exercise, eating disorders (such as anorexia nervosa), extreme physical or psychological stress, or a combination of these can disrupt the normal menstrual cycle.

With secondary amenorrhea:

- This problem is much more common than primary amenorrhea.
- Common causes include many of those listed for primary amenorrhea, as well as pregnancy, certain contraceptives, breastfeeding, mental stress, and certain medications.
- Hormonal problems involving the hypothalamus, pituitary, thyroid, ovary, or adrenal glands can also cause amenorrhea.
- Women who have very low body weight sometimes stop getting their periods as well.
- Women with premature ovarian failure stop getting regular their periods before natural menopause.

What is the treatment for amenorrhea?

Treatment for amenorrhea depends on the underlying cause. Sometimes lifestyle changes can help if weight, stress, or physical activity is causing the amenorrhea. Other times medications and oral contraceptives can help the problem. For more information, talk to your health care provider.

Section 12.3

Dysmenorrhea

Reprinted from "Dysmenorrhea," Walter Reed Army Medical Center. The text of this document is available online at http://www.wramc.army.mil/Patients/diseases/wh/c16/Pages/s2.aspx; accessed May 13, 2008.

Description

Severe, painful cramps during menstruation. Primary dysmenorrhea means pain has recurred regularly or within a year or two of the first period (puberty). Secondary dysmenorrhea means pain began years after periods started. Women with dysmenorrhea are generally fertile. Severity of symptoms varies greatly from woman to woman, and from one time to the next in the same woman. Dysmenorrhea usually is less severe after a woman has had a baby.

Frequent Signs and Symptoms

- Cramping and sometimes sharp pains in the lower abdomen, lower back, and thighs. The pain starts at onset of menses and lasts for hours to days.
- Nausea and vomiting (sometimes).
- Diarrhea (occasionally).
- Sweating.
- Lack of energy.
- Urinary frequency.
- Irritability, nervousness, depression.

Causes

- Strong or prolonged contractions of the muscular wall of the uterus. These may be caused by concentration of prostaglandins (hormones found in the cervix and uterus). Research shows that women with dysmenorrhea produce and excrete more prostaglandins than those who don't have as much discomfort.

- Dilation (stretching) of the cervix to allow passage of blood dots from the uterus to the vagina in cases where the cervix is narrowed or constricted.
- Other causes include pelvic infections; endometriosis, especially if dysmenorrhea begins after age twenty; adenomyosis (an abnormal benign growth of the endometrium); fibroids or other benign tumors of the uterus; or use of intrauterine device (IUD).

Risk Factors

Risk increases with the following:

- Use of caffeine or nicotine.
- Stress. The degree of dysmenorrhea may vary according to general health or mental state. While emotional or psychological factors don't cause the pain, they can worsen it or cause some women to be less responsive to treatment.
- Family history of dysmenorrhea.
- Lack of exercise; poor diet.

Preventive Measures

- Take female hormones that prevent ovulation, such as oral contraceptives.
- Treat the underlying cause.

Expected Outcome

- Symptoms can be controlled with treatment.
- Symptoms improve with age and with childbirth. Symptoms are rare in postmenopausal women.

Possible Complications

- Severe pain that regularly interferes with normal activity
- Infertility from underlying cause.

Treatment/Post-Procedure Care

General measures are as follows:

- Pelvic exam and a patient history may help suggest the cause of dysmenorrhea. Initial treatment aims are to relieve pain. Long-term goals of treatment involve treating any underlying cause with medication, counseling, or possibly surgery.
- Heat helps relieve pain. Use a heating pad or hot-water bottle on the abdomen or back, or take hot baths. Sit in a tub of hot water for ten to fifteen minutes as often as necessary.
- Transcutaneous electrical nerve stimulator (TENS) treatment may help relieve pain.
- Psychotherapy or counseling, if dysmenorrhea is stress related, may help.
- Hypnosis therapy may help.
- Treatment as required, for the cause for the secondary dysmenorrhea may also help.
- Surgery may be recommended for women whose pain cannot be controlled by medications.

Measures involving medication are as follows:

- For minor discomfort, use nonsteroidal anti-inflammatory drugs (NSAIDs) such as aspirin, ibuprofen, or naproxen.
- Other medications that may be prescribed are antiprostaglandins (for painful menstrual periods) and oral contraceptives, which prohibit ovulation.
- In severe cases, hormones (e.g., gonadotropin-releasing hormone [Gn-RH]) can stop ovary function and relieve pain.

Activity

- No restrictions. When resting in bed, elevate your feet or bend your knees and lie on your side.
- Regular, vigorous exercise reduces discomfort of future periods.

Diet

- Reduce or discontinue consumption of any caffeine-containing beverages or foods.
- You may be prescribed vitamin B supplements. These help relieve symptoms in some persons.

- Herbal teas may help reduce symptoms of dysmenorrhea for some women.

When to Notify Your Healthcare Provider

Notify your healthcare provider if:

- you or a family member has symptoms of dysmenorrhea that cannot be controlled;
- bleeding becomes excessive (you saturate a pad or tampon more frequently than once each hour);
- signs of infection develop, such as fever, a general ill feeling, headache, dizziness, or muscle aches; or
- new, unexplained symptoms develop. Drugs used in treatment may produce side effects.

Section 12.4

Menorrhagia

Reprinted from "Menorrhagia," Walter Reed Army Medical Center. The text of this document is available online at http://www.wramc.army.mil/Patients/diseases/wh/c16/Pages/s6.aspx; accessed May 13, 2008.

Description

A fairly common disorder that is characterized by an unusually heavy or prolonged period of menstrual flow. The average amount of blood loss during a normal menstrual period is about two ounces. With menorrhagia, a woman may lose three ounces or more. It rarely signifies a serious underlying disorder.

Frequent Signs and Symptoms

- Excessive menstrual flow (varies greatly from woman to woman)
- Menstrual period lasts for more than seven days

- Passing of large clots of blood
- Paleness and fatigue (anemia)

Causes

- Anovulation (failure to release an egg each month)
- Imbalance of female hormones (estrogen and progesterone)
- Fibroids (benign uterine tumors)
- Pelvic infection
- Endometrial disorder
- Intrauterine device (IUD)
- Hypothyroidism

Risk Factors

Risk increases with the following:

- Obesity
- Estrogen administration (without progestin)
- Young women who have not established a regular ovulation cycle
- Women approaching menopause

Preventive Measure

Annual pelvic examinations with a cervical smear test (Pap smear).

Expected Outcome

- Varies with cause of bleeding.
- Patients with hormonal causes usually respond to treatment.

Possible Complications

- Anemia due to excessive blood loss.
- Surgery may be required.

Treatment/Post Procedure Care

General measures are as follows:

- Special medical diagnostic tests (e.g., pregnancy test, endometrial biopsy, blood test) to help determine cause of bleeding may be performed.
- Treatment usually depends on the age of the woman, whether or not she desires future pregnancy, and any underlying disorder.
- Wear extra sanitary pads during excessive flow to prevent embarrassment.
- If using an IUD, consider a change to another method of contraception.
- Dilatation and curettage, often referred to as D & C (dilatation of the cervix and a scraping out of the uterus with a curette) may be performed.
- Hysterectomy may be considered in persistent cases where fertility is not desired.

Medication may also be used:

- Hormone therapy to control bleeding may be prescribed.
- If hormones cannot be taken for some reason, other medications to control the bleeding may be recommended.
- Iron replacement therapy may be prescribed for anemia.

Activity

Resting with feet up may be helpful.

Diet

No special diet is required.

When to Contact Your Doctor

Notify your healthcare provider if any of the following occur:

- You or a family member has signs or symptoms of menorrhagia.
- Symptoms worsen after treatment begins.
- New or unexplained symptoms develop. Drugs used in treatment may cause side effects.

Chapter 13

Ovarian Pain and Disorders of the Ovaries

Chapter Contents

Section 13.1

Mittelschmerz (Ovulation Pain)

Mittelschmerz is one-sided lower-abdominal pain that occurs in women at or around the time of ovulation.

Causes

About 20 percent of women experience mittelschmerz, or pain associated with ovulation. The pain may occur just before, during, or after ovulation.

There are several explanations for the cause of this pain. Just prior to ovulation, follicle growth may stretch the surface of the ovary, causing pain. At the time of ovulation, fluid or blood is released from the ruptured egg follicle and may cause irritation of the abdominal lining. Mittelschmerz may be felt on one side one month, then switch to the opposite side the next month, or it may be felt on the same side for several months in succession.

The pain is not harmful and does not signify the presence of disease. In fact, women who feel this pain may be at an advantage when planning or trying to avoid pregnancy. A woman is most likely to become pregnant just before ovulation, on the day of ovulation, or immediately after ovulation. However, birth control methods that rely solely on predicting ovulation are far from completely reliable.

Symptoms

Lower-abdominal pain that is:

- one-sided;
- recurrent or with similar pain in past;
- typically lasting minutes to a few hours, but may extend as long as twenty-four to forty-eight hours;
- usually sharp, cramping, distinctive pain;

- Severe (rare);
- may switch sides from month to month or from one episode to another; or
- begins midway through the menstrual cycle.

Exams and Tests

A pelvic examination shows no abnormalities. Other diagnostic procedures (such as an abdominal ultrasound) may be performed to rule out other causes of ovarian pain if ovulatory pain is prolonged.

Treatment

No treatment is usually necessary. Pain relievers (analgesics) may be needed in cases of prolonged or intense pain.

Outlook (Prognosis)

The outcome is expected to be excellent.

Possible Complications

There are usually no complications.

When to Contact a Medical Professional

Call for an appointment with your health care provider if mid-cycle ovulation pain seems to change or become unusually prolonged.

Prevention

Hormonal forms of contraception can be taken to prevent ovulation—and therefore ovulatory pain—but otherwise there is no known prevention.

References

Goldman L, Ausiello D. Cecil *Textbook of Medicine*, 22nd ed. Philadelphia, Pa: WB Saunders; 2004:1495.

Rakel RE. *Textbook of Family Practice*. 6th ed. Philadelphia, Pa: WB Saunders; 2002:679.

Section 13.2

Ovarian Cysts

Reprinted from "Ovarian Cysts," National Women's Health Information Center, January 2005.

What are ovaries?

The ovaries are a pair of organs in the female reproductive system. They are located in the pelvis, one on each side of the uterus, which is the hollow, pear-shaped organ where a baby grows. Each ovary is about the size and shape of an almond. The ovaries produce eggs and female hormones. Hormones are chemicals that control the way certain cells or organs function.

Every month, during the menstrual cycle, an egg is released from one ovary in a process called ovulation. The egg travels from the ovary through the fallopian tube to the uterus. The ovaries are also the main source of the female hormones estrogen and progesterone. These hormones influence the development of a woman's breasts, body shape, and body hair. They also regulate the menstrual cycle and pregnancy.

What are ovarian cysts?

A cyst is a fluid-filled sac, and can be located anywhere in the body. On the ovary, different types of cysts can form. The most common type of ovarian cyst is called a functional cyst, which often forms during the normal menstrual cycle. Each month, a woman's ovaries grow tiny cysts that hold the eggs. When an egg is mature, the sac breaks open to release the egg, so it can travel through the fallopian tube for fertilization. Then the sac dissolves. In one type of functional cyst, called a follicular cyst, the sac doesn't break open to release the egg and may continue to grow. This type of cyst usually disappears within one to three months. A corpus luteum cyst, another type of functional cyst, forms if the sac doesn't dissolve. Instead, the sac seals off after the egg is released. Fluid then builds up inside of it. This type of cyst usually goes away on its own after a few weeks. However, it can grow to almost four inches and may bleed or twist the ovary and cause pain.

Clomid® or Serophene®, which are drugs used to induce ovulation, can raise the risk of getting this type of cyst. These cysts are almost never associated with cancer.

There are also other types of cysts:

- **Endometriomas:** These cysts develop in women who have endometriosis, when tissue from the lining of the uterus grows outside of the uterus. The tissue may attach to the ovary and form a growth. These cysts can be painful during sexual intercourse and during menstruation.
- **Cystadenomas:** These cysts develop from cells on the outer surface of the ovary. They are often filled with a watery fluid or thick, sticky gel. They can become large and cause pain.
- **Dermoid cysts:** The cells in the ovary are able to make hair, teeth, and other growing tissues that become part of a forming ovarian cyst. These cysts can become large and cause pain.
- **Polycystic ovaries:** The eggs mature within the follicles, or sacs, but the sac doesn't break open to release the egg. The cycle repeats, follicles continue to grow inside the ovary, and cysts form.

What are the symptoms of ovarian cysts?

Many women have ovarian cysts without having any symptoms. Sometimes, though, a cyst will cause these problems:

- Pressure, fullness, or pain in the abdomen
- Dull ache in the lower back and thighs
- Problems passing urine completely
- Pain during sexual intercourse
- Weight gain
- Painful menstrual periods and abnormal bleeding
- Nausea or vomiting
- Breast tenderness

If you have these symptoms, get help right away:

- Pain with fever and vomiting
- Sudden, severe abdominal pain

- Faintness, dizziness, or weakness
- Rapid breathing

How are ovarian cysts found?

Since ovarian cysts may not cause symptoms, they are usually found during a routine pelvic exam. During this exam, your doctor is able to feel the swelling of the cyst on your ovary. Once a cyst is found, the doctor may perform an ultrasound, which uses sound waves to create images of the body. With an ultrasound, the doctor can see how the cyst is shaped; its size and location; and whether it's fluid-filled, solid, or mixed. A pregnancy test is also done. Hormone levels (such as luteinizing hormone [LH], follicle stimulating hormone [FSH], estradiol, and testosterone) may also be checked. Your doctor may want to do other tests as well.

To find out if the cyst might be cancerous, your doctor may do a blood test to measure a substance in the blood called CA-125. The amount of this protein is higher if a woman has ovarian cancer. However, some ovarian cancers do not make enough CA-125 to be detected by the test. There are also noncancerous diseases that increase the levels of CA-125, like uterine fibroids and endometriosis. These noncancerous causes of increased CA-125 are more common in women under thirty-five, while ovarian cancer is very uncommon in this age group. For this reason, the CA-125 test is recommended mostly for women over age thirty-five, who are at high risk for the disease and have a cyst that is partially solid.

How are cysts treated?

Watchful waiting: The patient waits and gets re-examined in one to three months to see if the cyst has changed in size. This is a common treatment option for women who are in their childbearing years, have no symptoms, and have a fluid-filled cyst. It also might be an option for postmenopausal women.

Surgery: If the cyst doesn't go away after several menstrual periods, has gotten larger, looks unusual on the ultrasound, causes pain, or you're postmenopausal, the doctor may want to remove it.

There are two main surgical procedures:

- *Laparoscopy:* If the cyst is small and looks benign on the ultrasound, your doctor may perform a laparoscopy. This procedure is done under general anesthesia. A very small incision is made above or below the navel, and a small instrument that acts like a telescope is inserted into the abdomen. If the cyst is small and looks benign, it can be removed.

- *Laparotomy:* If the cyst is large and looks suspicious, the doctor may perform a procedure called a laparotomy. This procedure involves making bigger incisions in the stomach to remove the cyst. While you are under general anesthesia, the doctor is able to have the cyst tested to find out if the tissue is cancerous. If it is cancerous, the doctor may need to remove the ovary and other tissues that may be affected, like the uterus or lymph nodes.

Birth control pills: If you frequently develop cysts, your doctor may prescribe birth control pills to prevent you from ovulating. This will lower the chances of forming new cysts.

Can ovarian cysts be prevented?

Ovarian cysts cannot be prevented. Fortunately, the vast majority of cysts don't cause any symptoms, are not related to cancer, and go away on their own. Talk to your doctor or nurse if you notice any changes in your period, pain in the pelvic area, or any of the major symptoms listed above. A pelvic exam, possibly with an ultrasound, can help determine if a cyst is causing the problem. If a woman is not seeking pregnancy and develops functional cysts, frequently, future cysts may be prevented by taking oral contraceptives, Depo-Provera, or Norplant.

When are women most likely to have ovarian cysts?

Functional ovarian cysts usually occur during the childbearing years. Most often, cysts in women of this age group are not cancerous. Women who are past menopause (ages fifty to seventy) with ovarian cysts have a higher risk of ovarian cancer. At any age, if you think you have a cyst, it's important to tell your doctor.

Section 13.3

Polycystic Ovary Syndrome

Reprinted from "Polycystic Ovary Syndrome (PCOS)," National Women's Health Information Center, April 2007.

What is polycystic ovary syndrome (PCOS)?

Polycystic ovary syndrome (PCOS) is a health problem that can affect a woman's menstrual cycle, ability to have children, hormones, heart, blood vessels, and appearance. With PCOS, women typically have:

- high levels of androgens (these are sometimes called male hormones, although females also make them);
- missed or irregular periods;
- many small cysts (fluid-filled sacs) in their ovaries.

How many women have polycystic ovary syndrome (PCOS)?

About one in ten women of childbearing age has PCOS. It can occur in girls as young as eleven years old. PCOS is the most common cause of female infertility (not being able to get pregnant).

What causes polycystic ovary syndrome (PCOS)?

The cause of PCOS is unknown. Most researchers think that more than one factor could play a role in developing PCOS. Genes are thought to be one factor. Women with PCOS tend to have a mother or sister with PCOS. Researchers also think insulin could be linked to PCOS. Insulin is a hormone that controls the change of sugar, starches, and other food into energy for the body to use or store. For many women with PCOS, their bodies have problems using insulin so that too much insulin is in the body. Excess insulin appears to increase production of androgen. This hormone is made in fat cells, the ovaries, and the adrenal gland. Levels of androgen that are higher than normal can lead to acne, excessive hair growth, weight gain, and problems with ovulation.

Does polycystic ovary syndrome (PCOS) run in families?

Most researchers think that PCOS runs in families. Women with PCOS tend to have a mother or sister with PCOS. Still, there is no proof that PCOS is inherited.

What are the symptoms of polycystic ovary syndrome (PCOS)?

Not all women with PCOS share the same symptoms. These are some of the symptoms of PCOS:

- Infrequent menstrual periods, no menstrual periods, and/or irregular bleeding
- Infertility (not able to get pregnant) because of not ovulating
- Increased hair growth on the face, chest, stomach, back, thumbs, or toes—a condition called hirsutism
- Ovarian cysts
- Acne, oily skin, or dandruff
- Weight gain or obesity, usually carrying extra weight around the waist
- Insulin resistance or type 2 diabetes
- High cholesterol
- High blood pressure
- Male-pattern baldness or thinning hair
- Patches of thickened and dark brown or black skin on the neck, arms, breasts, or thighs
- Skin tags, or tiny excess flaps of skin in the armpits or neck area
- Pelvic pain
- Anxiety or depression due to appearance and/or infertility
- Sleep apnea—excessive snoring and times when breathing stops while asleep

Why do women with polycystic ovary syndrome (PCOS) have trouble with their menstrual cycle?

The ovaries are two small organs, one on each side of a woman's uterus. A woman's ovaries have follicles, which are tiny sacs filled with liquid that hold the eggs. These sacs also are called cysts. Each month about twenty eggs start to mature, but usually only one matures fully. As this one egg grows, the follicle accumulates fluid in it. When that egg matures, the follicle breaks open to release it. The egg then travels through the fallopian tube for fertilization. When the single egg leaves the follicle, ovulation takes place.

In women with PCOS, the ovary doesn't make all of the hormones it needs for any of the eggs to fully mature. Follicles may start to grow and build up fluid. But no one follicle becomes large enough. Instead, some follicles may remain as cysts. Since no follicle becomes large enough and no egg matures or is released, ovulation does not occur and the hormone progesterone is not made. Without progesterone, a woman's menstrual cycle is irregular or absent. Plus, the cysts make male hormones, which also prevent ovulation.

Does polycystic ovary syndrome (PCOS) change at menopause?

Yes and no. Because PCOS affects many systems in the body, many symptoms persist even though ovarian function and hormone levels change as a woman nears menopause. For instance, excessive hair growth continues, and male pattern baldness or thinning hair gets worse after menopause. Also, the risks of complications from PCOS, such as heart attack, stroke, and diabetes, increase as a woman gets older.

What tests are used to diagnose polycystic ovary syndrome (PCOS)?

There is no single test to diagnose PCOS. Your doctor will take a medical history, perform a physical exam, and possibly take some tests to rule out other causes of your symptoms. During the physical exam the doctor will want to measure your blood pressure, body mass index (BMI), and waist size. He or she also will check out the areas of increased hair growth, so try to allow the natural hair growth for a few days before the visit. Your doctor might want to do a pelvic exam to see if your ovaries are enlarged or swollen by the increased number of small cysts. A vaginal ultrasound also might be used to examine the ovaries for cysts and check out the endometrium, the lining of the uterus. The uterine lining may become thicker if your periods are not regular. You also might have blood taken to check your hormone levels and to measure glucose (sugar) levels.

How is polycystic ovary syndrome (PCOS) treated?

Because there is no cure for PCOS, it needs to be managed to prevent problems. Treatment goals are based on your symptoms, whether or not you want to become pregnant, and lowering your chances of getting heart disease and diabetes. Many women will need a combination of treatments to meet these goals. Some treatments for PCOS are listed here.

Birth control pills: For women who don't want to become pregnant, birth control pills can control menstrual cycles, reduce male hormone levels, and help to clear acne. However, the menstrual cycle will become abnormal again if the pill is stopped. Women may also think about taking a pill that only has progesterone, like Provera®, to control the menstrual cycle and reduce the risk of endometrial cancer. But progesterone alone does not help reduce acne and hair growth.

Diabetes medications: The medicine metformin (Glucophage®) is used to treat type 2 diabetes. It also has been found to help with PCOS symptoms, although it is not FDA-approved for this use. Metformin affects the way insulin controls blood glucose (sugar) and lowers testosterone production. Abnormal hair growth will slow down, and ovulation may return after a few months of use. Recent research has shown metformin to have other positive effects, such as decreased body mass and improved cholesterol levels. Metformin will not cause a person to become diabetic.

Fertility medications: Lack of ovulation is usually the reason for fertility problems in women with PCOS. Several medications that stimulate ovulation can help women with PCOS become pregnant. Even so, other reasons for infertility in both the woman and man should be ruled out before fertility medications are used. Also, there is an increased risk for multiple births (twins, triplets) with fertility medications. For most patients, clomiphene citrate (Clomid®, Serophene®) is the first choice therapy to stimulate ovulation. If this fails, metformin taken with clomiphene is usually tried. When metformin is taken along with fertility medications, it may help women with PCOS ovulate on lower doses of medication. Gonadotropins also can be used to stimulate ovulation. These are given as shots. But gonadotropins are more expensive and there are greater chances of multiple births compared to clomiphene. Another option is in vitro fertilization (IVF). IVF offers the best chance of becoming pregnant in any one cycle and gives doctors better control over the chance of multiple births. But, IVF is very costly.

Medicine for increased hair growth or extra male hormones: Medicines called anti-androgens may reduce hair growth and clear acne. Spironolactone (Aldactone®), first used to treat high blood pressure, has been shown to reduce the impact of male hormones on hair growth in women. Finasteride (Propecia®), a medicine taken by men for hair loss, has the same effect. Anti-androgens often are combined with oral contraceptives.

Before taking Aldactone®, tell your doctor if you are pregnant or plan to become pregnant. Do not breastfeed while taking this medicine. Women who may become pregnant should not handle Propecia®.

Vaniqa® cream also reduces facial hair in some women. Other treatments such as laser hair removal or electrolysis work well at getting rid of hair in some women. A woman with PCOS can also take hormonal treatment to keep new hair from growing.

Surgery: "Ovarian drilling" is a surgery that brings on ovulation. It is sometimes used when a woman does not respond to fertility medicines. The doctor makes a very small cut above or below the navel and inserts a small tool that acts like a telescope into the abdomen. This is called laparoscopy. The doctor then punctures the ovary with a small needle carrying an electric current to destroy a small portion of the ovary. This procedure carries a risk of developing scar tissue on the ovary. This surgery can lower male hormone levels and help with ovulation. But these effects may only last a few months. This treatment doesn't help with loss of scalp hair and increased hair growth on other parts of the body.

Lifestyle modification: Keeping a healthy weight by eating healthy foods and exercising is another way women can help manage PCOS. Many women with PCOS are overweight or obese. Eat fewer processed foods and foods with added sugars and more whole-grain products, fruits, vegetables, and lean meats to help lower blood sugar (glucose) levels, improve the body's use of insulin, and normalize hormone levels in your body. Even a 10 percent loss in body weight can restore a normal period and make a woman's cycle more regular.

How does polycystic ovary syndrome (PCOS) affect a woman while pregnant?

There appears to be higher rates of miscarriage, gestational diabetes, pregnancy-induced high blood pressure (preeclampsia), and premature delivery in women with PCOS. Researchers are studying how the diabetes medicine metformin can prevent or reduce the chances of having these problems while pregnant. Metformin also lowers male hormone levels and limits weight gain in women who are obese when they get pregnant.

Metformin is a FDA pregnancy category B drug. It does not appear to cause major birth defects or other problems in pregnant women. But there have been no studies of metformin on pregnant women to confirm its safety. Talk to your doctor about taking metformin during pregnancy or if you are trying to become pregnant. Also, metformin is passed through milk in breastfeeding mothers. Talk with your doctor about metformin use if you are a nursing mother.

Does polycystic ovary syndrome (PCOS) put women at risk for other health problems?

Women with PCOS have greater chances of developing several serious, life-threatening diseases, including type 2 diabetes, cardiovascular disease (CVD), and cancer. Recent studies found the following things:

- More than 50 percent of women with PCOS will have diabetes or pre-diabetes (impaired glucose tolerance) before the age of forty.
- Women with PCOS have a four to seven times higher risk of heart attack than women of the same age without PCOS.
- Women with PCOS are at greater risk of having high blood pressure.
- Women with PCOS have high levels of low-density lipoprotein (LDL, or bad) cholesterol and low levels of high-density lipoprotein (HDL, or good) cholesterol.

The chance of getting endometrial cancer is another concern for women with PCOS. Irregular menstrual periods and the absence of ovulation cause women to produce the hormone estrogen, but not the hormone progesterone. Progesterone causes the endometrium to shed its lining each month as a menstrual period. Without progesterone, the endometrium becomes thick, which can cause heavy bleeding or irregular bleeding. Over time, this can lead to endometrial hyperplasia, when the lining grows too much, and cancer.

I have PCOS. What can I do to prevent complications?

Getting your symptoms under control at an earlier age can help to reduce your chances of having complications like diabetes and heart disease. Talk to your doctor about treating all your symptoms, rather than focusing on just one aspect of your PCOS, such as problems getting pregnant. Also, talk to your doctor about getting tested for diabetes regularly. Eating right, exercising, and not smoking also will help to reduce your chances of having other health problems.

How can I cope with the emotional affects of PCOS?

Having PCOS can be difficult. Many women are embarrassed by their appearance. Others may worry about being able to get pregnant. Some women with PCOS might get depressed. Getting treatment for PCOS can help with these concerns and help boost a woman's self-esteem. Support groups located across the United States and online also can help women with PCOS deal with the emotional affects.

Chapter 14

Endometriosis

What is endometriosis?

Endometriosis is a common, yet poorly understood disease that can strike women of any socioeconomic class or race. The name endometriosis comes from the word "endometrium," which is the tissue that lines the inside of the uterus. Normally, if a woman is not pregnant, this tissue builds up and is shed each month as menstrual flow (your period). Endometriosis occurs when this tissue grows outside the uterus on the surfaces of organs in the pelvic and abdominal areas where it does not normally grow. Tissues surrounding the area of endometriosis may become inflamed or swollen, leading to the development of scar tissue. After menopause, the abnormal implants shrink away and the symptoms subside.

In what places, outside of the uterus, do areas of endometriosis grow?

Most endometriosis is found in the pelvic cavity, including:

- on or under the ovaries;

"Facts about Endometriosis," reprinted courtesy of the Illinois Department of Public Health (www.idph.state.il.us). The text of this document is available online at http://www.idph.state.il.us/about/womenshealth/factsheets/endo.htm; accessed May 12, 2008.

- behind the uterus;
- on the tissues that hold the uterus in place;
- on the bowels or bladder.

In extremely rare cases, endometriosis areas can grow in the lungs or other parts of the body.

What are some symptoms of endometriosis?

Endometriosis can affect a menstruating woman, from the time of her first period to menopause. One of the most common symptoms of endometriosis is pain, mostly in the abdomen, lower back, and pelvic areas. The severity of pain a woman feels is not linked to the amount of endometriosis. Some women experience no pain even though their endometriosis is extensive, which means that the affected areas are large or there is scarring. Some women, on the other hand, have severe pain even though they have only a few small areas of endometriosis. The following are some symptoms of endometriosis:

- extremely painful (or disabling) menstrual cramps;
- lower back, intestinal, and pelvic pain;
- pain during or after sex;
- intestinal pain;
- painful bowel movements or painful urination during menstrual periods;
- heavy menstrual periods, or spotting or bleeding between periods;
- infertility.

What can raise my chances of getting endometriosis?

You are more likely to develop endometriosis is you:

- began getting your period at an early age;
- have heavy periods;
- have periods that last more than seven days;
- have a short monthly cycle (twenty-seven days or less);
- have a close relative (mother, aunt, sister) with endometriosis.

How can I reduce my chances of getting endometriosis?

Some studies suggest that you may lower your chances of developing endometriosis if you exercise regularly and avoid alcohol and caffeine.

Does endometriosis make you infertile?

Severe endometriosis with extensive scarring and organ damage may affect fertility. It is considered one of the three major causes of female infertility; about 30 percent to 40 percent of women with endometriosis are infertile. While the pregnancy rates for patients with endometriosis remain lower than those of the general population, most patients with endometriosis do not experience fertility problems. For those with endometriosis-related infertility, it is often treated successfully with hormones and surgery.

How do I know if I have endometriosis?

Currently, health care providers use a number of tests for endometriosis. The two most common are imaging tests—ultrasound, a machine that uses sound waves to produce images of organs and systems within the body, and magnetic resonance imaging (MRI), a machine that uses magnets and radio waves to provide an image. The only way to know for sure is by having surgery. The most common type is laparoscopy. The surgeon uses a small viewing instrument with a light, called a laparoscope, to look at the reproductive organs, intestines, and other surfaces to see if there is any endometriosis. The diagnosis can be confirmed by doing a biopsy, which involves taking a small tissue sample and studying it under a microscope.

What are the treatments for endometriosis?

There is no cure for endometriosis, but there are treatments. For patients who wish to become pregnant, doctors are advising that, depending on the age of the patient and the amount of pain associated with the disease, the best course of action is to have a trial period of unprotected intercourse for six months to one year. If pregnancy does not occur within that time, then further treatment may be needed. For patients not seeking to become pregnant the treatment may include:

- **Pain medication:** Works well if the pain or other symptoms are mild. These medications range from over-the-counter remedies to strong prescription drugs.

- **Hormone therapy:** Effective if your areas are small and/or you have minimal pain. Hormones can come in pill form, by shot or injection, or in a nasal spray. Common hormones used to treat endometriosis pain are progesterone, birth control pills, Danocrine, and gonadotropin-releasing hormone (GnRH).
- **Surgical treatment:** Usually the best choice if your endometriosis is extensive, or if you have more severe pain. Surgical treatments range from minor to major surgical procedures. You and your health care provider should talk about possible options for removing endometriosis before your surgery. Then, based on the findings and treatment at surgery, you and your health care provider can discuss medical treatment options for after surgery.

Chapter 15

Uterine Fibroids

What are uterine fibroids?

Uterine fibroids are tumors or lumps made of muscle cells and other tissue that grow within the wall of the uterus. Fibroids may grow as a single tumor or in clusters.

A single fibroid can be less than one inch in size or can grow to eight inches across or more. A bunch or cluster of fibroids can also vary in size.

Where do uterine fibroids grow?

Most fibroids grow within the wall of the uterus. Health care providers put fibroids into three groups based on where they grow:

- Submucosal fibroids grow just underneath the uterine lining.
- Intramural fibroids grow in between the muscles of the uterus.
- Subserosal fibroids grow on the outside of the uterus.

Some fibroids grow on stalks that grow out from the surface of the uterus, or into the cavity of the uterus. These are called pedunculated fibroids.

Excerpted from "Fast Facts about Uterine Fibroids," National Institute of Child Health and Human Development, National Institutes of Health, August 18, 2006.

What are the symptoms of uterine fibroids?

Many women don't feel any symptoms with uterine fibroids. But fibroids can cause the following symptoms:

- Heavy bleeding or painful periods
- Bleeding between periods
- Feeling "full" in the lower abdomen—sometimes called "pelvic pressure"
- Urinating often (results from a fibroid pressing on the bladder)
- Pain during sex
- Lower back pain
- Reproductive problems, such as infertility, multiple miscarriages, and early onset of labor during pregnancy

What causes uterine fibroids?

Currently, we know little about what causes uterine fibroids. Scientists have a number of theories, but none of these ideas explains fibroids completely. Most likely, fibroids are the end result of many factors interacting with each other. These factors could be genetic, hormonal, environmental, or a combination of all three. Once we know the cause or causes of fibroids, our efforts to find a cure or even prevent fibroids will move ahead more quickly.

Does having uterine fibroids mean that I will be infertile or unable to have children?

Most women who have fibroids do not have problems with fertility and are able to get pregnant. In some cases, fibroids can prevent a woman from getting pregnant through natural methods. However, advances in treatments for fibroids and infertility have greatly improved the chances for a woman to get pregnant, even if she has uterine fibroids.

Researchers are still looking into what role, if any, uterine fibroids play in infertility. Currently, though, there are few answers. One study's results suggest that only submucosal fibroids have a negative impact on fertility, but these results are not yet confirmed. The relationship between fibroids and infertility remains a very active research area.

Does having uterine fibroids mean I will need a hysterectomy?

Hysterectomy (removal of the uterus) is not the best option for every woman with uterine fibroids. If you want to have children, then you would want to avoid this treatment. Likewise, if you don't have symptoms of uterine fibroids, or your fibroids are small, you may have better results from pain medications or hormone treatments. Health care providers are also exploring less-invasive surgical treatments for fibroids that save the uterus.

In some cases, though, a hysterectomy is the best method of treatment. If you have uterine fibroids and are thinking about having a hysterectomy, make sure you talk over all features of the surgery with your doctor and your family. Having a hysterectomy means that you will no longer be able to have children. This process cannot be reversed, so be certain about your choice before having the surgery.

Keep in mind that the physical scars of the procedure may heal quickly, but some of the effects of hysterectomy are long lasting. You may want to talk to women who have had the procedure before you decide to have your surgery. Many health care centers, women's clinics, and hospitals offer support groups for women who have had, or are in the process of having hysterectomies.

Who gets uterine fibroids?

Most of the time, fibroids grow in women of childbearing age. Research studies estimate that doctors diagnose up to 30 percent of women of childbearing age with uterine fibroids; but, because some women show no symptoms of fibroids, as many as 77 percent of women of childbearing age could have the condition, without knowing it. We don't know exactly how many new cases of fibroids occur in a year, nor do we know how many women have fibroids at any one time.

There have also been reports of rare cases in which young girls who have not yet started their periods (pre-pubertal) had small fibroids. Researchers have also found that fibroids sometimes run in families.

Researchers now recognize several risk factors for uterine fibroids:

- Current statistics place African American women at three to five times greater risk than white women for fibroids.
- Women who are overweight or obese for their height (based on body mass index or BMI) are also at slightly higher risk for fibroids than women who are average weight for their height.

- Women who have given birth appear to be at lower risk for uterine fibroids.

But, because we don't know what causes fibroids, we also don't know what increases or decreases the risk.

How do I know that I have uterine fibroids?

Unless you start to have symptoms, you probably won't know that you have uterine fibroids.

Sometimes, health care providers find fibroids during a routine gynecological exam.

During this exam, the health care provider checks out the size of your uterus by putting two fingers of one hand into the vagina, while applying light pressure to your abdomen with the other hand.

If you have fibroids, your uterus may feel larger than normal; or, if you have fibroids, your uterus may extend into places it should not.

If your health care provider thinks that you have fibroids, he or she may use imaging technology—machines that create a "picture" of the inside of your body without surgery—to confirm the diagnosis. Some common types of imaging technology include the following:

- Ultrasound, which uses sound waves to form the picture
- Magnetic resonance imaging or MRI, which uses magnets and radio waves to build the picture
- X-rays, which use a form of electromagnetic radiation to "see" into the body
- Computed tomography (CT) or "cat" scan, which takes x-rays of the body from many angles to provide a more complete image

Sometimes, health care providers use a combination of these technologies.

Sometimes, however, the only way to confirm the presence of uterine fibroids is through surgery:

- Laparoscopy: In this procedure, the surgeon makes a small cut into the abdomen, after inflating it with a harmless gas; then, using a small viewing instrument with a light in it, the doctor can look for fibroids.

- Your health care provider may suggest a procedure called a hysteroscopy, which involves inserting a camera on a long tube through the vagina directly into the uterus to see the fibroids.

Keep in mind that because these are surgical procedures, you will need time to recover from them. However, the amount of recovery time you'll need may vary.

What are the treatments for uterine fibroids?

Health care providers consider a number of things when recommending treatment for fibroids, including the following:

- Does the woman have symptoms of uterine fibroids?
- Does she want to become pregnant?
- How large are the fibroids?
- What is the woman's age?

If you have uterine fibroids, but show no symptoms or have no problems, you may not need any treatment. Your health care provider will check the fibroids at your routine gynecological exam to see if they have grown. Also, because fibroids are dependent on hormones, your fibroids may decrease in size during or after menopause.

If you have pain now and then or feel mild symptoms, your health care provider may suggest pain medication, ranging from over-the-counter remedies to strong prescription drugs.

Medical therapy: If you have many symptoms or feel pain often, you may benefit from medical therapy—that is, therapy using certain medications rather than surgery. Keep in mind that many medications have side effects, some of them serious.

One way to reduce symptoms of uterine fibroids is using one of a group of hormones called gonadotropin releasing hormone agonists (GnRHa). These hormones block the body from making the hormones that cause women to menstruate or have their periods. If you have symptoms, have health conditions that make surgery less advisable, and are near menopause or do not want children, you may receive GnRHa therapy to treat your fibroids.

Antihormonal agents, like mifepristone, also slow or stop the growth of fibroids.

Medical therapy is often used before a woman has surgery for her fibroids.

This therapy offers only temporary relief from the symptoms of fibroids; once you go off the therapy, your fibroids may grow back.

Surgical therapy: If you have moderate symptoms of fibroids, surgery may be the best form of treatment. Talk to your doctor about the different types of surgery. Surgery can be a major or minor procedure. Also talk about the possible risks of the procedure and the side effects:

- Myomectomy removes only the fibroids and leaves the healthy areas of the uterus in place. This procedure can preserve a woman's ability to have children. Sometimes a laparoscope is used to see the inside the abdomen during a myomectomy. A hysteroscope may be used to see the size, shape, and location of fibroids inside the lining of the uterus. In some cases, surgeons may use the instrument to remove the fibroid.
- Hysterectomy is used if your fibroids are large, or you have heavy bleeding, and you are either near or past menopause, or you don't want children. Hysterectomy is the only sure way to cure uterine fibroids. In general, recovery time from a hysterectomy is one to two months. Health care providers now have hysterectomy options that differ in how invasive they are. If you are pre-menopausal, talk to your doctor about keeping your ovaries. The ovaries provide hormones that help maintain bone health and sexual health. Sometimes surgeons use a laparoscope to see inside the abdomen during a hysterectomy. Abdominal hysterectomy is a procedure that involves a cut into the abdomen to remove the uterus. Vaginal hysterectomy is less invasive because the doctor reaches the uterus through the vagina, instead of making a cut into the abdomen. This procedure may not be an option if the fibroids are very large.
- Uterine artery embolization (UAE), also called uterine fibroid embolization or UFE, is a newer treatment that cuts off the blood supply to the fibroids, making them shrink. Recovery time for UAE is much shorter than for hysterectomy. Because this procedure can affect how the ovaries function and can limit fertility, health care providers do not recommend UAE for women who still want to have children.

Are there any developing treatments for uterine fibroids?

Currently, researchers are looking into other methods of treating uterine fibroids. Keep in mind that these methods are not yet standard treatments for uterine fibroids, which means your health care provider may not offer them, or your insurance company may not pay for them. But, it's possible that research to confirm the safety and effectiveness of these "experimental" treatments may advance our ability to treat uterine fibroids. These developing treatments include the following:

- Magnetic resonance imaging (MRI)–guided ultrasound surgery uses a high-intensity ultrasound beam to send high temperatures to the fibroids to make them shrink. The MRI scanner helps visualize the fibroid and the ultrasound can then send sound waves to destroy the tissue.
- Some health care providers use lasers to remove a fibroid or to cut off the blood supply to the fibroid, making it shrink.

Do uterine fibroids lead to cancer?

Uterine fibroids are not cancerous. Fibroids are not associated with cancer; they rarely develop into cancer (in less than 0.1 percent of cases). Having fibroids does not increase your risk for uterine cancer.

Do uterine fibroids ever go away?

For the most part, fibroids stop growing or shrink once a woman passes menopause. However, this is not the case for all women. Some studies suggests a relationship between hormone replacement therapy or HRT, used to reduce the symptoms of menopause, and uterine fibroids, but the nature of this relationship is still unclear. More research is needed in this area.

Chapter 16

Vaginal and Pelvic Infections

Chapter Contents

Section 16.1

Bacterial Vaginosis

Reprinted from "Bacterial Vaginosis,"
National Institute of Allergy and Infectious Diseases,
National Institutes of Health, May 15, 2008.

Overview

According to the Centers for Disease Control and Prevention (CDC), bacterial vaginosis (BV) is the most common cause of vaginitis symptoms among women of childbearing age. It previously was called nonspecific vaginitis, or *Gardnerella*-associated vaginitis. Health experts are not sure what role sexual activity plays in developing BV.

Cause

BV is a sign of a change in the growth of vaginal bacteria. The resulting chemical imbalance occurs when different types of bacteria outnumber the normal "good," or beneficial, ones. Instead of *Lactobacillus* (a type bacteria that normally lives in the vagina) being most common, increased numbers of bacteria such as *Gardnerella vaginalis, Bacteroides, Mobiluncus*, and *Mycoplasma hominis* inhabit the vaginas of women with BV.

Transmission

Although health experts are not sure what role sexual activity plays in developing BV, a change in sexual partners or having multiple sexual partners may increase a woman's chances of getting the infection. Using an intrauterine device (IUD) and douching also may increase her risk of getting BV.

Symptoms

The main symptom of BV is an abnormal, foul-smelling vaginal discharge. Some women describe it as a fish-like odor that is most noticeable after having sex.

Other symptoms may include the following:

- Thin vaginal discharge, usually white or gray in color
- Pain during urination
- Itching around the vagina

Some women who have signs of BV, such as increased levels of certain harmful bacteria, have no symptoms. A health care provider who sees these signs during a physical examination can confirm the diagnosis by doing lab tests of vaginal fluid.

Diagnosis

A health care provider can examine a sample of vaginal fluid under a microscope, either stained or in special lighting, to look for bacteria associated with BV. Then, they can diagnose BV based on the following things:

- Absence of lactobacilli
- Presence of numerous "clue cells" (cells from the vaginal lining that are coated with BV germs)
- Fishy odor
- Change from normal vaginal fluid

Treatment

Health care providers use antibiotics such as metronidazole or clindamycin to treat women with BV. Generally, male sex partners will not be treated.

Complications

In most cases, BV causes no complications. There have been documented risks of BV, however, such as an association between BV and pelvic inflammatory disease (PID). PID is a serious disease in women that can cause infertility and tubal (ectopic) pregnancy.

BV also can cause other problems such as premature delivery and low-birth-weight babies. Therefore, some health experts recommend that all pregnant women who previously have delivered a premature baby be checked for BV, whether or not they have symptoms. A pregnant woman who has not delivered a premature baby should be treated if she has symptoms and laboratory evidence of BV.

BV also is associated with increased chances of getting one or more sexually transmitted infections, including chlamydia, gonorrhea, or human immunodeficiency virus (HIV) infection.

Section 16.2

Toxic Shock Syndrome

Reprinted from "Toxic Shock Syndrome,"
© 2008 A.D.A.M., Inc. Reprinted with permission.

Alternative Names

TSS; staphylococcal toxic shock syndrome

Definition

Toxic shock syndrome is a severe disease that involves fever, shock, and problems with the function of several body organs.

Causes

Toxic shock syndrome (TSS) is caused by a toxin produced by certain types of *Staphylococcus* bacteria. (A similar syndrome, called toxic shock–like syndrome (TSLS), can be caused by *Streptococcus* bacteria.)

Although the earliest described cases of TSS involved women who were using tampons during their periods (menstruation), only 55 percent of current cases are associated with menstruation. Toxic shock syndrome can also occur in children, postmenopausal women, and men.

Risk factors include:

- menstruation;
- use of barrier contraceptives such as a diaphragm or vaginal sponge;
- tampon use (particularly if you leave in for a long time);

- foreign bodies or packings (such as those used to stop nosebleeds);
- childbirth;
- surgery;
- current *Staphylococcus aureus* (*S. aureus*) infection.

Symptoms

- High fever, sometimes accompanied by chills
- Malaise (discomfort, ill feeling)
- Nausea
- Vomiting
- Diarrhea
- Widespread red rash resembling a sunburn
- Rash followed in one or two weeks by peeling of the skin, particularly on the palms of the hand or bottom of the feet
- Redness of eyes, mouth, throat
- Confusion
- Seizures
- Headaches
- Muscle aches
- Hypotension (low blood pressure)
- Organ failure (usually kidneys and liver)

Exams and Tests

There is no one diagnostic test for TSS. The diagnosis of toxic shock syndrome is based on several criteria: fever, low blood pressure, rash that peels after one to two weeks, and at least three organs with signs of dysfunction. In some cases, blood cultures may be positive for growth of *S. aureus*.

Treatment

Any foreign materials, such as tampons, vaginal sponges, or nasal packing, will be removed. Sites of infection (such as surgical wound) will be drained.

Treatments maintain important body functions (supportive measures) are essential. This may include:

- intravenous (IV) fluids;
- methods to control blood pressure;
- dialysis (if severe kidney problems are present);
- antibiotics for any infection (may be given through an IV).

Outlook (Prognosis)

Toxic shock syndrome may be deadly in up to 50 percent of cases. The condition may return in those that survive.

Possible Complications

- Severe organ dysfunction
    - Kidney failure
    - Heart failure
    - Liver failure
- Shock

When to Contact a Medical Professional

TSS is a medical emergency. You must seek immediate attention if you develop fever or rash, particularly during menstruation and tampon use, or if you have had recent surgery.

Prevention

Menstrual TSS can be prevented by avoiding the use of highly absorbent tampons. Risk can also be reduced by using less absorbent tampons, changing tampons more frequently, and using tampons only intermittently (not regularly) during menstruation.

References

Rakel P. *Conn's Current Therapy 2006*. 58th ed. Philadelphia, Pa: WB Saunders; 2006:103–6.

Goldman L, Ausiello D. *Cecil Textbook of Medicine*, 22nd ed. Philadelphia, Pa: WB Saunders; 2004:1785–86.

Section 16.3

Vaginal Yeast Infections

Reprinted from "Vaginal Yeast Infections," National Women's Health Information Center, April 2006.

What is a vaginal yeast infection?

A vaginal yeast infection is irritation of the vagina and the area around the vagina, called the vulva. It is caused by an overgrowth of the fungus or yeast *Candida*. Yeast normally live in the vagina in small numbers, but when the bacteria in the vagina become out of balance, too many yeast grow and cause an infection.

Vaginal yeast infections are very common. About 75 percent of women have a yeast infection during their lives. And almost half of women have two or more yeast infections.

What are the signs of a vaginal yeast infection?

The most common symptom of a yeast infection is extreme itchiness in and around the vagina. Other symptoms include the following:

- Burning, redness, and swelling of the vagina and the area around it
- Pain when urinating
- Pain or discomfort during sex
- A thick, white vaginal discharge that looks like cottage cheese and does not have a bad smell

You may only have a few of these symptoms and they may be mild or severe.

Should I call my doctor if I think I have a yeast infection?

Yes, you need to see your doctor to know for sure if you have a yeast infection, especially if you've never had one before. The signs of a yeast infection are similar to those of sexually transmitted diseases (STDs) like chlamydia and gonorrhea. So, it's hard to be sure you have a yeast infection and not something more serious.

If you've had vaginal yeast infections in the past, talk to your doctor about using over-the-counter medicines.

How is a vaginal yeast infection diagnosed?

Your doctor will do a pelvic exam to look for swelling and discharge. She may also use a swab to take a sample from the vagina. A quick look under the microscope or a lab test will show if yeast is causing the problem.

Why did I get a yeast infection?

Many things can change the acidity of the vagina and boost your chances of a vaginal yeast infection. These include the following:

- Stress
- Lack of sleep
- Sickness
- Poor diet, or extreme intake of sugary foods
- Pregnancy
- Having your period
- Taking birth control pills
- Taking antibiotics
- Taking steroid medicines
- Diseases such as poorly controlled diabetes and human immunodeficiency virus (HIV) infection

Can I get a yeast infection from having sex?

Yes, but it is rare. Women usually do not get yeast infections from sex. Instead, a weakened immune system is the most common cause of yeast infections.

How are yeast infections treated?

Yeast infections can be cured with antifungal medicines in the form of creams, tablets, ointments, or suppositories that are inserted into the vagina. These medicines include butoconazole, clotrimazole, miconazole, nystatin, tioconazole, and terconazole. These products can be bought over the counter at the drug store or grocery store. Your doctor can also prescribe you a single dose of oral fluconazole.

Infections that do not respond to these medicines are becoming more common. Using antifungal medicines when you don't really have a yeast infection can boost your risk of getting a hard-to-treat infection in the future.

Is it safe to use over-the-counter medicines for yeast infections?

Yes, but it is important to talk to your doctor first. Always call your doctor before treating yourself for a vaginal yeast infection if any of the following are true:

- You are pregnant
- You have never been diagnosed with a yeast infection
- You are having repeat yeast infections

Studies show that two-thirds of women who buy these products do not really have a yeast infection. Using these medicines incorrectly may lead to a hard-to-treat infection. Plus, treating yourself for a yeast infection when you really have another kind of infection may worsen the problem.

If you decide to use these over-the-counter medicines, be sure to read and follow the directions carefully. Some creams and inserts may weaken condoms and diaphragms.

If I have a yeast infection, does my sexual partner need to be treated?

Not unless he shows signs of a yeast infection. Rarely, men who have sex with women with yeast infections will get an itchy rash on their penis. If this happens, he should see his doctor.

What should I do if I get repeat yeast infections?

Call your doctor. About 5 percent of women develop four or more vaginal yeast infections in one year. This is called recurrent vulvovaginal candidiasis (RVVC). RVVC is more common in women with diabetes or weakened immune systems. Doctors normally treat this problem with antifungal medicine for up to six months.

How can I avoid getting another yeast infection?

To help prevent vaginal yeast infections, try the following:

- Don't use douches.
- Avoid scented hygiene products like bubble bath, sprays, pads, and tampons.
- Change tampons and pads often during your period.
- Don't wear tight underwear or clothes made of synthetic fibers.
- Wear cotton underwear and pantyhose with a cotton crotch.
- Change out of wet swimsuits and exercise clothes as soon as possible.

If you have repeat yeast infections, talk to your doctor.

Section 16.4

Sexually Transmitted Diseases

Reprinted from "STDs Today,"
Centers for Disease Control and Prevention, 2007.

Sexually transmitted diseases (STDs) affect men and women of all backgrounds and economic levels. In the United States, overall incidence of STDs has increased dramatically in recent years.[1] The Centers for Disease Control and Prevention (CDC) estimates that nineteen million new infections occur each year, almost half of them among young people ages fifteen to twenty-four.[2]

Despite the fact that STDs are extremely widespread and add an estimated $13 billion dollars to the nation's healthcare costs each year,[3] most people in the United States remain unaware of the risk and consequences of all but the most prominent STD—human immunodeficiency virus (HIV), the virus that causes acquired immunodeficiency syndrome (AIDS).

Common STDs and the Organisms That Cause Them

Many people are aware of the most prominent STD—HIV. However, many other STDs affect millions of men and women each year. Many of these STDs initially cause no symptoms, especially in women. Symptoms, when they do develop, may be confused with those of other diseases that are not transmitted through sexual contact. STDs can still be transmitted person to person even if they do not show symptoms. Also, health problems caused by STDs tend to be more severe for women than for men.

Below are descriptions of several of the most common STDs, including information about incidence, symptoms (if any), and treatment.

Acquired immunodeficiency syndrome (AIDS): AIDS was first reported in the United States in 1981. Since the beginning of the epidemic, an estimated 944,306 people have developed AIDS in the United States.[4] AIDS is caused by the human immunodeficiency virus (HIV), a virus that destroys the body's ability to fight off infection.

People who have AIDS are very susceptible to many life-threatening diseases, called opportunistic infections, and to certain forms of cancer. Transmission of the virus primarily occurs during unprotected sexual activity and by sharing needles used to inject intravenous drugs.

Chancroid: Chancroid is a bacterial infection caused by *Haemophilus ducreyi*, which is spread by sexual contact and results in genital ulcers. The disease is found primarily in developing and third world countries. Only a few hundred cases a year are diagnosed in the United States. The majority of individuals in the U.S. diagnosed with chancroid have traveled outside the country to areas where the disease is known to occur frequently.[5]

The infection begins with the appearance of painful open sores on the genitals, sometimes accompanied by swollen, tender lymph nodes in the groin. These symptoms occur within a week after exposure. Symptoms in women are often less noticeable and may be limited to painful urination or defecation, painful intercourse, rectal bleeding, or vaginal discharge. Chancroid lesions may be difficult to distinguish from ulcers caused by genital herpes or syphilis. A physician must therefore diagnose the infection by excluding other diseases with similar symptoms. Chancroid is one of the genital ulcer diseases that may be associated with an increased risk of transmission of the human immunodeficiency virus (HIV), the cause of AIDS.

People with chancroid can be treated effectively with one of several antibiotics.

Chlamydia: Chlamydial infection is a common sexually transmitted disease (STD) caused by the bacterium *Chlamydia trachomatis*. Chlamydia is the most frequently reported bacterial sexually transmitted disease in the United States. An estimated 2.8 million Americans are infected with chlamydia each year.[6] Under-reporting is substantial because most people with chlamydia are not aware of their infections and do not seek testing. The highest rates of chlamydial infection are in fifteen- to nineteen-year-old adolescents, regardless of demographics or location.[7] According to a 1997 report, the annual cost of chlamydial infection was estimated at over $2 billion.[8]

Chlamydia can be transmitted during vaginal, oral, or anal sexual contact with an infected partner. A pregnant woman may pass the infection to her newborn during delivery, with subsequent neonatal eye infection or pneumonia. Even though symptoms of chlamydia are usually mild or absent, it can damage a woman's reproductive organs and cause serious complications. Irreversible damage, including infertility, can occur "silently" before a woman ever recognizes a problem. Chlamydia also can cause discharge from the penis of an infected man, although complications among men are rare.

Pelvic inflammatory disease (PID), a serious complication of chlamydial infection, has emerged as a major cause of infertility among women of childbearing age.

Chlamydia can be easily treated and cured with antibiotics.

Genital herpes/HSV: Genital herpes is a contagious viral infection caused by the herpes simplex virus (HSV) which has affected an estimated one out of five (or forty-five million) Americans. There are two types of HSV, and both can cause genital herpes. Genital HSV-2 infection is more common in women (approximately one out of four women) than in men (almost one out of five). Doctors estimate that as many as 500,000 new cases may occur each year.[9]

HSV type 1 most commonly causes sores on the lips (known as fever blisters or cold sores), but it can cause genital infections through oral-genital or genital-genital contact. HSV type 2 most often causes genital sores, but it also can infect the mouth. Both HSV 1 and 2 can produce sores in and around the vaginal area, on the penis, around the anal opening, and on the buttocks or thighs. Occasionally, sores also appear on other parts of the body where broken skin has come into contact with HSV. The virus remains in certain nerve cells of the body for life, causing periodic symptoms in some people.

Genital herpes infection usually is acquired by sexual contact with someone who unknowingly is having an asymptomatic outbreak of herpes sores in the genital area. People with oral herpes can transmit the infection to the genital area of a partner during oral-genital sex. Herpes infections also can be transmitted by a person who is infected with HSV who has noticeable symptoms. The virus is spread only rarely, if at all, by contact with objects such as a toilet seat or hot tub.

There is no treatment that can cure herpes, but antiviral medications can shorten and prevent outbreaks during the period of time the person takes the medication.

Genital human papillomavirus (HPV) infection: HPV is one of the most common causes of sexually transmitted disease (STD) in the world. Experts estimate that as many as twenty-four million Americans are infected with HPV, and the frequency of infection and disease appears to be increasing. At least 50 percent of sexually active men and women acquire genital HPV infection at some point in their lives. By age fifty, at least 80 percent of women will have acquired genital HPV infection.[10]

Human papillomavirus is the name of a group of viruses that includes more than one hundred different strains or types. More than thirty of these viruses are sexually transmitted, and they can infect the genital area of men and women including the skin of the penis, vulva (area outside the vagina), or anus, and the linings of the vagina, cervix, or rectum. Low-risk types of HPV cause genital warts, the most recognizable sign of genital HPV infection. Other high-risk types of HPV cause cervical cancer and other genital cancers.[11]

One study sponsored by the National Institute of Allergy and Infectious Diseases (NIAID) reported that almost half of the women infected with HPV had no obvious symptoms. Because the viral infection persists, individuals may not be aware of their infection or the potential risk of transmission to others and of developing complications.[12] Most people who become infected with HPV will not have any symptoms and will clear the infection on their own.

There is no "cure" for HPV infection, although in most women the infection goes away on its own.

In June 2006, the Advisory Committee on Immunization Practices (ACIP) voted to recommend the first vaccine developed to prevent cervical cancer and other diseases in females caused by certain types of genital human papillomavirus (HPV). The vaccine, Gardasil®, protects against four HPV types, which together cause 70 percent of cervical cancers and 90 percent of genital warts.[13]

Gonorrhea: Gonorrhea is caused by *Neisseria gonorrhoeae*, a bacterium that can grow and multiply easily in the warm, moist areas of the reproductive tract. CDC estimates that more than seven hundred thousand persons in the United States get new gonorrheal infections each year. Only about half of these infections are reported to CDC.[14]

The most common symptoms of infection are a discharge from the vagina or penis and painful or difficult urination. The most common and serious complications occur in women and, as with chlamydial infection, these complications include pelvic inflammatory disease (PID), ectopic pregnancy, and infertility.

Gonorrhea can grow in the cervix (opening to the womb), uterus (womb), and fallopian tubes (egg canals) in women, and in the urethra (urine canal) in women and men. The bacterium can also grow in the mouth, throat, eyes, and anus. If it spreads to the blood or joints it can be life threatening. In addition, people with gonorrhea can more easily contract HIV, the virus that causes AIDS. HIV-infected people with gonorrhea are more likely to transmit HIV to someone else.

Several antibiotics can successfully cure gonorrhea in adolescents and adults. However, drug-resistant strains of gonorrhea are increasing in many areas of the world, including the United States, and successful treatment of gonorrhea is becoming more difficult. New antibiotics or combinations of drugs must be used to treat these resistant strains.

Syphilis: Syphilis is caused by the bacterium *Treponema pallidum*. The incidence of syphilis has increased and decreased dramatically in recent years, and in the United States, health officials reported over thirty-two thousand cases of syphilis in 2002. Between 2001 and 2002, the number of reported primary and secondary (P & S) syphilis cases increased 12.4 percent. Rates in women continued to decrease, and overall, the rate in men was 3.5 times that in women. This, in conjunction with reports of syphilis outbreaks in men who have sex with men (MSM), suggests that rates of syphilis in MSM are increasing.[15]

Syphilis is passed from person to person through direct contact with a syphilis sore. The first symptoms of syphilis infection may go undetected because they are very mild and disappear spontaneously. The initial symptom is a chancre (genital sore); it is usually a painless open sore that most often appears on the penis or around or in the vagina.

It can also occur near the mouth, anus, or on the hands. Transmission of the organism occurs during vaginal, anal, or oral sex. Pregnant women with the disease can pass it to the babies they are carrying.

If untreated, syphilis may go on to more advanced stages, including a transient rash and, eventually, can cause serious involvement of the brain, nerves, eyes, heart, blood vessels, liver, bones, and joints. Chancres caused by syphilis make it easier to transmit and acquire HIV infection sexually. There is an estimated two- to fivefold increased risk of acquiring HIV infection when syphilis is present.[16] The full course of the disease can take years.

Penicillin remains the most effective drug to treat people with syphilis.

Trichomoniasis: Trichomoniasis is caused by the single-celled protozoan parasite *Trichomonas vaginalis*. It is the most common curable STD in young, sexually active women, and it affects men as well although symptoms are most common in women. An estimated 7.4 million new cases occur each year.[17]

The vagina is the most common site of infection in women, and the urethra (urine canal) is the most common site of infection in men. The parasite is sexually transmitted through penis-to-vagina intercourse or vulva-to-vulva (the genital area outside the vagina) contact with an infected partner. Women can acquire the disease from infected men or women, but men usually contract it only from infected women.

Most men with trichomoniasis do not have signs or symptoms; however, some men may temporarily have an irritation inside the penis, mild discharge, or slight burning after urination or ejaculation. Some women have signs or symptoms of infection which include a frothy, yellow-green vaginal discharge with a strong odor. The infection also may cause discomfort during intercourse and urination, as well as irritation and itching of the female genital area.

Trichomoniasis can usually be cured with the prescription drug metronidazole, given by mouth in a single dose.

Viral hepatitis: Hepatitis A is a liver disease caused by the hepatitis A virus (HAV). Hepatitis A virus is spread from person to person by putting something in the mouth that has been contaminated with the stool of a person with hepatitis A. This type of transmission is called "fecal-oral." Fewer than 5 percent of infections are transmitted through fecal-oral contact during sexual intercourse. Two products are used to prevent hepatitis A virus infection: immune globulin and hepatitis A vaccine.

Hepatitis B is a serious disease caused by a virus that attacks the liver. The virus, which is called hepatitis B virus (HBV), can cause lifelong infection, cirrhosis (scarring) of the liver, liver cancer, liver failure, and death. HBV is spread when blood from an infected person enters the body of a person who is not infected. For example, HBV is spread through having sex with an infected person without using a condom (the efficacy of latex condoms in preventing infection with HBV is unknown, but their proper use might reduce transmission), by sharing drugs, needles, or "works" when "shooting" drugs, through needle sticks or sharps exposures on the job, or from an infected mother to her baby during birth. Of approximately two hundred thousand new HBV infections in the United States each year, approximately half are transmitted through sexual intercourse. Preliminary data from a large U.S. multisite study indicate that approximately one third of persons with acute hepatitis B virus infections in 1995 had a history of another STD.[18]

Hepatitis C is a liver disease caused by the hepatitis C virus (HCV). HCV is spread primarily by direct contact with human blood, including sharing of needles for injection drug use and sex with someone with HCV. There is no vaccine to prevent hepatitis C.

Hepatitis D (delta) is a liver disease caused by the hepatitis D virus (HDV), a defective virus that needs the hepatitis B virus to exist. Hepatitis D virus (HDV) is found in the blood of persons infected with the virus. Infection occurs when blood from an infected person enters the body of a person who is not immune. Hepatitis B vaccine should be given to prevent HBV/HDV co-infection.

Hepatitis E is a liver disease caused by the hepatitis E virus (HEV) transmitted in much the same way as hepatitis A virus. Hepatitis E, however, does not occur often in the United States. HEV is found in the stool (feces) of persons and animals with hepatitis E and spread by eating or drinking contaminated food or water.

At present, there are no specific treatments for the acute symptoms of viral hepatitis. Doctors recommend bed rest, a healthy diet, and avoidance of alcoholic beverages. A genetically engineered form of a naturally occurring protein, interferon alpha, is used to treat people with chronic hepatitis C. Studies supported by the National Institutes of Health led to the approval of interferon alpha for the treatment of those with chronic HBV as well.

Other STDs: Other diseases that may be sexually transmitted include bacterial vaginosis, scabies, pubic lice, and pelvic inflammatory disease (PID).

Who Is Being Infected?

In the United States alone, an estimated nineteen million new cases of STDs are reported each year.[19] Table 16.1 shows the incidence and prevalence of some of the most common STDs.

Variations in Risk

STDs affect men and women of all backgrounds and economic levels. However, STDs disproportionately affect women, infants of infected mothers, adolescents and young adults, and communities of color. Although fifteen- to twenty-four-year-olds represent only one-quarter of the sexually active population, they account for nearly half of all new STDs each year.[30]

Some contributing factors in the rise of STDs, particularly among young people, are that teenagers are increasingly likely to have more sex partners at earlier ages, and sexually active teenagers often are reluctant to obtain STD services, or they may face serious obstacles when trying to obtain them. In addition, health care providers often are uncomfortable discussing sexuality and risk reduction with their patients, thus missing opportunities to counsel and screen young people for STDs.[31]

Table 16.1. Incidence and Prevalence of Common STDs

STD	Incidence*	Prevalence**
Chlamydia	2,800,000[20]	***
Gonorrhea	700,000[21]	***
Syphilis	32,000[22] (reported)	***
Herpes (HSV)	1,000,000[23]	45,000,000[24]
Hepatitis B (HBV)	60,000[25]	1,250,000[26]
Genital Warts/Human Papillomavirus (HPV)	6,200,000[27]	20,000,000[28]
Trichomoniasis	7,400,000[29]	***

*Estimated number of new cases each year

**Estimated number of people currently infected

***No recent surveys on national prevalence for gonorrhea, syphilis, or trichomoniasis have been conducted.

What Are Some Health Risks of STD Infection?

STDs can result in irreparable lifetime damage, including blindness, bone deformities, mental retardation, and death for infants infected by their mothers during gestation or birth.

In women, STDs can lead to pelvic inflammatory disease (PID), infertility, potentially fatal ectopic pregnancies, and cancer of the reproductive tract.

References

1. *State of the Nation Report 2005: Challenges Facing STD Prevention in Youth* American Social Health Association.
2. Weinstock H, Berman S, Cates W. Sexually transmitted diseases among American youth: incidence and prevalence estimates, 2000. *Perspectives on Sexual and Reproductive Health* 2004;36(1):6–10, cited in CDC Trends in Reportable Sexually Transmitted Diseases in the United States, 2004.
3. HW Chesson, JM Blandford, TL Gift, G Tao, KL Irwin. The estimated direct medical cost of STDs among American youth, 2000. Abstract P075. 2004 National STD Prevention Conference. Philadelphia, PA. March 8-11, 2004, cited in CDC Trends in Reportable Sexually Transmitted Diseases in the United States, 2004.
4. Basic Statistics from *HIV/AIDS Surveillance Report, 2004*. Vol. 16. Atlanta: US Department of Health and Human Services, Centers for Disease Control and Prevention; 2005.
5. Chancroid, Medline Plus, U.S. National Library of Medicine, and the National Institutes of Health.
6. Chlamydia, CDC.
7. Healthy People 2010, Sexually Transmitted Diseases.
8. CDC Media Release.
9. Genital Herpes, CDC.
10. Genital HPV Infection, CDC.
11. Genital HPV Infection, CDC.
12. Human Papillomavirus and Genital Warts, National Institute of Allergy and Infectious Diseases (NIAID).

13. HPV Vaccine Questions and Answers, CDC.

14. Gonorrhea, CDC.

15. Syphilis, CDC.

16. Syphilis, CDC.

17. Trichomoniasis, CDC.

18. Alter and Mast, 1994; CDC, 1994b; Goldstein et al., 1996, cited in The Hidden Epidemic: Confronting Sexually Transmitted Diseases (1997), Institute of Medicine (IOM).

19. Trends in Reportable Sexually Transmitted Diseases in the United States, 2004, CDC.

20. Weinstock H, Berman S, Cates W. Sexually transmitted diseases among American youth: incidence and prevalence estimates, 2000. Perspectives on Sexual and Reproductive Health 2004;36(1):6–10, cited in CDC Trends in Reportable Sexually Transmitted Diseases in the United States, 2004.

21. Gonorrhea, CDC.

22. Syphilis, CDC.

23. Tracking the Hidden Epidemics 2000.

24. Genital Herpes, CDC.

25. Viral Hepatitis B Fact Sheet, CDC.

26. Viral Hepatitis B Fact Sheet, CDC.

27. Genital HPV Infection, CDC.

28. Genital HPV Infection, CDC.

29. Trichomoniasis, CDC.

30. Weinstock H et al., Sexually transmitted diseases among American youth: incidence and prevalence estimates, 2000, *Perspectives on Sexual and Reproductive Health*, 2004, 36(1): 6–10, cited in Guttmacher Institute Facts on American Teens' Sexual and Reproductive Health.

31. Healthy People 2010, Sexually Transmitted Diseases.

Section 16.5

Pelvic Inflammatory Disease

Reprinted from "Pelvic Inflammatory Disease (PID),"

Alternative Names

PID; oophoritis; salpingitis; salpingo-oophoritis; salpingo-peritonitis

Definition

Pelvic inflammatory disease (PID) is a general term for infection of the lining of the uterus, the fallopian tubes, or the ovaries.

Causes

The majority of pelvic inflammatory disease cases are caused by the same bacteria that lead to sexually transmitted diseases (such as chlamydia, gonorrhea, mycoplasma, staph, strep).

Although PID most commonly spreads through sex, bacteria may also enter the body after gynecological procedures such as the insertion of an intrauterine device (IUD), childbirth, miscarriage, therapeutic or elective abortion, and endometrial biopsy.

In the United States, nearly one million women develop PID each year. It is estimated that one in eight sexually active adolescent girls will develop PID before reaching age twenty. Since PID is frequently underdiagnosed, statistics are probably greatly underestimated.

Risk factors include:

- sexual activity during adolescence;
- multiple sexual partners;
- past history of PID;
- past history of any sexually transmitted disease;
- insertion of an IUD.

Birth control pills are thought in some cases to lead to cervical ectropion, a condition that allows easier access to tissue where bacteria may grow. However, birth control pills may protect against PID by stimulating the body to produce a thicker cervical mucous, which makes it harder for semen to carry bacteria to the uterus.

Symptoms

The most common symptoms of PID include:

- vaginal discharge with abnormal color, consistency, or odor;
- abdominal pain;
- fever (not always present; may come and go).

Other nonspecific symptoms that may be seen with PID include:

- chills;
- irregular menstrual bleeding or spotting;
- increased menstrual cramping;
- menstruation, absent;
- increased pain during ovulation;
- sexual intercourse, painful;
- bleeding after intercourse;
- low back pain;
- fatigue;
- lack of appetite;
- nausea, with or without vomiting;
- frequent urination;
- pain with urination;
- tenderness.

Note: There may be no symptoms. People who experience ectopic pregnancies (pregnancies where the embryo implants in the fallopian tubes instead of the uterus) or infertility are often found to have silent PID, which is usually caused by chlamydia infection.

Exams and Tests

You may have a fever and abdominal tenderness. A pelvic examination may show that you have cervical discharge, pain with movement of the cervix during the exam, a cervix that bleeds easily, or uterine or ovarian tenderness.

Tests and procedures may include:

- white blood cell count (WBC);
- erythrocyte sedimentation rate (ESR);
- wet prep or wet mount microscopic examination;
- serum human chorionic gonadotropin (HCG)—pregnancy test;
- endocervical culture for gonorrhea, chlamydia, or other organisms;
- laparoscopy;
- pelvic ultrasound or computed tomography (CT) scan.

Treatment

If you are diagnosed with mild PID, you may be given antibiotics and told to closely follow up with your health care provider.

More severe cases may require you to stay in the hospital. Antibiotics are first given by intravenous (IV) line, and then later by mouth. Surgery may be considered for complicated, persistent cases that do not respond to antibiotics. Any sexual partner(s) must also be treated. The use of condoms during treatment is essential.

Possible Complications

PID infections can cause scarring and adhesions of the pelvic organs, possibly leading to infertility, ectopic pregnancy, and chronic pelvic pain.

When to Contact a Medical Professional

Call your health care provider if you have symptoms of PID. Also call if you think you have been exposed to a sexually transmitted disease or if treatment of a current STD does not seem to be working.

Prevention

Preventive measure include:

- practicing safer sex behaviors;
- following your doctor's recommendations after gynecological procedures;
- getting prompt treatment for sexually transmitted diseases.

The risk of PID can be reduced by getting regular STD screening exams. Couples can be tested for STDs before beginning sexual relations. Testing can detect STDs that may not be producing symptoms yet.

Chapter 17

Disorders of the Cervix

Chapter Contents

Section 17.1

Cervical Dysplasia

Reprinted from "Cervical Dysplasia," Walter Reed Army Medical Center. The text of this document is available online at http://www.wramc.army.mil/Patients/diseases/wh/c5/Pages/s2.aspx; accessed May 13, 2008.

Description

Dysplasia is abnormal growth and development of the cells of the lining of the cervix. It can range from mild to moderate or severe depending on the spread of the abnormal cells. The degree of abnormality is considered a precancerous condition, but does not represent cancer of the cervix. The diagnosis may be medically classified as cervical intraepithelial neoplasia (CIN) I, II, or III; or low-grade squamous intraepithelial lesion (SIL) or high-grade SIL. These classifications help define the extent of the abnormal growth and to determine the appropriate treatment. Dysplasia occurs in females age fifteen and over, and most often in those age twenty-five to thirty-five.

Frequent Signs and Symptoms

Usually no signs or symptoms occur. The suspected diagnosis results from a routine Pap smear evaluation.

Causes

There is an association with human papillomaviruses (genital warts) or similar viruses

Risk Factors

Risk increases with the following:

- Repeated infections
- Smoking
- Immunosuppression
- Multiple pregnancies and pregnancy before age twenty

- Multiple sexual partners
- Long-term oral contraceptive use

Preventive Measures

- Sexual monogamy of both partners
- Yearly Pap smears (will not prevent dysplasia, but will aid in early diagnosis)
- Stopping smoking
- Use of a diaphragm by the female or a condom by the male for sexual intercourse

Expected Outcome

With early diagnosis and treatment, when necessary, the outlook is excellent. Spontaneous regression (reversal) occurs in a significant number of patients.

Possible Complications

Some severe dysplasia may progress to cancer of the cervix. Recurrence is possible, especially in the first two years following treatment. If a woman has completed childbearing, recurrent dysplasia can be treated with a hysterectomy. Rarely, complications can result from the treatment, such as excessive bleeding or infection.

Treatment/Post-Procedure Care

General measures: To confirm the diagnosis, a colposcopy (examination of the cervix with a colposcope, a slender optical instrument with a lighted tip) is usually performed and combined with a biopsy. Treatment measures will vary depending on the degree and extent of the cervical dysplasia. Possibilities include cryotherapy (freezing), laser therapy, loop resection, conization of the cervix, or cone biopsy. Be sure you under- stand the treatment options and any risk factors involved. Follow-up care will depend on the treatment method used. Follow-up Pap smears every three to six months for a year may be recommended to verify the success of treatment and to detect any recurrence.

Medication: Prescription pain medication should generally be required only for two to seven days following the procedure. You may use nonprescription drugs, such as acetaminophen, for minor pain.

Activity: To help recovery and aid your well-being, resume daily activities, including work, as soon as you are able. Delay sexual relations until a follow-up medical examination determines that healing is complete.

Diet: No special diet.

When to Notify Your Healthcare Provider

Notify your healthcare provider if any of the following occur:

- Pain, swelling, redness, drainage, or bleeding increases in the surgical area
- You develop signs of infection: headache, muscle aches, dizziness, or a general ill feeling and fever
- Vaginal discharge increases or begins to have an unpleasant odor

Section 17.2

Cervical Polyps

Reprinted from "Cervical Polyps," Walter Reed Army Medical Center. The text of this document is available online at http://www.wramc.army.mil/Patients/diseases/wh/c5/Pages/s3.aspx; accessed May 13, 2008.

Description

Small, fragile, bulbous growths on stalks protruding through the cervix (lower third of the uterus) from the lining inside the uterus (endometrium). They may be single or numerous.

Frequent Signs and Symptoms

- Unexpected spotting of blood between monthly menstrual periods
- Spotting of blood after sexual intercourse or bowel movements
- Vaginal discharge

Causes

Cervical polyps are caused by cervix inflammation from infection, erosion, or ulceration. They frequently accompany chronic infections in the vagina or cervix, although they are not contagious. The small growths are usually benign, but in very rare cases, they represent early cancer of the cervix.

Risk Factors

Risk increases with the following:

- Diabetes mellitus
- Recurrent vaginitis or cervicitis

Preventive Measures

To prevent vaginal or cervix infections that can precede cervical polyps:

- Wear cotton underpants or pantyhose with a cotton crotch to prevent accumulation of excess heat and moisture, which can make you susceptible to vaginal and cervical infections.
- Avoid contracting sexually transmitted diseases by having your sexual partner wear a condom during intercourse.

Expected Outcome

Usually curable with minor surgery. You may feel brief, mild pain during the procedure and have mild to moderate cramps for several hours. Spotting of blood from the vagina may occur for one or two days.

Possible Complications

- Bleeding and some mild pain with removal of the polyps.
- In very rare instances, cervical polyps may become malignant.

Treatment/Post-Procedure Care

General measures: Surgery to remove cervical polyps with a wire snare, electrocautery, or liquid nitrogen. This can often be done in a simple office procedure. The cervix may be cauterized after removing the polyp to prevent regrowth of the same or another polyp. Don't douche unless it is recommended. Use small sanitary pads to protect your clothing from creams or suppositories. A polyp that accompanies cervicitis (inflammation or infection of the cervix) may require more extensive surgery.

Medication: Usually no medications are necessary for this disorder.

Activity: No restrictions. Delay sexual relations until a follow-up pelvic examination determines that healing is complete.

Diet: No special diet.

When to Notify Your Healthcare Provider

Notify your healthcare provider if any of the following occur:

- You have symptoms of cervical polyps
- Discomfort persists longer than one week after treatment
- Symptoms recur
- Unexplained vaginal bleeding or swelling develops

Section 17.3

Cervicitis

Reprinted from "Cervicitis," Walter Reed Army Medical Center. The text of this document is available online at http://www.wramc.army.mil/Patients/diseases/wh/c5/Pages/s4.aspx; accessed May 13, 2008.

Description

Inflammation or infection of the cervix There are two types and either may be contagious: Acute cervicitis, which is usually a bacterial or viral infection with specific symptoms, and chronic cervicitis, which is a long-term infection that may not have symptoms.

Frequent Signs and Symptoms

Acute cervicitis:

- Thick yellow vaginal discharge

Chronic cervicitis:

- Slight, sometimes unnoticeable vaginal discharge
- Backache
- Discomfort with urination
- Discomfort with sexual intercourse

Extensive chronic cervicitis:

- Profuse vaginal discharge
- Bleeding between menstrual periods
- Spotting or bleeding after sexual intercourse

Causes

Acute cervicitis is usually caused by the organisms *Neisseria gonorrhoeae* or *Chlamydia trachomatis*. Herpesvirus can also be a cause.

Chronic cervicitis is caused by repeated episodes of acute cervicitis, or one episode that is not treated long enough to heal completely.

Risk Factors

Risk increases with the following:

- Multiple sexual partners
- Diabetes mellitus
- Acute or recurrent vaginitis

Preventive Measures

- Have an annual pelvic examination and Pap smear.
- Wear cotton underpants or pantyhose with a cotton crotch.
- Avoid underpants made from nonventilating materials.
- Synthetic materials hold in vaginal wetness and warmth, which may trigger vaginal or cervical infections.
- Avoid contracting sexually transmitted diseases by having your sexual partner wear a condom for intercourse.
- If cervicitis is caused by a sexually transmitted infection, your sexual partner also needs treatment.

Expected Outcome

Mild cervicitis will heal without treatment. Acute cervicitis caused by venereal disease is contagious through sexual intercourse and is curable with medication. Most other cases of cervicitis can be cured with treatment. All women with cervicitis need regular checkups until the condition heals.

Possible Complications

- Cervical polyps
- Pelvic inflammatory disease
- Malignant change in cervix cells (rare)

Treatment/Post-Procedure Care

General measures: Diagnostic tests may include a culture of the vaginal discharge and laboratory blood studies. Use sanitary pads instead of tampons during treatment. Don't douche unless it is recommend. Treatment may involve destruction of abnormal cells with silver nitrate (chemical used for cautery); cryosurgery (destruction of abnormal tissue by applying freezing temperatures, usually with liquid nitrogen); or electrocautery (destruction of tissue by heat applied with a controlled electric current). Surgery (hysterectomy) may be considered for widespread tissue destruction (rare).

Medication: Oral antibiotics may be used if infectious cervicitis is suspected. Antiviral or antibiotic vaginal creams or suppositories to fight infection may be prescribed.

Activity: No restrictions, except to avoid sexual relations until determination that the infection has healed.

Diet: No special diet.

When to Notify Your Healthcare Provider

Notify your healthcare provider if any of the following occur:

- You or a family member has symptoms of cervicitis.
- During treatment, discomfort persists longer than one week or symptoms worsen.
- Unexplained vaginal bleeding or swelling develops during or after treatment.
- New, unexplained symptoms develop. Drugs used in treatment may produce side effects.

Chapter 18

Vulval Disorders

Chapter Contents

Section 18.1

Vulvitis

Definition

Vulvitis is inflammation of the external female genitalia (vulva).

Causes

Vulvitis can be caused by a number of conditions. These include chronic dermatitis, seborrhea or eczema, and allergies, particularly to soaps, colored toilet paper, vaginal sprays, laundry detergents, bubble bath, or fragrances. It can also be caused by infections such as fungal and bacterial infections, pediculosis, or scabies.

Vulvitis can affect women of all ages. In young girls and postmenopausal women, the condition may be caused by low estrogen levels.

Symptoms

- Redness and swelling of the vulvar skin
- Burning or itching of the vulvar skin
- Thickening of the vulvar skin
- Possible small cracks in the vulvar skin
- Possible vaginal discharge

Exams and Tests

A pelvic examination often reveals redness and thickening and may reveal cracks or skin lesions on the vulva.

If there is any vaginal discharge, a wet prep inspection may reveal vaginal infection such as vulvovaginitis or vaginitis as the source.

Treatment

Discontinue the use of any potential irritants. An over-the-counter cortisone cream may be used two or three times a day on the affected area for up to one week. If these measures do not relieve symptoms, see your health care provider.

If discharge from a vaginal infection is the cause of vulvitis, the source of the vaginal infection should be treated. Cortisone cream may be used to decrease vulvar itching.

If treatment of vulvitis does not work, further evaluation may include biopsy of the skin to rule out the potential of vulvar dystrophy (a chronic vulvar skin condition) or vulvar dysplasia, a precancerous condition. A biopsy may also be necessary if any skin lesions are present.

Outlook (Prognosis)

Itching may be hard to control, but after the cause is identified and treated, it should go away in several weeks.

Possible Complications

Itching of the vulva may be a sign of genital warts (HPV—human papillomavirus), vulvar dystrophy, or vulvar dysplasia (a precancerous condition).

Sexually transmitted diseases (STDs), which can cause vulvitis, may lead to other problems, such as infertility. STDs should be treated appropriately.

When to Contact a Medical Professional

Call for an appointment with your health care provider if symptoms occur and do not respond to self-care measures, or if vaginal discharge accompanies the symptoms. Also call if skin lesions are noted on the vulva.

Prevention

Since one of the main causes of vulvitis is exposure of the vulva to chemicals (bubble bath, douches, detergents, fabric softeners, perfumes, etc.) or other irritating materials (wool, fibrous, or "itchy" materials), daily cleansing with mild soap, adequate rinsing, and thorough drying of the genital area is one of the best ways to avoid it. Also, avoid using feminine hygiene sprays, fragrances, or powders in the genital area.

Avoid wearing extremely tight-fitting pants or shorts, which may cause irritation by constantly rubbing against the skin and by holding in heat and restricting air circulation. Underwear made of silk or nylon is not very absorbent and also restricts air circulation. This can increase sweating in the genital area, which can cause irritation and may provide a more welcoming environment for infectious organisms.

Wearing cotton underwear or pantyhose that have a cotton crotch allows better air circulation and can decrease the amount of moisture in the area. For the above-mentioned reasons, you should also avoid wearing sweaty exercise clothing for prolonged periods. Not wearing underwear while sleeping will also allow more air circulation.

Those infections that may be spread by intimate or sexual contact may be prevented or minimized by practicing abstinence or using safer sexual behaviors, especially condom use.

Section 18.2

Vulvodynia

Excerpted from "Frequently Asked Questions about Vulvodynia," National Institutes of Health Office of Research on Women's Health, 2007.

What is vulvodynia?

Vulvodynia is chronic unexplained pain or discomfort of the vulva. The vulva is the area of the female genitals surrounding the vaginal opening and includes the labia, the vestibule, and the perineum. Some women refer to it as "the pain down there" or as "feminine pain." It affects all women, including racial and ethnic minorities, women with disabilities, sexual minorities, and those in rural and urban areas.

What are the symptoms of vulvodynia?

Women with vulvodynia often experience burning, stinging, irritation, rawness, or stabbing pain in their genitals, with no apparent explanation. The pain or discomfort can be chronic or intermittent, and generalized or localized to one area of the vulva. Some women also report itching. For many women, sexual intercourse, and even tampon insertion or wearing clothes (such as underwear or trousers) is very uncomfortable or painful.

What causes vulvodynia? Do I have an infection or disease?

While a number of causes have been proposed, researchers still don't know why vulvodynia happens to some women. Most likely, there is no single cause. Because of this, vulvodynia remains difficult to assess and diagnose. Many health care providers are not aware of the existence of vulvodynia, so aren't always able to diagnose it. As a result, many women may go for a long period of time without diagnosis.

How is vulvodynia diagnosed?

You should share with your health care provider information about your symptoms and related problems you are experiencing. In turn, your health care provider should talk to you about these symptoms and raise questions about your lifestyle, medications you may be taking, and your sexual and family history, in order to better understand the possible causes of your pain. Your health care provider should also do an examination of your pelvic area, including your vulva and vagina and laboratory tests to rule out other causes of your pain and discomfort. These causes could include endometriosis, a yeast infection, a sexually transmitted infection, or dermatitis. The diagnosis of vulvodynia can be established after ruling out other causes of your pain and discomfort.

Is there a treatment or cure for vulvodynia?

While there is no cure, there are a number of treatment options for vulvodynia. These can include advice on general vulvar care, topical and/or oral medications, physical therapy exercises, injections, biofeedback, or even surgery in some specific cases. Although no single treatment is effective for all cases, a multifaceted approach to prevent and reduce symptoms can improve quality of life. You and your health care provider should work together to develop a strategy of treatment that works best for you. Many women find that wearing only cotton underwear; not wearing panty hose, or tight-fitting jeans or other clothes around their pelvic area; using only white, unbleached toilet tissue and 100 percent cotton sanitary products (tampons and pads); and washing their genitals frequently with water and avoiding using creams, soaps, douches, or deodorants on their vulva also helps. What is important is to find a low-stress strategy for you that reduces the pain and discomfort.

How may vulvodynia affect my personal relationships?

For many women, vulvodynia may result in sexual activity being very uncomfortable and even painful. Because of this, vulvodynia may also cause emotional stress for women whose intimate partner may not fully understand the effects of this condition. Women should be encouraged to discuss vulvodynia openly and honestly with their partner and should not feel obligated to engage in sexual activity if it is painful.

Did my partner give this to me? Can I give this to my partner?

There does not appear to be a link between sexually transmitted infections and vulvodynia; thus it cannot be shared among sexual partners. However, because vulvodynia can interfere with a woman's enjoyment of sexual activity, women should discuss vulvodynia openly and honestly with their partner.

Is there something a woman can do to prevent it?

This is still unknown. Further research is needed to assess the causes and underlying factors that contribute to vulvodynia.

How do I talk to my health care provider about vulvodynia?

For many women, talking about pain or discomfort that occurs in or around their genitals can be very uncomfortable and difficult. Women may feel embarrassed, or worry that they might have a sexually transmitted infection. Others may worry that their health care provider won't take them seriously and dismiss their concerns as unimportant. Some may have raised this with other providers, and felt frustrated by their responses. Nevertheless, it is very important that women tell their health care providers about any pain and discomfort they are experiencing, being specific about where the pain and discomfort occurs, when it started, and whether or not the pain and discomfort is episodic in nature. Be open about what sort of home remedies you may have tried, and whether or not there have been other changes in your medical history. While you may indeed have vulvodynia, it is entirely possible that there may be another cause for your pain and discomfort, and you and your health care provider will want to determine that as well. If your health care provider does not respond to your concerns you should raise the possibility of vulvodynia with him or her, or seek another opinion.

Why did it take so long for my health care provider to diagnose it?

Many health care providers are unaware that vulvodynia is a diagnosis. Further, most health care providers will want to make sure that your vulvar pain doesn't have another organic cause.

What research is being done about vulvodynia?

Researchers continue to explore better clinical definitions of vulvodynia, better methods of identifying conditions that coexist with vulvodynia, the etiology of the condition, risk factors associated with its development, and more comprehensive clinical management tools for vulvodynia.

Chapter 19

Pelvic Floor Disorders

Chapter Contents

Section 19.1

Uterine Prolapse

Excerpted from "Uterine Prolapse,"

Uterine prolapse is falling or sliding of the uterus from its normal position in the pelvic cavity into the vaginal canal.

Causes

The uterus is normally supported by pelvic connective tissue and the pubococcygeus muscle, and held in position by special ligaments. Weakening of these tissues allows the uterus to descend into the vaginal canal. Tissue trauma sustained during childbirth, especially with large babies or difficult labor and delivery, is typically the cause of muscle weakness.

The loss of muscle tone and the relaxation of muscles, which are both associated with normal aging and a reduction in the female hormone estrogen, are also thought to play an important role in the development of uterine prolapse. Descent can also be caused by a pelvic tumor, however, this is fairly rare.

Uterine prolapse occurs most commonly in women who have had one or more vaginal births, and in Caucasian women.

Other conditions associated with an increased risk of developing problems with the supportive tissues of the uterus include obesity and chronic coughing or straining. Obesity places additional strain on the supportive muscles of the pelvis, as does excessive coughing caused by lung conditions such as chronic bronchitis and asthma. Chronic constipation and the pushing associated with it causes weakness in these muscles.

Symptoms

- Sensation of heaviness or pulling in the pelvis
- A feeling as if "sitting on a small ball"

- Low backache
- Protrusion from the vaginal opening (in moderate to severe cases)
- Difficult or painful sexual intercourse

Exams and Tests

A pelvic examination (with the woman bearing down) reveals protrusion of the cervix into the lower part of the vagina (mild prolapse), past the vaginal introitus/opening (moderate prolapse), or protrusion of the entire uterus past the vaginal introitus/opening (severe prolapse).

These signs are often accompanied by protrusion of the bladder and front wall of the vagina (cystocele) or rectum and back wall of the vagina (rectocele) into the vaginal space. The ovaries and bladder may also be positioned lower in the pelvis than usual.

A mass may be noted on pelvic exam if a tumor is the cause of the prolapse (rare).

Treatment

Uterine prolapse can be treated with a vaginal pessary or surgery.

A vaginal pessary is an object inserted into the vagina to hold the uterus in place. It may be used as a temporary or permanent form of treatment. Vaginal pessaries are fitted for each individual woman.

Pessaries may cause an irritating and abnormal smelling discharge, and they require periodic cleaning, usually done by the physician. In some women they rub on and irritate the vaginal mucosa, and in some cases may erode and cause ulcerations. Some types of pessaries may interfere with normal sexual intercourse by limiting the depth of penetration.

If the woman is obese, attaining and maintaining optimal weight is recommended. Heavy lifting or straining should be avoided.

There are some surgical procedures that can be done without removing the uterus, such as a sacral colpopexy. This procedure involves the use of surgical mesh for supporting the uterus.

Most surgery should be deferred until symptoms are significant enough to outweigh the risks. The surgical approach depends on:

- the woman's age and general health;
- desire for future pregnancies;

- preservation of vaginal function;
- degree of prolapse;
- associated conditions.

When indicated, a vaginal hysterectomy is performed. Any sagging of the vaginal walls, urethra, bladder, or rectum can be surgically corrected at the same time.

Outlook (Prognosis)

With proper precautions (periodic check-ups and cleaning) vaginal pessaries can be effective for many women with uterine prolapse. Surgery, if done, usually provides excellent results, however, some women may require treatment again in the future for recurrent prolapse of the vaginal walls.

Possible Complications

Urinary tract infections and other urinary symptoms may occur due to the frequently associated cystocele. Constipation and hemorrhoids may also occur as a result of the associated rectocele. Ulceration and infection may occur in more severe cases of prolapse.

When to Contact a Medical Professional

Call for an appointment with your health care provider if symptoms of uterine prolapse occur.

Prevention

Prenatal and postpartum Kegel exercises (tightening of the pelvic floor musculature as if trying to interrupt urine flow) help to strengthen the muscles and reduces the risk.

How an episiotomy and other obstetric procedures affect the later development of uterine prolapse is unclear. Estrogen replacement therapy in postmenopausal women tends to help maintain muscle tone.

Section 19.2

Cystocele

Reprinted from "Cystocele (Fallen Bladder)," National Institute of Diabetes and Digestive and Kidney Diseases, National Institutes of Health, NIH Publication No. 07-4557, August 2007.

What is a cystocele?

A cystocele occurs when the wall between a woman's bladder and her vagina weakens and allows the bladder to droop into the vagina. This condition may cause discomfort and problems with emptying the bladder.

A bladder that has dropped from its normal position may cause two kinds of problems—unwanted urine leakage and incomplete emptying of the bladder. In some women, a fallen bladder stretches the opening into the urethra, causing urine leakage when the woman coughs, sneezes, laughs, or moves in any way that puts pressure on the bladder.

A cystocele is mild—grade 1—when the bladder droops only a short way into the vagina. With a more severe—grade 2—cystocele, the bladder sinks far enough to reach the opening of the vagina. The most advanced—grade 3—cystocele occurs when the bladder bulges out through the opening of the vagina.

What causes a cystocele?

A cystocele may result from muscle straining while giving birth. Other kinds of straining—such as heavy lifting or repeated straining during bowel movements—may also cause the bladder to fall. The hormone estrogen helps keep the muscles around the vagina strong. When women go through menopause—that is, when they stop having menstrual periods—their bodies stop making estrogen, so the muscles around the vagina and bladder may grow weak.

How is a cystocele diagnosed?

A doctor may be able to diagnose a grade 2 or grade 3 cystocele from a description of symptoms and from physical examination of the vagina because the fallen part of the bladder will be visible. A voiding cystourethrogram is a test that involves taking x-rays of the bladder during urination. This x-ray shows the shape of the bladder and lets the doctor see any problems that might block the normal flow of urine. Other tests may be needed to find or rule out problems in other parts of the urinary system.

How is a cystocele treated?

Treatment options range from no treatment for a mild cystocele to surgery for a serious cystocele. If a cystocele is not bothersome, the doctor may only recommend avoiding heavy lifting or straining that could cause the cystocele to worsen. If symptoms are moderately bothersome, the doctor may recommend a pessary—a device placed in the vagina to hold the bladder in place. Pessaries come in a variety of shapes and sizes to allow the doctor to find the most comfortable fit for the patient. Pessaries must be removed regularly to avoid infection or ulcers.

Large cystoceles may require surgery to move and keep the bladder in a more normal position. This operation may be performed by a gynecologist, a urologist, or a urogynecologist. The most common procedure for cystocele repair is for the surgeon to make an incision in the wall of the vagina and repair the area to tighten the layers of tissue that separate the organs, creating more support for the bladder. The patient may stay in the hospital for several days and take four to six weeks to recover fully.

Section 19.3

Rectocele

"Rectocele," reprinted with permission of the University of Michigan Health System, Michigan Bowel Control Program, September 2008.

What is a rectocele?

A rectocele can be described as a bulge in the wall of the rectum into the vagina. The wall of the rectum becomes thin and weak. It may balloon out into the vagina when you have a bowel movement.

There are other structures that may also balloon into the vagina. The bladder bulging into the vagina is a cystocele. The small intestine pushing down on the vagina from above is an enterocele. The uterus bulging into the vagina is called uterine prolapse.

How does it occur?

The wall that lies between the rectum (front wall of the rectum) and the vagina (back wall of the vagina) is called the rectovaginal septum. The thinning of the rectovaginal septum and weakening of the pelvic support structures is the underlying cause of a rectocele.

The most common cause is childbirth and chronic constipation. The muscles and ligaments in the pelvis that hold up and support the female organs and vagina become stretched and weakened during straining. The more babies you have, the more the support tissues are stretched and weakened. Not everyone who has a baby will develop a rectocele. Some women have stronger supporting tissue in the pelvis and may not have as much of a problem as others.

Other conditions that can cause a rectocele include chronic constipation, a chronic cough, a lot of heavy lifting, and obesity. Older women may have this problem because the loss of female hormones causes the vaginal tissue to become weaker.

What are the symptoms?

There may not be any symptoms. If you do have symptoms, they may include:

- pelvic pressure in the rectal area;
- protrusion of the lower part of the vagina through the opening of the vagina;
- constipation and trapping of the stool, making it difficult to have a bowel movement (you may have to press on the lower part of your vagina to help push the stool out of your rectum, this is called splinting);
- a rapid urge to have a bowel movement after leaving the bathroom, caused by stool returning to the lower rectum that was trapped in the rectocele;
- incontinence especially after having a bowel movement.

How is it diagnosed?

Your health care provider will ask about your symptoms and perform a pelvic exam. Your provider will ask you to bear down, pushing like you are having a bowel movement so he or she can see how far the lower part of the vagina protrudes into the vagina and possibly outside of the vagina. Your provider will also ask you to contract the muscles of your pelvis (like you are stopping the stream in the middle of urinating) to determine the strength of your pelvic muscles. Your provider may also do a rectal exam. You may also be asked to have a defecography. A defecography is a special x-ray that looks at the pelvic organs while you are straining like you are trying to have a bowel movement.

How is it treated?

- If the rectocele is not causing any symptoms, it need not be treated. Constipation should always be avoided. Eating a diet rich in fiber and drinking six to eight glasses of decaffeinated fluid every day can assist in keeping bowel movements soft.
- Avoid prolonged straining. If the bowels will not completely empty after a bowel movement, get up and return later. A pessary (a ring that is inserted in the vagina) may be used to assist in supporting pelvic organs.
- Avoiding heavy lifting, and lifting correctly (with your legs, not with your waist or back).
- Treating a chronic cough or bronchitis.

- Not smoking.
- Avoiding too much weight gain.
- Doing Kegel exercises, especially after you have a baby.
- Splinting: This is inserting a tampon or two fingers inside the vagina and pushing back.
- Surgical repair may be indicated if the rectocele is severe. A rectocele repair may be performed through the anus, vagina, perineum (between the anus and vagina), the abdomen, or may be a combined repair.
- Often a combination of nonsurgical and surgical treatments is needed to correct the problem.

Chapter 20

Gynecological Procedures

Chapter Contents

Section 20.1

Screening, Diagnostic, and Therapeutic Procedures for Common Gynecological Concerns

Reprinted from "Screening and Diagnostic Procedures," "Therapeutic Procedures," and "Combination Procedures (Diagnostic and Therapeutic)," Reprinted with permission.

Screening and Diagnostic Procedures

Biopsy: A biopsy involves removing a small piece of tissue from the body for microscopic examination and testing.

Bone density test: Bone density measurements are done to determine if you have low bone mass (osteopenia or osteoporosis). It predicts your risk of future fractures and helps doctors determine if you will need drug therapy.

Breast biopsy: This test is done when a mammogram reveals an abnormality in the breast and it cannot be confirmed as benign (noncancerous). It involves removing all or part of the abnormal tissue and may be done by open surgery (with a scalpel) or by one of four needle aspiration techniques: fine needle aspiration, core needle biopsy, vacuum-assisted biopsy, or large core biopsy.

Cervical biopsy: A cervical biopsy is performed to evaluate abnormal cervical tissue found during a Pap test or colposcopy. A punch biopsy is most commonly done. A cervical conization (cone biopsy) is a more extensive form of cervical biopsy.

Cervical conization: See "Combination Procedures."

Cone biopsy: See cervical conization in "Combination Procedures."

Colposcopy: This test is usually done if the cervix looks abnormal during a routine examination or if a Pap test shows abnormal cells.

Your doctor may also order it if you have genital warts or if your mother took diethylstilbestrol (DES) when pregnant with you. A colposcope is placed in the vagina and used to magnify the area of the cervix where an abnormality is suspected. If abnormal cells are found, your doctor may do a biopsy of the area.

Endocervical curettage (ECC): This procedure is frequently done in conjunction with a cervical biopsy. It involves taking a sample of the tissue just past the opening of the cervix as a precaution against missing any abnormal tissue.

Endometrial or uterine biopsy: This test, done to obtain a sample of the endometrial lining of the uterus, may be used to investigate abnormal menses (heavy bleeding, bleeding between periods, post-menopausal bleeding), infertility, and chronic infections. It is useful in detecting uterine polyps, uterine fibroids, uterine cancer, and adenomyosis.

Hysterosalpingography: During this x-ray procedure, dye is injected into the uterus to outline any irregularities of the uterine wall. The dye may or may not travel through the fallopian passages so they can be evaluated as well. Selective salpingography is a more extensive form of hysterosalpingography.

Mammogram: This low-dose x-ray provides a picture of the internal structure of the breast. It is used to detect tumors and cysts.

Magnetic resonance imaging (MRI): An MRI scan may be used to identify the location of uterine fibroids. When there is a question about whether you have fibroids or adenomyosis, an MRI can usually tell the difference.

Pelvic ultrasound: This test produces an image of your pelvic organs by bouncing sound waves off them. Both transabdominal (the ultrasound wand is moved across the abdomen) and transvaginal (the ultrasound wand is placed in the vagina) ultrasound scans may be done. It is used to evaluate conditions such as uterine fibroids and ovarian cysts. Also see fluid-contrast ultrasound below.

Toluidine blue dye test: This test is used to evaluate abnormal changes in the vulva. The dye is applied on the vulva and causes skin with precancerous or cancerous changes to turn blue.

Sonohysteroscopy: See fluid-contrast ultrasound below.

Fluid-contrast ultrasound (FCUS): This procedure is an adaptation of standard pelvic ultrasound. It is used to evaluate the lining of the uterus and the uterine cavity. It can measure the thickness of the uterine lining (endometrium) and reveal the texture of its surface and any abnormalities such as polyps or fibroids. A small catheter is inserted through the cervix into the uterus and an ultrasound wand is placed in the vagina. A sterile solution is slowly injected through the catheter into the uterine cavity and the area is imaged with the ultrasound.

Vaginal culture: This test involves collecting cervical mucus to identify the cause of an infection.

Therapeutic Procedures

Adhesiolysis: This is also called lysis of adhesions. Cutting of adhesions (scar tissue).

Colporrhaphy: Surgical repair of the vaginal wall. Used to repair enteroceles (hernias).

Endometrial ablation: This procedure is used to treat abnormal bleeding in women who do not plan to become pregnant but may not need a hysterectomy. A hysteroscope is passed through the cervix into the uterus and one of a number of types of energy—electrical, laser, or thermal—is used to destroy the endometrial layer of the uterus.

Hysterectomy: This procedure is removal of the uterus. It can be a partial hysterectomy (removal of the upper portion of the uterus, leaving the cervix); a total hysterectomy (removal of the entire uterus and cervix); or a radical hysterectomy (removal of the uterus, the tissue on both sides of the cervix, and the upper part of the vagina). The fallopian tubes and ovaries may also be removed at the time of hysterectomy. When the ovaries are also removed, a hysterectomy can relieve the pain of endometriosis. A hysterectomy may be done through open abdominal surgery, laparoscopic surgery, or hysteroscopic surgery.

Myomectomy: This procedure is done to remove uterine fibroids without hysterectomy for women who wish to become pregnant or do not want to lose their uterus. Myomectomies may be performed through conventional open abdominal surgery, with laparoscopic techniques, or hysteroscopically, depending on the location of the fibroids.

Oophorectomy: Oophorectomy is the surgical removal of one ovary, both ovaries, or a part of an ovary. It is performed to treat ovarian cancer, pelvic inflammatory disease, and endometriosis or remove cysts or abscesses. It may also be done to remove the main source of estrogens that stimulate the growth of some breast cancers. If one ovary is removed, a woman may continue to menstruate and have children. If both ovaries are removed, menstruation stops and a woman loses the ability to bear children.

Trachelectomy: Surgical removal of the cervix (but not the rest of the uterus). A radical trachelectomy is when the cervix and surrounding tissue is removed, along with some pelvic lymph nodes.

Suspensions: Uterine or vaginal vault.

Tubal surgeries: Removal of fallopian tubes, tubal ligation, correction of tubal pregnancy, reanastomosis (reconnection of the fallopian tubes), or wire guide cannulation to open a blocked tube.

Uterine artery embolization (UAE): See uterine fibroid embolization below.

Uterine fibroid embolization (UFE): This procedure blocks the arteries carrying blood to the fibroids.

Vulvectomy: Simple or radical.

Combination Procedures (Diagnostic and Therapeutic)

Dilatation and curettage (D&C): During a D&C procedure, the cervix is dilated (widened) to allow the insertion of an instrument called a curette into the uterus. The curette is used to scrape lining of the uterus (endometrium) and collect the tissue from inside the uterus. It may be performed to remove tissue for diagnostic examination, to remove small tumors, or to treat abnormal uterine bleeding. A D&C may also be performed to remove remaining material after an incomplete miscarriage or abortion. This is called an aspiration or suction D&C and removes tissue from the uterus with a vacuum device.

Cervical conization: Also called cone biopsy, this is a more extensive form of cervical biopsy and is performed to follow up when colposcopy or a cervical biopsy have failed to provide enough information for a definitive diagnosis. A cone-shaped wedge of tissue from the cervix is removed by one of several methods depending on your circumstance:

- *Cold knife conization:* Performed with a scalpel.
- *Laser conization:* The cone of tissue may be removed or destroyed by vaporization.
- *Loop electrosurgical excision procedure (LEEP):* A thin wire loop that emits a low-voltage high-frequency radio wave is used to remove tissue.
- *Large loop excision of transformation zone (LLETZ).*
- *Combined conization:* A procedure started with one technique, such as the use of a laser, may be completed with another, such as a cold-knife technique.
- *Harmonic scalpel (HS) conization:* Ultrasonic mechanical vibrations are used to cut and coagulate.

In some cases, the cone biopsy treats the problem because all the diseased tissue is removed.

Cone biopsy: See cervical conization above.

Fluoroscopic tubal catheterization: See selective salpingography below.

Hysteroscopy: This procedure is done to look for uterine abnormalities. A thin, telescope-like instrument (a fiber optic endoscope called a hysteroscope) is inserted through the vagina and cervix into the uterus. If an abnormality is detected during a diagnostic procedure, a surgical procedure can often be performed immediately by substituting a surgical hysteroscope (one that allows operating instruments to be inserted through it to the uterus). Surgical procedures may include:

- Removal of polyps, fibroid tumors, scar tissue, or tissue overgrowth (hyperplasia);
- Opening blocked fallopian tubes (recanalization);
- Treating abnormal bleeding with endometrial ablation.

Pelviscopy (pelvic laparoscopy): This procedure is done to examine and treat abdominal and pelvic organs through a small surgical viewing instrument (laparoscope) inserted into the abdomen at the navel.

Selective salpingography: This x-ray test is used to identify fallopian tube disease or obstructions. A fine catheter is passed into the fallopian tube, then dye is injected to look for abnormalities or obstructions. Occasionally, the pressure of the dye may be all that is needed to open a blocked fallopian tube. If not, a wire guide canalization or transcervical balloon tuboplasty can be performed during your salpingography test.

Section 20.2

Dilatation and Curettage (D&C)

From "Dilatation and Curettage (D&C) Operation: Treatment Summary," © 2007 Spire Healthcare. For additional information, contact Spire Healthcare at P.O. Box 62647, 120 Holborn, London EC19 1JH; telephone in London: 0800-434-6600; or visit http://www.spirehealthcare.com.

What Is Involved?

Dilatation (or dilation) means "stretching" the entrance of the cervix (neck of the womb). Curettage means "scraping" the lining of the uterus. Dilatation and curettage (D&C) is a procedure used to diagnose and treat conditions affecting the uterus (womb) such as abnormal bleeding, or to help detect cancer or noncancerous growths of the womb.

If you have had a miscarriage, or if some of your placenta has stayed inside your womb after giving birth, you may need to have a type of D&C called an ERPC (evacuation of retained products of conception). This is to remove any remaining tissue and reduce your risk of developing an infection.

Usually, D&C is done as part of a procedure called a hysteroscopy. A hysteroscopy is an examination of the inside of the womb using a narrow, tube-like telescope called a hysteroscope.

D&C is usually done under general anesthesia, which means you will be asleep throughout the procedure and will not feel any pain. The procedure is normally carried out with no overnight stay in hospital.

Your doctor will explain the risks and benefits of having a D&C, and will also discuss the alternatives to the treatment.

About the Procedure

After the anesthesia has taken effect, your consultant will place an instrument called a speculum into your vagina so that he or she can see the cervix (the neck of your womb). Your cervix will then be gradually opened (dilated) using a series of rods of increasing thickness (dilators).

A D&C is usually done using a hysteroscope. This is an instrument that is passed gently through the cervix and into the womb. The hysteroscope has a small light and camera lens at its tip, which sends pictures from the inside of the womb to a video screen.

Once the cervix has been opened, tissue from the endometrium (the lining of the womb) can be removed, either with an instrument called a curette or with suction. If the D&C is being carried out to help with a diagnosis, the tissue that has been removed will be sent to a laboratory for examination. The results will usually be ready several days later and will be sent in a report to the doctor who recommended the test.

If you have had a miscarriage, the tissue that is removed during the treatment will be disposed of sensitively. Please let your doctor or nurse know if you have particular wishes about disposing of the tissue. The procedure usually lasts about ten minutes.

Afterwards, you may have some slight abdominal pain, similar to period pain, and there may be some vaginal bleeding for several days. Occasionally, the bleeding and discharge continue for up to a month.

A D&C is a commonly performed and generally safe surgical procedure. For most women, the benefits are greater than the disadvantages. However, like all medical procedures, there is an element of risk.

The main possible complications of any procedure include bleeding during or soon after the procedure, infection, and an unexpected reaction to the anesthetic.

Very occasionally, the womb is perforated or damaged during the D&C. This can lead to bleeding and infection. Most perforations heal without any treatment, but in some cases further surgery may be needed. It is also possible for the cervix to be damaged during the procedure.

The chance of complications depends on the exact type of operation you are having and other factors such as your general health. Ask your doctor to explain how any risks apply to you.

Section 20.3

Hysterectomy

Reprinted from "Hysterectomy," National Women's Health Information Center, July 2006.

What is a hysterectomy?

A hysterectomy is an operation to remove a woman's uterus (womb). The uterus is where a baby grows when a woman is pregnant. In some cases, the ovaries and fallopian tubes also are removed. These organs are located in a woman's lower abdomen. The cervix is the lower end of the uterus. The ovaries are organs that produce eggs and hormones. The fallopian tubes carry eggs from the ovaries to the uterus.

There are several types of hysterectomies:

- **Complete or total:** Removes the cervix as well as the uterus. (This is the most common type of hysterectomy.)
- **Partial or subtotal:** Removes the upper part of the uterus and leaves the cervix in place.
- **Radical:** Removes the uterus, the cervix, the upper part of the vagina, and supporting tissues. (This is done in some cases of cancer.)

Often one or both ovaries and fallopian tubes are removed at the same time a hysterectomy is done.

If you haven't reached menopause (when you haven't had a period for twelve months in a row), a hysterectomy will stop your monthly bleeding (periods). You also won't be able to get pregnant. And you may have menopausal symptoms, such as hot flashes and vaginal dryness. If both ovaries are removed as well, you will suddenly enter menopause.

How common are hysterectomies?

A hysterectomy is the second most common surgery among women in the United States. (The most common is cesarean section delivery.) Each year, more than six hundred thousand are done. One in three women in the United States has had a hysterectomy by age sixty.

How is a hysterectomy performed?

Hysterectomies are done through a cut in the abdomen (abdominal hysterectomy) or the vagina (vaginal hysterectomy). Sometimes an instrument called a laparoscope is used to help see inside the abdomen during vaginal hysterectomy. The type of surgery that is done depends on the reason for the surgery. Abdominal hysterectomies are more common and usually require a longer recovery time.

How long does it take to recover from a hysterectomy?

Recovering from a hysterectomy takes time. You will stay in the hospital from one to two days for postsurgery care. Some women may stay in the hospital up to four days. Recovery times for the different types of hysterectomy are as follows:

- **Abdominal:** Complete recovery usually takes four to eight weeks. You will gradually be able to increase your activities.
- **Vaginal or laparoscopic:** Most women are able to return to normal activity in one to two weeks.

For both, by the sixth week, you should be able to take tub baths and resume sexual activities.

Why do women have hysterectomies?

Hysterectomy is used to treat the following conditions:

- **Fibroids:** More hysterectomies are done because of fibroids than any other problem of the uterus. For many women with fibroids, symptoms are minimal and require no treatment. Also, the fibroids often shrink after menopause. But fibroids can cause heavy bleeding or pain in some women.

- **Endometriosis:** This happens when the tissue lining the inside of your uterus grows outside the uterus on your ovaries, fallopian tubes, or other pelvic or abdominal organs. When medication and surgery do not cure endometriosis, a hysterectomy often is performed.
- **Uterine prolapse:** This is when the uterus moves from its usual place down into the vagina. This can lead to urinary problems, pelvic pressure, or difficulty with bowel movements.
- **Cancer:** If you have cancer of the uterus, cervix, or ovary a hysterectomy may be part of the treatment your doctor recommends.
- **Persistent vaginal bleeding:** If your periods are heavy, not regular, or last for many days each cycle and nonsurgical methods have not helped to control bleeding, a hysterectomy may bring relief.
- **Chronic pelvic pain:** Surgery is a last resort for women who have chronic pelvic pain that clearly comes from the uterus. However, many forms of pelvic pain aren't cured by a hysterectomy, and so this approach can be a permanent mistake.

Are there any risks?

A hysterectomy involves some major and minor risks. Most women do not have problems during or after the operation. Some risks are as follows:

- Heavy blood loss that requires blood transfusion
- Bowel injury
- Bladder injury
- Anesthesia problems (such as breathing or heart problems)
- Need to change to abdominal incision during surgery
- Wound pulling open

Can a hysterectomy lower my sexual desire?

Women who have had a hysterectomy, in which one or both ovaries are removed, can have lowered sexual desire and decreased pleasure and orgasm. If you have problems with sexual desire or functioning, talk to your doctor.

Do options other than a hysterectomy exist?

If you have cancer, a hysterectomy might be the only option. But if you have uterine fibroids, endometriosis, or uterine prolapse, there are other treatments you can try first:

- **Drug therapy:** Certain medications may lighten heavy uterine bleeding or correct uterine bleeding that is not regular. Certain medications can help with endometriosis.
- **Endometrial ablation:** If you have heavy or irregular uterine bleeding, this procedure might ease your symptoms. With a special device, a doctor uses electricity, heat, or cold to destroy the lining of your uterus and stop uterine bleeding.
- **Uterine artery embolization:** For treating fibroid, this procedure involves blocking the blood supply to the tumors. Without blood, the fibroids shrink over time, which can reduce pain and heavy bleeding.
- **Myomectomy:** If you have fibroid tumors, this surgical procedure removes the tumors while leaving your uterus intact. There's a risk that the tumors could come back.
- **Vaginal pessary:** This is an object inserted into the vagina to hold the womb in place. It may be used as a temporary or permanent form of treatment. Vaginal pessaries come in many shapes and sizes, and they must be fitted for each woman individually.

Talk to your doctor about nonsurgical treatments to try first. Doing so is really important if the recommendation for a hysterectomy is for a reason other than cancer.

What should I do if I am told that I need a hysterectomy?

- Talk to your doctor about your options. Ask about other treatments for your condition.
- Consider getting a second opinion from another doctor.
- Ask about possible complications of surgery.

- Keep in mind that every woman is different and every situation is different. A good treatment choice for one woman may not be good for another.

If my cervix was removed in my hysterectomy, do I still need to have Pap tests?

Ask your doctor if you need to have periodic Pap tests. Regardless of whether you need a Pap test or not, all women who have had a hysterectomy must continue to have regular gynecologic exams.

Chapter 21

Menopause

Chapter Contents

Section 21.1

The Signs and Changes of Menopause

Excerpted from "Menopause," National Institute on Aging, National Institutes of Health, May 2005.

What is menopause?

Menopause is a normal part of life, just like puberty. It is the time of your last period, but symptoms can begin several years before that. And these symptoms can last for months or years after. Some time around forty, you might notice that your period is different—how long it lasts, how much you bleed, or how often it happens may not be the same. Or, without warning, you might find yourself feeling very warm during the day or in the middle of the night. Changing levels of estrogen and progesterone, which are two female hormones made in your ovaries, might lead to these symptoms.

This time of change, called perimenopause by many women and their doctors, often begins several years before your last menstrual period. It lasts for one year after your last period, the point in time known as menopause. A full year without a period is needed before you can say you have been "through menopause." Postmenopause follows menopause and lasts the rest of your life.

Menopause doesn't usually happen before you are forty, but it can happen any time from your thirties to your mid-fifties or later. The average age is fifty-one. Smoking can lead to early menopause. Some types of surgery can bring on menopause. For example, removing your uterus (hysterectomy) before menopause will make your periods stop, but your ovaries will still make hormones. That means you could still have symptoms of menopause like hot flashes when your ovaries start to make less estrogen. But, when both ovaries are also removed (oophorectomy), menopause symptoms can start right away, no matter what your age is, because your body has lost its main supply of estrogen.

What are the signs of menopause?

Women may have different signs or symptoms at menopause. That's because estrogen is used by many parts of your body. So, changes in how much estrogen you have can cause assorted symptoms. But, that doesn't mean you will have all, or even most, of them. In fact, some of the signs that happen around the time of menopause may really be a result of growing older, not changes in estrogen.

Changes in your period: This might be what you notice first. Your period may no longer be regular. How much you bleed could change. It could be lighter than normal. Or, you could have a heavier flow. Periods may be shorter or last longer. These are all normal results of changes in your reproductive system as you grow older. But, just to make sure there isn't a problem, see your doctor if any of the following are true:

- Your periods are coming very close together.
- You have heavy bleeding.
- You have spotting.
- Your periods are lasting more than a week.

Hot flashes: These are very common around the time of menopause because they are related to changing estrogen levels. They may last a few years after menopause. A hot flash is a sudden feeling of heat in the upper part or all of your body. Your face and neck become flushed. Red blotches may appear on your chest, back, and arms. Heavy sweating and cold shivering can follow. Flashes can be as mild as a light blush or severe enough to wake you from a sound sleep (called night sweats). Most hot flashes last between thirty seconds and ten minutes.

Problems with the vagina and bladder: Changing estrogen levels can cause your genital area to get drier and thinner. This could make sexual intercourse uncomfortable. You could have more vaginal or urinary infections. You might find it hard to hold urine long enough to get to the bathroom. Sometimes your urine might leak during exercise, sneezing, coughing, laughing, or running.

Sex: Around the time of menopause you may find that your feelings about sex have changed. You could be less interested. Or, you could feel freer and sexier after menopause. You can stop worrying about becoming pregnant after one full year without a period. But, remember you can't ever stop worrying about sexually transmitted diseases (STDs), such as human immunodeficiency virus (HIV)/acquired immunodeficiency syndrome (AIDS) or gonorrhea. If you think you might be at risk for an STD, make sure your partner uses a condom each time you have sex.

Sleep problems: You might start having trouble getting a good night's sleep. Maybe you can't fall asleep easily, or you wake too early. Night sweats might wake you up. You might have trouble falling back to sleep if you wake during the night.

Mood changes: You might find yourself more moody, irritable, or depressed around the time of menopause. It's not clear why this happens—is there is a connection between changes in estrogen levels and emotions or not? It's possible that stress, family changes such as growing children or aging parents, or always feeling tired could be causing these mood changes.

Changes in your body: You might think your body is changing. Your waist could get larger. You could lose muscle and gain fat. Your skin could get thinner. You might have memory problems, and your joints and muscles could feel stiff and achy. Are these a result of having less estrogen or just related to growing older? We don't know.

What about my heart and bones?

Two common health problems can start to happen at menopause, and you might not even notice.

Osteoporosis: Day in and day out your body is busy breaking down old bone and replacing it with new healthy bone. Estrogen helps control bone loss. So losing estrogen around the time of menopause causes women to begin to lose more bone than is replaced. In time, bones can become weak and break easily. This condition is called osteoporosis. Talk to your doctor to see if you should have a bone density test to find out if you are at risk for this problem. Your doctor can also suggest ways to prevent or treat osteoporosis.

Heart disease: After menopause, women are more likely to have heart disease. Changes in estrogen levels may be part of the cause. But, so is getting older. As you age, you may develop other problems, like high blood pressure or weight gain, that put you at greater risk for heart disease. Be sure to have your blood pressure and levels of triglycerides, fasting blood glucose, and low-density lipoprotein (LDL), high-density lipoprotein (HDL), and total cholesterol checked regularly. Talk to your health care provider to find out what you should do to protect your heart.

How can I stay healthy after menopause?

Staying healthy after menopause may mean making some changes in the way you live:

- Don't smoke. If you do use any type of tobacco, stop—it's never too late to benefit from quitting smoking.
- Eat a healthy diet—one low in fat, high in fiber, with plenty of fruits, vegetables, and whole-grain foods, as well as all the important vitamins and minerals.
- Make sure you get enough calcium and vitamin D—in your diet or in vitamin/mineral supplements.
- Learn what your healthy weight is, and try to stay there.
- Do weight-bearing exercise, such as walking, jogging, or dancing, at least three days each week for healthy bones. But try to be physically active in other ways for your general health.

Are you bothered by hot flashes? Menopause is not a disease that has to be treated. But you might need help with symptoms like hot flashes. Here are some ideas that have helped some women:

- Try to keep track of when hot flashes happen—a diary can help. You might be able to use this information to find out what triggers your flashes and then avoid it.
- When a hot flash starts, go somewhere cool.
- If night sweats wake you, try sleeping in a cool room or with a fan on.
- Dress in layers that you can take off if you get too warm.
- Use sheets and clothing that let your skin "breathe."
- Have a cold drink (water or juice) when a flash is starting.

You could also talk to your doctor about whether there are any medicines to manage hot flashes. Gabapentin, megestrol acetate, and certain antidepressants seem to be helpful to some women.

What about those lost hormones?

These days you hear a lot about whether you should use hormones to help relieve some menopause symptoms. It's hard to know what to do.

During perimenopause, some doctors suggest birth control pills to help with very heavy, frequent, or unpredictable menstrual periods. These pills might also help with symptoms like hot flashes, as well as prevent pregnancy.

As you get closer to menopause, you might be bothered more by symptoms like hot flashes, night sweats, or vaginal dryness. Your doctor might then suggest taking estrogen (as well as progesterone, if you still have a uterus). This is known as menopausal hormone therapy (MHT). Some people still call it hormone replacement therapy or HRT. Taking these hormones will probably help with menopause symptoms and prevent the bone loss that can happen at menopause. However, there is a chance your symptoms will come back when you stop MHT.

Also, menopausal hormone therapy has risks. That is why the U.S. Food and Drug Administration suggests that women who want to try MHT to manage their hot flashes or vaginal dryness use the lowest dose that works, for the shortest time it's needed.

Right now, there is a lot that is unknown about taking hormones around menopause.

Do phytoestrogens help?

Phytoestrogens are estrogen-like substances found in some cereals, vegetables, legumes (beans), and herbs. They might work in the body like a weak form of estrogen. They might relieve some symptoms of menopause, but they could also carry risks like estrogen. We don't know. Be sure to tell your doctor if you decide to try eating a lot more foods that contain phytoestrogens or to try using an herbal supplement. Any food or over-the-counter product that you use for its drug-like effects could change how other prescribed drugs work or cause an overdose.

How do I decide what to do?

Talk to your health care provider for help deciding how to best manage menopause. You can see a gynecologist, geriatrician, general practitioner, or internist. Talk about your symptoms and whether they bother you. Make sure the doctor knows your medical history and your family medical history. This includes whether you are at risk for heart disease, osteoporosis, and breast cancer. Remember that your decision is never final. You can—and should—review it with your doctor during a checkup. Your needs may change, and so might what we know about menopause.

Section 21.2

Stages of Menopause

Reprinted from "Menopause and Hormone Therapy: Stages of Menopause," National Women's Health Information Center, June 2007.

Menopause is only one of several stages in the reproductive life of a woman. The whole menopause transition is divided into the following stages:

- **Premature menopause:** Menopause that happens before the age of forty, whether it is natural or induced.
- **Premenopause:** Refers to the entirety of a woman's life from her first to her last regular menstrual period. It is best defined as a time of "normal" reproductive function in a woman.
- **Perimenopause:** This means "around menopause" and is a transitional stage of two to ten years before complete cessation of the menstrual period and is usually experienced by women from thirty-five to fifty years of age. This stage of menopause is characterized by hormone fluctuations, which cause the typical menopause symptoms, such as hot flashes.
- **Menopause:** Represents the end stage of a natural transition in a woman's reproductive life. Menopause is the point at which estrogen and progesterone production decreases permanently to very low levels. The ovaries stop producing eggs and a woman is no longer able to get pregnant naturally.
- **Postmenopause:** This refers to a woman's time of life after menopause has occurred. It is generally believed that the post-menopausal phase begins when twelve full months have passed

since the last menstrual period. From here a woman will be postmenopausal for the rest of her life.

Male menopause: Women may not be the only ones who suffer the effects of changing hormones. Some doctors are noticing that their male patients are reporting some of the same symptoms that women experience in menopause.

Section 21.3

Premature Menopause

Reprinted from "Menopause and Hormone Therapy: Premature Menopause," National Women's Health Information Center, June 2007.

Premature menopause is menopause that happens before the age of forty—whether it is natural or induced. Women who enter menopause early get symptoms similar to those of natural menopause, like hot flashes, emotional problems, vaginal dryness, and decreased sex drive. For some women with early menopause, these symptoms are severe. Also, women who have early menopause tend to get weaker bones faster than women who enter menopause later in life. This raises their chances of getting osteoporosis and breaking a bone. Premature menopause can happen for the following reasons:

- **Chromosome defects:** Defects in the chromosomes can cause premature menopause. For example, women with Turner syndrome are born without a second X chromosome or born without part of the chromosome. The ovaries don't form normally, and early menopause results.
- **Genetics:** Women with a family history of premature menopause are more likely to have early menopause themselves.
- **Autoimmune diseases:** The body's immune system, which normally fights off diseases, mistakenly attacks a part of its own reproductive system. This hurts the ovaries and prevents them from making female hormones. Thyroid disease and rheumatoid arthritis are two diseases in which this can happen.

- **Surgery to remove the ovaries:** Surgical removal of both ovaries, also called a bilateral oophorectomy, puts a woman into menopause right away. She will no longer have periods, and hormones decline rapidly. She may have menopausal symptoms right away, like hot flashes and diminished sexual desire. Women who have a hysterectomy, but have their ovaries left in place, will not have induced menopause because their ovaries will continue to make hormones. But because their uterus is removed, they no longer have their periods and cannot get pregnant. They might have hot flashes since the surgery can sometimes disturb the blood supply to the ovaries. Later on, they might have natural menopause a year or two earlier than expected.
- **Chemotherapy or pelvic radiation treatments for cancer:** Cancer chemotherapy or pelvic radiation therapy for reproductive system cancers can cause ovarian damage. Women may stop getting their periods, have fertility problems, or lose their fertility. This can happen right away or take several months. With cancer treatment, the chances of going into menopause depend on the type of chemotherapy used, how much was used, and the age of the woman when she gets treatment. The younger a woman is, the less likely she will go into menopause.

How to Find Out If You Have Premature Menopause

Your doctor will ask you if you've had changes typical of menopause, like hot flashes, irregular periods, sleep problems, and vaginal dryness. Normally, menopause is confirmed when a woman hasn't had her period for twelve months in a row.

However, with certain types of premature menopause, these signs may not be enough for a diagnosis. A blood test that measures follicle-stimulating hormone (FSH) can be done. Your ovaries use this hormone to make estrogen. FSH levels rise when the ovaries stop making estrogen. When FSH levels are higher than normal, you've reached menopause. However, your estrogen levels vary daily, so you may need this test more than once to know for sure.

You may also have a test for levels of estradiol (a type of estrogen) and luteinizing hormone (LH). Estradiol levels fall when the ovaries fail. Levels lower than normal are a sign of menopause. LH is a hormone that triggers ovulation. If you test above normal levels, you've gone through menopause.

Section 21.4

Perimenopause

Reprinted from "Perimenopause," National Women's Health Information Center, March 2006.

What is perimenopause?

Perimenopause is the time leading up to menopause when you start to notice menopause-related changes—plus the year after menopause. Perimenopause is what some people call "being in menopause" or "going through menopause." But menopause itself is only one day—the day you haven't had a period for twelve months in a row. During perimenopause, your ovaries start to shut down, making less of certain hormones (estrogen and progesterone), and you begin to lose the ability to become pregnant. This change is a natural part of aging that signals the ending of your reproductive years.

When does perimenopause start?

Women normally go through perimenopause between ages forty-five and fifty-five, but some women start perimenopause earlier, even in their thirties. When perimenopause starts, and how long it lasts varies from woman to women. You will likely notice menopause-related symptoms, such as changes in periods.

What are some of the signs and symptoms?

Menopause affects every woman differently. Your only symptom may be your period stopping. You may have other symptoms, too. Many symptoms at this time of life are because of just getting older. But some are due to approaching menopause. Menopause-related symptoms you might have during perimenopause include the following:

- Changes in pattern of periods (can be shorter or longer, lighter or heavier, more or less time between periods)
- Hot flashes (sudden rush of heat in upper body)

- Night sweats (hot flashes that happen while you sleep), often followed by a chill
- Trouble sleeping through the night (with or without night sweats)
- Vaginal dryness
- Mood changes, feeling crabby (probably because of lack of sleep)
- Trouble focusing, feeling mixed-up or confused
- Hair loss or thinning on your head, more hair growth on your face

When you visit your doctor, take along a diary about what's happening with your period. For a few months before your visit, record when your period starts and stops each month, and indicate whether it is light or heavy. Also note any other symptoms you have.

Is there any treatment for perimenopause? What can I do?

Some women take oral contraceptives (birth control pills, or "the pill") to ease perimenopausal symptoms—even if they don't need them for birth control. These hormone treatments of combined estrogen and progestin can help keep your periods regular plus ease all the symptoms listed above. Talk with your doctor to see if this option is for you. If you are over thirty-five, you should not take birth control pills if you smoke or have a history of blood clots. You need a prescription to get oral contraceptives.

After a woman reaches menopause, if she still needs treatment for menopause symptoms, she should switch from birth control pills to menopause hormone therapy (HT). HT contains much lower doses of hormones, and thus has less risk for bad side effects.

Making some changes in your life can also help ease your symptoms and keep you healthy:

- **Eat healthy:** A healthy diet is more important now than before because your risks of osteoporosis (extreme bone loss) and heart disease go up at this stage of life. Eat lots of whole-grain foods, vegetables, and fruits. Add calcium-rich foods (milk, cheese, yogurt) or take a calcium supplement to obtain your recommended daily intake. Get adequate vitamin D from sunshine or a supplement. Avoid alcohol or caffeine, which also can trigger hot flashes in some women.
- **Get moving:** Regular exercise helps keep your weight down, helps you sleep better, makes your bones stronger, and boosts

your mood. Try to get at least thirty minutes of exercise most days of the week, but let your doctor recommend what's best for you.

- **Find healthy ways to cope with stress:** Try meditation or yoga—both can help you relax, as well as handle your symptoms more easily.

Can I get pregnant while in perimenopause?

Yes, you can get pregnant until you've gone twelve months in a row without a period. Talk to your doctor about your birth control options. Keep in mind that birth control pills, shots, implants, or diaphragms will not protect you from sexually transmitted diseases (STDs) or human immunodeficiency virus (HIV). If you use one of these methods, be sure also to use a latex condom or dental dam (used for oral sex) correctly every time you have sexual contact. Be aware that condoms don't provide complete protection against STDs and HIV—the only sure protection is abstinence (not having sex of any kind). But making sure to always use—and correctly use—latex condoms and other barrier methods can help protect you from STDs.

Section 21.5

Treating the Symptoms of Menopause

Excerpted from "Menopause and Menopause Treatments," National Women's Health Information Center, March 1, 2006.

How do I manage menopause? What are my options?

Eating a healthy diet and exercising at menopause and beyond are important to feeling your best. Most women do not need any special treatment for menopause. But some women may have menopause symptoms that need treatment. Several treatments are available. It's a good idea to talk about the treatments with your doctor so you can choose what's best for you. There is no one treatment that is good for all women. Sometimes menopause symptoms go away over time without treatment, but there's no way to know when.

Hormone therapy (HT): If used properly, hormone therapy (once called hormone replacement therapy or HRT) is one way to deal with the more difficult symptoms of menopause. It's the only therapy that is approved by the government for treating more difficult hot flashes and vaginal dryness. Hormone therapy should *not* be used solely to prevent heart or bone disease, stroke, memory loss, or Alzheimer disease. There are many kinds of hormone therapies, so your doctor can suggest what's best for you. As with all treatments, HT has both possible benefits and possible risks; it is important to talk about these issues with your doctor. If you decide to use HT, use the lowest dose that helps and for the shortest time needed. Check with your doctor every six months to see if you still need HT.

HT can help with menopause by:

- reducing hot flashes;
- treating vaginal dryness;
- slowing bone loss;
- improving sleep (and thus decreasing mood swings).

For some women, HT may increase their chance of:

- blood clots;
- heart attack;
- stroke;
- breast cancer;
- gall bladder disease.

Who should not *take HT for menopause?*

Women who:

- think they are pregnant;
- have problems with vaginal bleeding;
- have had certain kinds of cancers (such as breast and uterine cancer);
- have had a stroke or heart attack;
- have had blood clots;
- have liver disease;
- have heart disease.

HT can also cause these side effects:

- Vaginal bleeding
- Bloating
- Breast tenderness or swelling
- Headaches
- Mood changes
- Nausea

Be sure to see your doctor if you have any of these side effects while using HT.

What about so-called natural treatments for menopause?

Some women decide to take herbal or other plant-based products to help relieve hot flashes. Some of the most common ones are as follows:

- **Soy:** Soy contains phytoestrogens (chemicals that are like estrogen). But, there is no proof that soy—or other sources of phytoestrogens—really do make hot flashes better. And the risks of taking soy—mainly soy pills and powders—are not known. The best sources of soy are foods such as tofu, tempeh, soy milk, and soy nuts. These soy products are more likely to work on mild hot flashes.
- **Other sources of phytoestrogens:** These include herbs such as black cohosh, wild yam, dong quai, and valerian root. Again, there is no proof that these herbs (or pills or creams containing these herbs) help with hot flashes.

Products that come from plants may sound like they are safe, but there is no proof they really are. There also is no proof that they are better at helping symptoms of menopause. Make sure to discuss these types of products with your doctor before taking them. You also should tell your doctor about other medicines you are taking, since some plant products can be harmful when combined with other drugs.

What about "bioidentical" hormone therapy?

This term means different things to different people. It's really hormones that are just the same as the hormones the body makes.

There are several products with hormone like this that are on the market and are well tested. But some people use this term to mean drugs that are custom-made from a doctor's order. There is no proof that these custom-made products are better or safer than hormone therapy that's on the market.

How much physical activity should I do?

A woman should first talk to her doctor to see what's best for her. The goal is to exercise regularly so you can lower the risk of serious disease (such as heart disease or diabetes) and maintain a healthy weight. This usually takes at least thirty minutes of exercise (such as brisk walking) on most days of the week.

How else can I help my symptoms?

Hot flashes: Some women report that eating or drinking hot or spicy foods, alcohol, or caffeine, feeling stressed, or being in a hot place can bring on hot flashes. Try to avoid any triggers that bring on your hot flashes. Dress in layers, and keep a fan in your home or workplace. Regular exercise might also ease hot flashes, but sometimes exercise can cause a hot flash. If hot flashes continue and HT is not an option, ask your doctor about taking an antidepressant or epilepsy medicine. There is proof that these can relieve hot flashes for some women.

Vaginal dryness: A water-based, over-the-counter vaginal lubricant (like KY® Jelly) can be helpful if sex is painful. A vaginal moisturizer (also over-the-counter) can provide lubrication and help keep needed moisture in vaginal tissues. Really bad vaginal dryness may need HT. If vaginal dryness is the only reason for considering HT, an estrogen product for the vagina is the best choice. Vaginal estrogen products (creams, tablet, ring) treat only the vagina.

Problems sleeping: One of the best ways to get a good night's sleep is to get at least thirty minutes of physical activity on most days of the week. But, don't exercise close to bedtime. Also avoid large meals, smoking, and working right before bedtime. Caffeine and alcohol should be avoided after noon. Drinking something warm before bedtime, such as herbal tea (no caffeine) or warm milk, might help you to feel sleepy. Keep your bedroom dark, quiet, and cool, and use your bedroom only for sleeping and sex. Avoid napping during the day, and try to go to bed and get up at the same times every day. If you wake during the night and can't get back to sleep, get up and read until you're sleepy. Don't just lie there. If hot flashes are the cause of sleep problems, treating the hot flashes will usually improve sleep.

Mood swings: Some women report mood swings or "feeling blue" as they reach menopause. Women who had mood swings (PMS) before their periods or postpartum depression after giving birth may have more mood swings around menopause. These are women who are sensitive to hormone changes. Often the mood swings will go away with time. If a woman is using HT for hot flashes or another menopause symptom, sometimes her mood swings will get better, too. Also, getting enough sleep and staying physically active will help you to feel your best. Mood swings are not the same as depression.

Memory problems: As people age, their memory is not as good as it once was. Some women say they have "fuzzy thinking" as they reach menopause. This may be caused by changing hormones and can improve over time. Getting enough sleep and keeping physically active can help. If memory problems are really bad, talk to your doctor right away. This is not caused by menopause.

I'm having a hysterectomy soon. Will this cause me to reach menopause?

Sometimes, younger women need a hysterectomy to treat health problems such as endometriosis or cancer. A hysterectomy is an operation to remove a woman's uterus (womb). Often one or both ovaries (the female organs that produce eggs and hormones) are removed at the same time the hysterectomy is done. If you haven't reached menopause, a hysterectomy will stop your period. But you will reach menopause only if both ovaries are removed, called surgical menopause. Because surgical menopause is instant menopause, it can cause more severe symptoms than natural menopause (menopause that occurs as part of the natural aging process). You should talk with your doctor about how to best manage these symptoms.

Women who have a hysterectomy but have their ovaries left in place will not reach menopause at the time of surgery because their ovaries will continue to make hormones. But because the uterus is removed, they will no longer have their periods and they cannot become pregnant. Later on, they might reach natural menopause a year or two earlier than expected.

Section 21.6

The Benefits and Risks of Hormone Replacement Therapy

Excerpted from "Hormones and Menopause: Tips from the National Institute on Aging," July 2006.

A hormone is a chemical substance made by a gland or organ to regulate various body functions. To help control the symptoms of menopause some women can take hormones, called menopausal hormone therapy (MHT). MHT used to be called hormone replacement therapy or HRT. Some women should not use MHT. There are many things to learn about hormones before you make the choice that is right for you.

Which hormones are used for menopause?

During perimenopause, the months or years right before menopause, levels of two female hormones, estrogen and progesterone, in a woman's body go up and down irregularly. This happens as the ovaries struggle to keep up with the body's needs. The symptoms of menopause might result from these changing hormone levels. After menopause, when a woman's ovaries make much less estrogen and progesterone, the symptoms of menopause may continue. Menopausal hormone therapy may help control these symptoms. A woman whose uterus has been removed can use estrogen alone to control her symptoms. But a woman who still has a uterus must take progesterone or a progestin (a synthetic progesterone) along with the estrogen. This will prevent unwanted thickening of the lining of the uterus and also cancer of the uterus, an uncommon but possible result of using estrogen alone.

Why take these hormones? Why not?

Menopause is a normal part of life. It is not a disease that has to be treated. Women may decide to use menopausal hormone therapy because of its benefits, but there are also side effects and risks to consider. Two good reasons to think about menopausal hormone therapy are as follows:

- Treating some of the bothersome symptoms of menopause
- Preventing or treating osteoporosis

But for some women there are noticeable side effects:

- Breast tenderness
- Spotting or a return of monthly periods
- Cramping
- Bloating

By changing the type or amount of the hormones, the way they are taken, or the timing of the doses, your doctor may be able to control these side effects. Or, over time, they may go away on their own.

For some women there are also serious risks (see Table 21.1). These risks are why you need to think a lot before deciding to use menopausal hormone therapy.

Although the risks are small for any one woman, you need to take them into account. Much of the following table on benefits and risks is based on one important clinical trial, the Women's Health Initiative (WHI). This study looked at estrogen (conjugated equine estrogens) used alone or with a particular progestin (medroxyprogesterone acetate). Some other types of estrogen, progesterone, or progestin may have been tested in smaller clinical trials to see if they have an effect on heart disease, breast cancer, or dementia. Others have not.

What are the benefits and risks of menopausal hormone therapy?

Here is what scientists can say right now about the benefits and risks of MHT. Remember—which hormones you use, the way you take them, and the dose—might affect these benefits and risks.

Because the average age of women participating in the trial was sixty-three, more than ten years past the average age of menopause, some experts now question whether the WHI results apply to women around the time of menopause. The WHI study found that in every ten thousand women using estrogen plus progestin, there would be seven more heart attacks than in every ten thousand women not using these hormones. Other research has suggested that if MHT is begun around the time of menopause, it might provide protection from heart disease, but not if a woman waits too long. This is a subject for further study.

How would I use the hormones?

Estrogen comes in many forms and dosages. You could use a skin patch or vaginal tablet or cream, take a pill, or get an implant, shot, or vaginal ring insert. Progesterone or progestin is often taken as a pill, sometimes in the same pill as the estrogen. It also comes as a patch, shot, IUD (intrauterine device), vaginal gel, or suppository.

The form your doctor suggests may depend on your symptoms. For example, patches or pills can relieve hot flashes, night sweats, and vaginal dryness. They will also slow or prevent bone loss and help delay osteoporosis while you are using them. Other forms—vaginal creams, tablets, or rings—are used for vaginal dryness. The vaginal ring insert might also help some urinary tract symptoms. But, the dose found in these other forms is probably too low to relieve hot flashes.

What are natural hormones?

The natural hormones some menopausal women use are estrogen and progesterone made from plants such as soy or yams. Some people also call them bioidentical hormones because they are supposed to be chemically the same as the hormones naturally made by a woman's body. So-called natural hormones are put together (compounded) by a compounding pharmacist. This pharmacist follows a formula decided on by your doctor.

Drug companies also make estrogens and progesterone from plants like soy and yams. Some of these are also chemically identical to the hormones made by your body. You get these from any pharmacy with a prescription from your doctor.

One difference between the natural hormones prepared by a compounding pharmacist and those made by a drug company is that the compounded natural hormones are not regulated and approved by the U.S. Food and Drug Administration (FDA). So, we don't know much about how safe or effective they are or how the quality varies from batch to batch. Hormones made by drug companies are regulated and approved by the FDA.

There are also "natural" treatments for the symptoms of menopause that are available over-the-counter, without a prescription. Some of these are also made from soy or yams. They are not regulated or approved by the FDA.

There is very little reliable scientific information from clinical trials about the safety of bioidentical hormones, how well they control the symptoms of menopause, and whether they are as good or better to use than FDA-approved estrogens, progesterone, and progestins.

What's right for me?

There is no "one size fits all" answer for all women who are trying to decide whether to use menopausal hormone therapy (MHT). You have to look at your own needs and weigh your own risks.

Ask yourself and your doctor these questions:

- How much are you bothered by menopausal symptoms such as hot flashes or vaginal dryness? Like many women your hot flashes or night sweats will likely go away over time, but vaginal dryness may not. MHT can help if your symptoms are troubling you.
- Are you at risk for developing osteoporosis? Estrogen might protect bone mass while you use it. However, there are other drugs that can protect your bones without the same risks as MHT.
- Do you have a history of heart disease? Using estrogen and progestin can increase your risk.

Table 21.1. Benefits and Risks of Menopausal Hormone Therapy

	Women with a Uterus (Estrogen + Progestin)	Women Without a Uterus (Estrogen Only)
Benefits		
Relieves hot flashes/night sweats	Yes	Yes
Relieves vaginal dryness	Yes	Yes
Reduces risk of bone fractures	Yes	Yes
Improves cholesterol levels	Yes	Yes
Reduces risk of colon cancer	Yes	Don't know
Risks		
Increases risk of stroke	Yes	Yes
Increases risk of serious blood clots	Yes	Yes
Increases risk of heart attack	Yes	No
Increases risk of breast cancer	Yes	Possibly
Increases risk of dementia, when begun by women age 65 and older	Yes	Yes
Unpleasant side effects, such as bloating and tender breasts	Yes	Yes
Pill form can raise level of triglycerides (a type of fat in the blood)	Yes	Yes

- Do you or others in your family have a history of breast cancer? If you have a family history of breast cancer, check with your doctor about your risk.
- Do you have a history of gall bladder disease or high levels of triglycerides? Some experts think that using a patch will not make your triglyceride (a type of fat in the blood) level go up or increase your chance of gall bladder problems. Using an estrogen pill might.
- Do you have liver disease or a history of stroke or blood clots in your veins? MHT might not be safe for you to use.
- Are you over age sixty-five and thinking about using MHT to prevent dementia? Estrogen and progestin could actually increase your risk of dementia. Estrogen alone might do that also.

Then, talk to your doctor about how best to treat or prevent your symptoms or the diseases for which you are at risk. Ask about your other choices. Remember, these too may have risks and benefits. If you decide to use MHT, the FDA suggests that you use the lowest dose that works, for the shortest time needed.

If you are already using menopausal hormone therapy and think you would like to stop, first ask your health care provider how to do that. Some doctors suggest tapering off slowly.

Whatever decision you make now about using MHT is not final. You can start or end the treatment at any time. If you stop, your risks will probably lessen over time, but so will the protection. Discuss your decision about menopausal hormone therapy each year with your doctor at your annual checkup.

Don't forget at your checkup to ask your doctor about any new study results. Research on menopause is ongoing. Scientists are looking for answers to questions such as the following:

- How long can a woman safely use menopausal hormone therapy?
- Are some types of estrogen or progesterone safer than others?
- Is one form of hormone therapy (patch, pill, or cream, for example) better than another?
- Is MHT safer if you start it around the time of menopause instead of when you are older?

For now, we know that each woman is different, and the decision for each one will probably also be different. But almost every study gives women and their doctors more information to answer the question: Is menopausal hormone therapy right for me?

Part Three

Sexual and Reproductive Concerns

Chapter 22

Understanding Your Sexuality

Sexuality

All people are sexual beings from birth to death. Our sexuality includes:

- our bodies;
- our biological sex;
- our gender—our biological, social, and legal status as girls and boys, women and men;
- our gender identities—how we feel about our gender;
- our sexual orientations—straight, lesbian, gay, bisexual;
- our values about life, love, and the people in our lives.

Our sexuality also includes feelings, attitudes, relationships, self-image, ideals, and behaviors, and it influences how we experience the world.

Being Sexual

Sex and Love in the Real World

Sex seems to be everywhere. It is used to sell everything, from cars to magazines. With all those messages, we can be confused about what sex means to us.

Some of the most difficult decisions in life are about sex. They can affect our plans for school, career, our lifestyles, relationships, and families. Whatever sexual decisions you make, choose ones that help you feel proud of yourself.

Of course we don't always have sex when we're feeling sexy. When to have sex is a personal choice. We usually make better decisions when we think through the possible benefits and risks. A good sex life is one that keeps in balance with everything else in your life—your health, education and career goals, relationships with other people, and your feelings about yourself.

We all have our own sexual values. What are yours? Are they about finding a life partner? Are they about satisfying a physical need? Are they about developing a relationship? Are they about waiting until marriage? Are they about all of these concerns? Your answers may change over your lifetime.

There's a difference between sexual desire and love. Sexual desire is a strong physical excitement. Love is a powerful caring for someone else. Love can exist without sexual desire, and vice versa. Many people are happiest when both love and sexual desire are shared by both partners.

Sex involves responsibility. Sex partners need to share responsibility for birth control. They should also protect each other from infections like human immunodeficiency virus (HIV), gonorrhea, herpes, genital warts, and chlamydia.

Communication is very important. Sex can mean different things to different people. But it is not a good substitute for conversation. Some people expect sexual intercourse to bring them closer. But sex can get in the way of intimacy—especially if you and your partner aren't talking. Sometimes, one partner is having sex just to have sex while the other expects a long-term relationship. We need to talk with our partners to be sure we are clear with each other.

Sexual Attraction

Some people have a lot of sexual desire. Some have less. And some have very little. Some women are attracted to men. Some are not. They may be interested in relationships with other women. Some men are attracted to women. Some are not. They may be interested in relationships with other men. Some people are attracted to both women and men. No one knows for sure what makes people gay, lesbian, bisexual, or straight. Sexual orientation develops naturally—beginning even before birth.

Although sexual orientation may seem to shift for some people in the course of a lifetime, it is not something that people can decide for themselves or others.

Except for pregnancy, the benefits and risks of sexual relationships are much the same, regardless of sexual orientation. However, gay, lesbian, and bisexual people are often subjected to harassment and discrimination based on their sexual orientation.

Enjoying Your Body and Sexuality

What is sexy? The media tells us that only certain body images are sexy. Remember—they are trying to sell a product or service. Being sexy depends more on personality—how we think of ourselves, present ourselves, take care of ourselves, and respect ourselves and other people.

Sexual stereotypes are dangerous. Society sends confusing messages about what it means to be male and female.

Women and men who struggle to look like models or celebrities may injure their health. They may develop eating disorders, exercise to excess, or abuse steroids. But differences in body type, height, and weight are normal and healthy.

Enjoying your body and understanding what gives you sexual pleasure can improve sex with a partner. Every woman and man has different feelings about sexual pleasure—many of us learn about what we like and don't like through masturbation. And many women and men will masturbate all their lives—whether or not they are in relationships.

Sexual Relationships

Self-respect is the key to a healthy and rewarding sex life. Being your own person means doing what you know is right for you. It's important to be honest with yourself about what you want and what you don't want.

In happy and healthy relationships, partners try not to hurt each other. Healthy relationships help us feel better about ourselves and about our place in the world. They make us feel safe. But some people put up with abuse to protect their relationships—this is unhealthy and dangerous. Emotional and verbal abuse are unhealthy. Physical and sexual abuse is wrong and illegal, in any relationship.

Avoid regrets—trust your feelings about becoming sexually involved. Our society doesn't always help people understand their real feelings about sex. It's okay to ignore the pressure to be sexually active. Just be true to yourself.

The benefits and risks of sexual relationships are much the same for all women. However, people who are perceived as gay, lesbian, or bisexual are often subjected to discrimination.

What Do I Feel about Sex?

Thinking about your answers to these questions may help you understand your feelings:

- What are my sexual desires?
- What are my sexual limits—am I clear with myself about what I will do and won't do?
- Do I want to have sex?
- What do I want to get out of it?
- What does my partner want? Why?
- Do we want the same thing?
- Could I get hurt or hurt my partner?
- Will we be honest, equal, respectful, and responsible?
- Have I considered the possible physical or emotional outcome?

It is wrong for a partner to pressure you, ask you to take risks, or ignore your feelings. It is not a good sign if your partner keeps secrets from you.

Chapter 23

Sexual Dysfunction

Chapter Contents

Section 23.1

The Four Categories of Sexual Dysfunction in Women

Reprinted with permission from "Sexual Dysfunction in Women," January 2008, http://familydoctor.org/online/famdocen/home/women/reproductive/sex-dys/612.html.

What is sexual dysfunction?

When you have problems with sex, doctors call it "sexual dysfunction." Both men and women can have it. There are four kinds of sexual problems in women:

- **Desire disorders:** When you are not interested in having sex or have less desire for sex than you used to.
- **Arousal disorders:** When you don't feel a sexual response in your body or you cannot stay sexually aroused.
- **Orgasmic disorders:** When you can't have an orgasm or you have pain during orgasm.
- **Sexual pain disorders:** When you have pain during or after sex.

What causes sexual dysfunction?

Many things can cause problems in your sex life. Certain medicines (such as oral contraceptives and chemotherapy drugs), diseases (such as diabetes or high blood pressure), excessive alcohol use, or vaginal infections can cause sexual problems. Depression, relationship problems, or abuse (current or past abuse) can also cause sexual dysfunction.

You may have less sexual desire during pregnancy, right after childbirth, or when you are breastfeeding. After menopause many women feel less sexual desire, have vaginal dryness, or have pain during sex due to a decrease in estrogen (a hormone in the body).

The stresses of everyday life can also affect your ability to have sex. Being tired from a busy job or caring for young children may affect your sexual desire. You may also be bored by a longstanding sexual routine.

How do I know if I have a problem?

Up to 70 percent of couples have a problem with sex at some time in their relationship. Most women will have sex that doesn't feel good at some point in her life. This doesn't necessarily mean you have a sexual problem.

If you don't want to have sex or it never feels good, you might have a sexual problem. Discuss your concerns with your doctor. Remember that anything you tell your doctor is private and that your doctor can help you find a reason and possible treatment for your sexual dysfunction.

What can I do?

If desire is the problem, try changing your usual routine. Try having sex at different times of the day, or try a different sexual position.

Arousal disorders can often be helped if you use a vaginal cream or sexual lubricant for dryness. If you have gone through menopause, talk to your doctor about taking estrogen or using an estrogen cream.

If you have a problem having an orgasm, you may not be getting enough foreplay or stimulation before actual intercourse begins. Extra stimulation (before you have sex with your partner) with a vibrator may be helpful. You might need rubbing or stimulation for up to an hour before having sex. Many women don't have an orgasm during intercourse. If you want an orgasm with intercourse, you or your partner may want to gently stroke your clitoris. Masturbation may also be helpful, as it can help you learn what techniques work best for you.

If you're having pain during sex, try different positions. When you are on top, you have more control over penetration and movement. Emptying your bladder before you have sex, using extra lubrication, or taking a warm bath before sex all may help. If you still have pain during sex, talk to your doctor. There are a variety of causes of pain during sex, so talk with your doctor. He or she can help you find the cause of your pain and decide what treatment is best for you.

Can medicine help?

If you have gone through menopause or have had your uterus and/or ovaries removed, taking the hormone estrogen may help with sexual problems. If you're not already taking estrogen, ask your doctor if this is an option for you.

You may have heard that taking sildenafil (Viagra®) or the male hormone testosterone can help women with sexual problems. There have not been many studies on the effects of Viagra or testosterone on women, so doctors do not know whether these things can help or not. Both Viagra and testosterone can have serious side effects, so using them is probably not worth the risk.

What else can I do?

Learn more about your body and how it works. Ask your doctor about how medicines, illnesses, surgery, age, pregnancy, or menopause can affect sex.

Practice "sensate focus" exercises where one partner gives a massage, while the other partner says what feels good and requests changes (example: "lighter," "faster," etc.). Fantasizing may increase your desire. Squeezing the muscles of your vagina tightly (called Kegel exercises) and then relaxing them may also increase your arousal. Try sexual activity other than intercourse, such as massage, oral sex, or masturbation.

What about my partner?

Talk with your partner about what each of you like and dislike, or what you might want to try. Ask for your partner's help. Remember that your partner may not want to do some things you want to try, and you may not want to try what your partner wants. You should respect each other's comforts and discomforts. This helps you and your partner have a good sexual relationship. If you feel you can't talk to your partner, your doctor or a counselor may be able to help you.

If you feel like your partner is abusing you, tell your doctor.

How can my doctor help?

Your doctor can suggest ways to treat your sexual problems or can refer you to a sex therapist or counselor if needed.

Section 23.2

Dyspareunia

Excerpted from "Sexual Intercourse—Painful,"

For both men and women, pain can occur in the pelvic area during or soon after sexual intercourse. It can happen at any time during sex—for example, at the time of penetration, erection, or ejaculation. Eventually, if pain from intercourse is ongoing, you could lose interest in any sexual activity.

The medical term for this is dyspareunia.

Causes

- Intercourse too soon after surgery or childbirth
- Vaginal dryness or inadequate lubrication (for example, from insufficient foreplay)
- Menopause (vaginal lining loses its normal moisture and becomes dry)
- Vaginal infection
- Reaction to the latex of a diaphragm or condom
- Prostatitis—inflammation of the prostate
- Genital irritation from soaps, detergents, douches, or feminine hygiene products
- Herpes sores, genital warts, or other sexually transmitted diseases
- Urinary tract infections
- Endometriosis
- Vaginismus—involuntary contraction of the vaginal muscles; this may be a result of ongoing painful intercourse as well as a cause
- Ill-fitting diaphragm

- Sexual abuse or rape
- Hemorrhoids
- Certain medications

Home Care

For painful intercourse in women after pregnancy:

- Wait at least six weeks after childbirth before resuming sexual relations.
- Be gentle and patient.

For vaginal dryness/inadequate lubrication:

- Try water-based lubricants.
- If you are going through menopause and lubricants don't work, talk to your doctor about estrogen creams or other prescription medications.

For painful intercourse caused by prostatitis:

- Soak in a warm bath.
- Drink plenty of fluids, but avoid alcohol and caffeine.
- Take acetaminophen or ibuprofen.
- Take antibiotics as prescribed.

For hemorrhoids, try stool softeners. Antibiotics may be required for urinary tract infections, sexually transmitted diseases, or vaginal infections.

Other causes of painful intercourse may require prescription medications or, rarely, surgery.

Sex therapy may be helpful, especially if no underlying medical cause is identified. Guilt, inner conflict, or unresolved feelings about past abuse may be involved which need to be worked through in therapy. It may be best for your partner to see the therapist with you.

When to Contact a Medical Professional

Call your doctor if:

- home remedies are not working;

- you have other symptoms with painful intercourse, like bleeding, genital lesions, irregular periods, discharge from penis or vagina, or involuntary vaginal muscle contraction.

If you are a victim of a sexual assault, report the crime to the police and go to the emergency room immediately. Get a trusted friend to accompany you. *Do not* change, bathe, shower, or even wash your hands before the emergency room (ER) evaluation. The temptation to do so will be great, but it is important to not lose any evidence in order to help find, charge, and convict the perpetrator.

What to Expect at Your Office Visit

Your doctor will take your medical history and perform a physical examination.

Medical history questions may include:

- When did the pain begin or has intercourse always been painful?
- Is intercourse painful every time that it is attempted?
- Is it painful for your partner as well?
- At what point during (or after) intercourse does the pain begin? Upon entry/penetration? During ejaculation?
- Where, specifically, is the pain?
- Does anything make the pain better?
- Do you have any other symptoms?
- What are your attitudes towards sex in general?
- Have you had a significant traumatic event in the past (rape, child abuse, or similar)?
- What medications do you take?
- What illnesses, diseases, and disorders are you being treated for?
- Have you had a significant emotional event recently?
- Have you ever had pain-free sex with this partner? With any partner?

It may be best to see the doctor together with your partner. Physical examination may include a pelvic examination (for women), a prostate examination (for men), and a rectal examination. If a physical problem is suspected, appropriate tests will be ordered.

Antibiotics, painkillers, or hormones are amongst the treatment options that may be considered.

Prevention

- Good hygiene and routine medical care will help to some degree.
- Adequate foreplay and stimulation will help to ensure proper lubrication of the vagina.
- The use of a water-soluble lubricant like K-Y Jelly may also help. Vaseline should not be used as a sexual lubricant because it is not compatible with latex condoms (it causes them to break), it is not water soluble, and it may encourage vaginal infections.
- Practicing safe sex can help prevent sexually transmitted diseases.

References

National Institutes of Health. National Institutes of Health State-of-the-Science Conference statement: management of menopause-related symptoms. *Ann Intern Med*. 2005;142(12 Pt 1):1003–13.

Klein MC, Kaczorowski J, Firoz T, Hubinette M, Jorgensen S, Gauthier R. A comparison of urinary and sexual outcomes in women experiencing vaginal and Caesarean births. *J Obstet Gynaecol Can*. 2005; 27(4): 332–39.

Mahutte NG. Medical management of endometriosis-associated pain. *Obstet Gynecol Clin North Am*. 2003; 30(1): 133–50.

Section 23.3

Vaginismus

Vaginismus is an involuntary spasm of the muscles surrounding the vagina. The spasms close the vagina.

Causes

Vaginismus is considered a disorder of sexual dysfunction. It has several possible causes, including past sexual trauma or abuse, psychological factors, or a history of discomfort with sexual intercourse. Sometimes no cause can be found.

Vaginismus is an uncommon condition, occurring in less than 2 percent of women in the United States.

Women with varying degrees of vaginismus often develop anxiety regarding sexual intercourse. The condition causes penetration to be difficult and painful, or even impossible. However, this does not mean the woman cannot become sexually aroused. Many women may have orgasms when the clitoris is stimulated.

Symptoms

- Vaginal penetration during sex is difficult or impossible.
- Vaginal pain is common during sexual intercourse or an attempted pelvic exam.

Exams and Tests

A pelvic exam can confirm the diagnosis of vaginismus. A medical history and complete physical exam is important to rule out other causes of pain with sexual intercourse (dyspareunia).

Treatment

Treatment involves extensive therapy that combines education, counseling, and behavioral exercises. Such exercises include pelvic floor muscle contraction and relaxation (Kegel exercises).

Vaginal dilation exercises are recommended using plastic dilators. This should be done under the direction of a sex therapist or other health care provider. Such therapy should involve the partner, and can gradually include more intimate contact, ultimately resulting in intercourse.

Educational resources should be provided. This includes information about sexual anatomy, physiology, the sexual response cycle, and common myths about sex.

Outlook (Prognosis)

When treated by a specialist in sex therapy, success rates are generally very high.

Possible Complications

Vaginismus may lead to unsatisfying sex activity and tension in intimate relationships.

When to Contact a Medical Professional

If you have pain associated with intercourse or difficulties with successful vaginal penetration, contact your health care provider.

Chapter 24

Birth Control

Chapter Contents

Section 24.1

Birth Control Methods and Effectiveness

Reprinted from "Birth Control Methods," National Women's Health Information Center, July 2005.

What is the best method of birth control (or contraception)?

All women and men should have control over if and when they become parents. Making decisions about birth control, or contraception, is not easy—there are many things to think about. Learning about birth control methods you or your partner can use to prevent pregnancy and talking with your doctor are two good ways to get started.

There is no "best" method of birth control. Each method has its own pros and cons. Some methods work better than others do at preventing pregnancy. Researchers are always working to develop or improve birth control methods.

The birth control method you choose should take into account the following:

- Your overall health
- How often you have sex
- The number of sexual partners you have
- If you want to have children
- How well each method works (or is effective) in preventing pregnancy
- Any potential side effects
- Your comfort level with using the method

Bear in mind that *no* method of birth control prevents pregnancy all of the time. Birth control methods can fail, but you can greatly increase a method's success rate by using it correctly all of the time. The only way to be sure you never get pregnant is to not have sex (abstinence).

What are the different birth control methods that I can use?

There are many methods of birth control that a woman can use. Talk with your doctor or nurse to help you figure out what method is best for you. You can always try one method and if you do not like it, you can try another one.

Keep in mind that most birth control does *not* protect you from human immunodeficiency virus (HIV) or other sexually transmitted diseases (STDs) like gonorrhea, herpes, and chlamydia. Other than not having sex, the best protection against STDs and HIV is the male latex condom. The female condom may give some STD protection.

Don't forget that all of the methods we talk about below work best if used correctly. Be sure you know the correct way to use them. Talk with your doctor or nurse and don't feel embarrassed about talking with her or him again if you forget or don't understand.

Know that learning how to use some birth control methods can take time and practice. Sometimes doctors do not explain how to use a method because they may think you already know how. For example, some people do not know that you can put on a male condom "inside out." Also, not everyone knows that you need to leave a "reservoir" or space at the tip of the condom for the sperm and fluid when a man ejaculates, or has an orgasm.

The more you know about the correct way to use birth control, the more control you will have over deciding if and when you want to become pregnant.

Here is a list of birth control methods with estimates of effectiveness, or how well they work in preventing pregnancy when used correctly, for each method.

Continuous abstinence: This means not having sexual intercourse (vaginal, anal, or oral intercourse) at any time. It is the only sure way to prevent pregnancy and protect against HIV and other STDs. This method is 100 percent effective at preventing pregnancy and STDs.

Periodic abstinence or fertility awareness methods: A woman who has a regular menstrual cycle has about seven or more fertile days or days when she is able to get pregnant each month. Periodic abstinence means you do not have sex on the days that you may be fertile. These fertile days are approximately five days before ovulation, the day of ovulation, and one or more days after ovulation. Fertility awareness means that you can be abstinent or have sex but you use a "barrier" method of birth control to keep sperm from getting to the egg. Barrier methods include condoms, diaphragms, or cervical caps, used together with spermicides, which kill sperm. These methods are 75 to 99 percent effective at preventing pregnancy.

Keep in mind that to practice these methods, you need to learn about your menstrual cycle (or how often you get your period). To learn about your cycle, keep a written record of when you get your period, what it is like (heavy or light blood flow), and how you feel (sore breasts, cramps). You also check your cervical mucus and take your basal body temperature daily, and record these in a chart. This is how you learn to predict, or tell, which days you are fertile or "unsafe." You can ask your doctor or nurse for more information on how to record and understand this information.

The male condom: Condoms are called barrier methods of birth control because they put up a block, or barrier, which keeps the sperm from reaching the egg. Only latex or polyurethane (because some people are allergic to latex) condoms are proven to help protect against STDs, including HIV. "Natural" or "lambskin" condoms made from animal products also are available, but lambskin condoms are not recommended for STD prevention because they have tiny pores that may allow for the passage of viruses like HIV, hepatitis B and herpes. Male condoms are 84 to 98 percent effective at preventing pregnancy. Condoms can only be used once. You can buy them at a drugstore. Condoms come lubricated (which can make sexual intercourse more comfortable and pleasurable) and non-lubricated (which can also be used for oral sex). It is best to use lubrication with non-lubricated condoms if you use them for vaginal or anal sex. You can use KY jelly or water-based lubricants, which you can buy at a drugstore. Oil-based lubricants like massage oils, baby oil, lotions, or petroleum jelly will weaken the condom, causing it to tear or break. Always keep condoms in a cool, dry place. If you keep them in a hot place (like a billfold, wallet, or glove compartment), the latex breaks down, causing the condom to tear or break. Latex or polyurethane condoms are the only method other than abstinence that can help protect against HIV and other sexually transmitted diseases (lambskin condoms do not).

Oral contraceptives: Also called "the pill," these contain the hormones estrogen and progestin and are available in different hormone dosages. A pill is taken daily to block the release of eggs from the ovaries. Oral contraceptives lighten the flow of your period and can reduce the risk of pelvic inflammatory disease (PID), ovarian cancer, benign ovarian cysts, endometrial cancer, and iron deficiency anemia. They do not protect against STDs or HIV. The pill may add to your risk of heart disease, including high blood pressure, blood clots, and blockage of the arteries, especially if you smoke. If you are over age thirty-five and smoke, or have a history of blood clots or breast, liver, or endometrial cancer, your doctor may advise you not to take the pill. The pill is 95 to 99.9 percent effective at preventing pregnancy. Some antibiotics may reduce the effectiveness of the pill in some women. Talk to your doctor or nurse about a backup method of birth control if she or he prescribes antibiotics.

Most oral contraceptives are swallowed in a pill form. One brand, called Ovcon 35®, can either be swallowed or chewed. If it is chewed, you must drink a full glass of liquid immediately after to make sure you get the full dose of medication. There are also extended cycle pills, brand name Seasonale®, which have twelve weeks of pills that contain hormones (active) and one week of pills that don't contain hormones (inactive). While taking Seasonale, women only have their period four times a year, when they are taking the inactive pills. There are many different types of oral contraceptives available, and it is important to talk to your doctor or nurse about which one is best for you. You will need a prescription for oral contraceptives.

The mini-pill: Unlike the pill, the mini-pill only has one hormone, progestin, instead of both estrogen and progestin. Taken daily, the mini-pill thickens cervical mucus to prevent sperm from reaching the egg. It also prevents a fertilized egg from implanting in the uterus (womb). The mini-pill also can decrease the flow of your period and protect against PID and ovarian and endometrial cancer. Mothers who breastfeed can use it because it will not affect their milk supply. The mini-pill is a good option for women who can't take estrogen, are over thirty-five, or have a risk of blood clots. The mini-pill does not protect against STDs or HIV. Mini-pills are 92 to 99.9 percent effective at preventing pregnancy if used correctly. The mini-pill needs to be taken at the same time each day. A backup method of birth control is needed if you take the pill more than three hours late. Some antibiotics may reduce the effectiveness of the pill in some women. Talk to your doctor or nurse about a backup method of birth control if she or he prescribes antibiotics. You will need to visit you doctor for a prescription and to make sure you are not having problems.

Copper T IUD (intrauterine device): An IUD is a small device that is shaped in the form of a "T." Your health care provider places it inside the uterus. The arms of the Copper T IUD contain some copper, which stops fertilization by preventing sperm from making their way up through the uterus into the fallopian tubes. If fertilization does occur, the IUD would prevent the fertilized egg from implanting in the lining of the uterus. The Copper T IUD can stay in your uterus for up to twelve years. It does not protect against STDs or HIV. This IUD is 99 percent effective at preventing pregnancy. You will need to visit your doctor to have it inserted and to make sure you are not having any problems. Not all doctors insert IUDs so check first before making your appointment.

Progestasert® IUD (intrauterine device): This IUD is a small plastic T- shaped device that is placed inside the uterus by a doctor. It contains the hormone progesterone, the same hormone produced by a woman's ovaries during the monthly menstrual cycle. The progesterone causes the cervical mucus to thicken so sperm cannot reach the egg, and it changes the lining of the uterus so that a fertilized egg cannot successfully implant. The Progestasert IUD can stay in your uterus for one year. This IUD is 98 percent effective at preventing pregnancy. You will need to visit your doctor to have it inserted and to make sure you are not having any problems. Not all doctors insert IUDs so check first before making your appointment.

Intrauterine system or IUS (Mirena): The IUS is a small T-shaped device like the IUD and is placed inside the uterus by a doctor. Each day, it releases a small amount of a hormone similar to progesterone called levonorgestrel that causes the cervical mucus to thicken so sperm cannot reach the egg. The IUS stays in your uterus for up to five years. It does not protect against STDs or HIV. The IUS is 99 percent effective. The Food and Drug Administration approved this method in December 2000. You will need to visit your doctor to have it inserted and to make sure you are not having any problems. Not all doctors insert the IUS so check first before making your appointment.

The female condom: Worn by the woman, this barrier method keeps sperm from getting into her body. It is made of polyurethane, is packaged with a lubricant, and may protect against STDs, including HIV. It can be inserted up to twenty-four hours prior to sexual intercourse. Female condoms are 79 to 95 percent effective at preventing pregnancy. There is only one kind of female condom, called Reality, and it can be purchased at a drugstore.

Depo-Provera: With this method women get injections, or shots, of the hormone progestin in the buttocks or arm every three months. It does not protect against STDs or HIV. Women should not use Depo-Provera for more than two years in a row because it can cause a temporary loss of bone density that increases the longer this method is used. The bone does start to grow after this method is stopped, but it may increase the risk of fracture and osteoporosis if used for a long time. It is 97 percent effective at preventing pregnancy. You will need to visit your doctor for the shots and to make sure you are not having any problems.

Diaphragm, cervical cap, or shield: These are barrier methods of birth control, where the sperm are blocked from entering the cervix and reaching the egg. The diaphragm is shaped like a shallow latex cup. The cervical cap is a thimble-shaped latex cup. The cervical shield is a silicone cup that has a one-way valve that creates suction and helps it fit against the cervix. The diaphragm and cervical cap come in different sizes and you need a doctor to "fit" you for one. The cervical shield comes in one size and you will not need a fitting. Before sexual intercourse, you use them with spermicide (to block or kill sperm) and place them up inside your vagina to cover your cervix (the opening to your womb). You can buy spermicide gel or foam at a drugstore. Some women can be sensitive to an ingredient called nonoxynol-9 and need to use spermicides that do not contain it. The diaphragm is 84 to 94 percent effective at preventing pregnancy. The cervical cap is 84 to 91 percent effective at preventing pregnancy for women who have not had a child and 68 to 74 percent effective for women who have had a child. The cervical shield is 85 percent effective at preventing pregnancy. Barrier methods must be left in place for six to eight hours after intercourse to prevent pregnancy and removed by twenty-four hours after intercourse for the diaphragm and forty-eight for the cap and shield. You will need to visit your doctor for a proper fitting for the diaphragm or cervical cap and a prescription for the cervical shield.

Contraceptive sponge: This is a barrier method of birth control that was re-approved by the Food and Drug Administration in 2005. It is a soft, disk shaped device, with a loop for removal. It is made out of polyurethane foam and contains the spermicide nonoxynol-9. Before intercourse, you wet the sponge and place it, loop side down, up inside your vagina to cover the cervix. The sponge is 84 to 91 percent effective at preventing pregnancy in women who have not had a child and 68 to 80 percent effective for women who have had a child. The sponge is effective for more than one act of intercourse for up twenty-four hours. It needs to be left in for at least six hours after intercourse to prevent pregnancy and must be removed within thirty hours after it is inserted. There is a risk of getting toxic shock syndrome or TSS if the sponge is left in for more than thirty hours. The sponge does not protect against STDs or HIV. There is only one kind of contraceptive sponge for sale in the United States, called the Today Sponge, and it can be purchased at a drugstore. Women who are sensitive to the spermicide nonoxynol-9 should not use this birth control method.

The patch (Ortho Evra®): This is a skin patch worn on the lower abdomen, buttocks, or upper body. It releases the hormones progestin and estrogen into the bloodstream. You put on a new patch once a week for three weeks, and then do not wear a patch during the fourth week in order to have a menstrual period. The patch is 98 to 99 percent effective at preventing pregnancy, but appears to be less effective in women who weigh more than 198 pounds. It does not protect against STDs or HIV. You will need to visit your doctor for a prescription and to make sure you are not having problems.

The hormonal vaginal contraceptive ring (NuvaRing®): The NuvaRing is a ring that releases the hormones progestin and estrogen. You squeeze the ring between your thumb and index finger and insert it into your vagina. You wear the ring for three weeks, take it out for the week that you have your period, and then put in a new ring. The ring is 98 to 99 percent effective at preventing pregnancy. You will need to visit your doctor for a prescription and to make sure you are not having problems. This birth control method is not recommended while breastfeeding because the hormone estrogen may decrease breast milk production.

Surgical sterilization (tubal ligation or vasectomy): These surgical methods are meant for people who want a permanent method of birth control. In other words, they never want to have a child or they do not want more children. Tubal ligation or "tying tubes" is done on the woman to stop eggs from going down to her uterus where they can be fertilized. The man has a vasectomy to keep sperm from going to his penis, so his ejaculate never has any sperm in it. They are 99.9 percent effective at preventing pregnancy.

Nonsurgical sterilization (Essure® permanent birth control system): This is the first nonsurgical method of sterilizing women. A thin tube is used to thread a tiny spring-like device through the vagina and uterus into each fallopian tube. Flexible coils temporarily anchor it inside the fallopian tube. A Dacron-like mesh material embedded in the coils irritates the fallopian tubes' lining to cause scar tissue to grow and eventually permanently plug the tubes. It can take about three months for the scar tissue to grow, so it is important to use another form of birth control during this time. Then you will have to return to your doctor for a test to see if scar tissue has fully blocked your tubes. After three years of follow-up studies, Essure has been shown to be 99.8 percent effective in preventing pregnancy.

Emergency contraception: This is *not* a regular method of birth control and should never be used as one. Emergency contraception, or emergency birth control, is used to keep a woman from getting pregnant when she has had unprotected vaginal intercourse. "Unprotected" can mean that no method of birth control was used. It can also mean that a birth control method was used but did not work—like a condom breaking. Or, a woman may have forgotten to take her birth control pills, or may have been abused or forced to have sex when she did not want to. Emergency contraception consists of taking two doses of hormonal pills taken twelve hours apart and started within three days after having unprotected sex. These are sometimes wrongly called the "morning after pill." The pills are 75 to 89 percent effective at preventing pregnancy. Another type of emergency contraception is having the Copper T IUD put into your uterus within seven days of unprotected sex. This method is 99.9 percent effective at preventing pregnancy. Neither method of emergency contraception protects against STDs or HIV. You will need to visit your doctor for either a prescription for the pills or for the insertion of the IUD, and to make sure you are not having problems.

Are there any foams or gels that I can use to keep from getting pregnant?

You can purchase what are called spermicides in drugstores. They work by killing sperm and come in several forms—foam, gel, cream, film, suppository, or tablet. They are inserted or placed in the vagina no more than one hour before intercourse. If you use a film, suppository, or tablet wait at least fifteen minutes before having intercourse so the spermicide can dissolve. Do not douche or rinse out your vagina for at least six to eight hours after intercourse. You will need to use more spermicide before each act of intercourse. You may protect yourself more against getting pregnant if you use a spermicide with a male condom, diaphragm, or cervical cap. There are spermicidal products made specifically for use with the diaphragm and cervical cap. Check the package to make sure you are buying what you want.

All spermicides have sperm-killing chemicals in them. Some spermicides also have an ingredient called nonoxynol-9 that may increase the risk of HIV infection when used frequently because it irritates the tissue in the vagina and anus, which can cause the virus to enter the body more freely. Some women are sensitive to nonoxynol-9 and need to use spermicides without it. Spermicides alone are about 74 percent effective at preventing pregnancy. Medications for vaginal yeast infections may decrease effectiveness of spermicides.

How effective is withdrawal as a birth control method?

Withdrawal is not the most effective birth control method. It works much better when a male condom is used.

Withdrawal is when a man takes his penis out of a woman's vagina (or "pulls out") before he ejaculates, or has an orgasm. This stops the sperm from going to the egg. "Pulling out" can be hard for a man to do and it takes a lot of self-control. When you use withdrawal, you can also be at risk getting pregnant *before* the man pulls out. When a man's penis first becomes erect, there can be fluid called pre-ejaculate fluid on the tip of the penis that has sperm in it. This sperm can get a woman pregnant. Withdrawal also does not protect you from STDs or HIV.

Everyone I know is on the pill. Is it safe?

Today's pills have lower doses of hormones than earlier birth control pills. This has greatly lowered the risk of side effects; however, there are both benefits and risks with taking birth control pills. Benefits include having more regular and lighter periods, fewer menstrual cramps; and a lower risk for ovarian and endometrial cancer and pelvic inflammatory disease (PID). Serious side effects include an increased chance, for some women, of developing heart disease, high blood pressure, and blood clots. Minor side effects include nausea, headaches, sore breasts, weight gain, irregular bleeding, and depression. Many of these side effects go away after taking the pill for a few months. Women who smoke, are over age thirty-five, or have a history of blood clots or breast or endometrial cancer are more at risk for dangerous side effects and may not be able to take the pill. Talk with your doctor or nurse about whether the pill is right for you.

Will birth control pills protect me from HIV, the virus that causes acquired immunodeficiency syndrome (AIDS), and other STDs?

Some people wrongly believe that if they take birth control pills, they are protecting themselves not only from getting pregnant but also from infection with HIV and other sexually transmitted diseases (STDs). Birth control pills or other types of birth control, such as intrauterine devices (IUDs), Depo-Provera, or tubal ligation, will *not* protect you from HIV and other STDs.

The male latex condom is the only birth control method that is proven to help protect you from HIV and other STDs. If you are allergic to latex, there are condoms made of polyurethane that you can use. Condoms come lubricated (which can make sexual intercourse more comfortable and pleasurable) and nonlubricated (which can be used for oral sex).

It is important to only use latex or polyurethane condoms to protect against HIV and other STDs. “Natural” or “lambskin” condoms have tiny pores that may allow for the passage of viruses like HIV, hepatitis B, and herpes. If you use nonlubricated condoms for vaginal or anal sex, you can add lubrication with water-based lubricants (like KY jelly) that you can buy at a drugstore. Never use oil-based products, such as massage oils, baby oil, lotions, or petroleum jelly, to lubricate a condom. These will weaken the condom, causing it to tear or break.

It is very important to use a condom correctly and consistently—which means every time you have vaginal, oral, or anal sex. If you do not know how to use a condom, talk with your doctor or nurse. Don’t be embarrassed. Also, do not assume that your partner knows how to use a condom correctly. Many men have never had anyone show them how. The biggest reason condoms fail is due to incorrect use. Male condoms can only be used once. Research is being done to find out how effective the female condom is in preventing HIV and other STDs.

I’ve heard my girlfriends talking about dental dams and I thought they were something only dentists used during oral surgery—what are they?

The dental dam is a square piece of rubber that is used by dentists during oral surgery and other procedures. It is not a method of birth control. But it can be used to help protect people from STDs, including HIV, during oral and anal sex. It is placed over the opening to the vagina before having oral sex. Dental dams can be purchased at surgical supply stores.

Section 24.2

Emergency Contraception

Reprinted from "Emergency Contraception," National Women's Health Information Center, May 2006.

What is emergency contraception (or emergency birth control)?

Emergency contraception, or emergency birth control, is used to help keep a woman from getting pregnant after she has had unprotected sex (sex without using birth control).

Use emergency contraception if:

- you didn't use birth control;
- you were forced to have sex;
- the condom broke or came off;
- he didn't pull out in time;
- you missed two or more birth control pills in a row;
- you were late getting your shot.

Emergency contraception should not be used as regular birth control. Other birth control methods are much better at keeping women from becoming pregnant. Talk with your doctor to decide which one is right for you.

How does emergency contraception work?

Emergency contraception can keep you from becoming pregnant by:

- keeping the egg from leaving the ovary; or

- keeping the sperm from meeting the egg; or
- keeping the fertilized egg from attaching to the uterus (womb).

If you are already pregnant, emergency contraception will *not* work.

What are the types of emergency contraception?

There are two types:

- emergency contraceptive pills (ECPs)
- intrauterine devices (IUDs)

ECPs contain higher doses of the same hormones in some brands of regular birth control pills. Some ECPs are "combined ECPs" with progestin and estrogen. Others are progestin-only. If you are breast-feeding or if you can't take estrogen, you should use progestin-only ECPs. You should always take ECPs as soon as you can after having sex, but they can work up to five days later. There are two types of ECPs:

- **Plan B (progestin-only):** Made for use as emergency contraception. The two pills can be taken in two doses (one pill right away, and the next pill twelve hours later), or both pills can be taken at the same time. Some women feel sick and throw up after taking ECPs. Taking both pills at the same time will not increase your chances of having these side effects. If you throw up after taking ECPs, call your doctor or pharmacist.
- **Higher dose of regular birth control pills:** The number of pills in a dose is different for each pill brand, and not all brands can be used for emergency contraception. The pills are taken in two doses (one dose right away, and the next dose twelve hours later). Always use the same brand for both doses. Some women feel sick and throw up after taking ECPs. If you throw up after taking ECPs, call your doctor or pharmacist.

The other type of emergency contraception is the IUD. The IUD is a T-shaped, plastic device placed into the uterus (womb) by a doctor within five days after having sex.

The IUD works by:

- keeping the sperm from meeting the egg; or

- keeping the egg from attaching to the uterus (womb).

Your doctor can remove the IUD after your next period. Or, it can be left in place for up to ten years to use as your regular birth control.

Are emergency contraceptive pills (ECPs) the same thing as the "morning after pill"?

Yes. ECPs are often called the "morning after pill," which is wrong because ECPs are never taken as only one pill and they don't have to be taken the morning after. You should always take ECPs as soon as you can after having unprotected sex (sex without using birth control), but they can work up to five days later.

How do I get emergency contraceptive pills (ECPs)?

Plan B (progestin-only) was recently approved to be sold over-the-counter to women who are eighteen years of age or older. Women under the age of eighteen will need a prescription. Women will have to show proof of age to buy Plan B. Plan B will be sold at pharmacies or stores that have a licensed pharmacist on staff.

Can I get emergency contraceptive pills (ECPs) before I need them?

Yes. Your doctor should bring up ECPs at your annual exam (when you have a pap smear or pap test). If your doctor does not talk about emergency contraception at your next exam, ask for it.

Will ECPs protect me from sexually transmitted diseases (STDs)?

No. ECPs can only keep you from becoming pregnant. Always use condoms to lower your risk of getting a sexually transmitted disease.

What do I need to do after I take emergency contraceptive pills (ECPs)?

Take the ECPs exactly as your doctor or pharmacist tells you to. If you see another doctor or nurse for any reason after taking ECPs, tell him/her that you have taken ECPs.

Some women feel sick and throw up after taking ECPs. This side effect happens more often with pills that contain both estrogen and progestin. Your doctor or pharmacist can give you medication to help control sickness. If you throw up after taking ECPs, call your doctor or pharmacist. After you have taken ECPs, your next period may come sooner or later than normal. Your period also may be heavier, lighter, or more spotty than normal. Use another birth control method if you have sex any time before your next period starts.

If you do not get your period in three weeks or if you think you might be pregnant after taking ECPs, consider getting a pregnancy test just to make sure you're not pregnant.

Does emergency contraception work all the time?

No. Emergency contraceptive pills (ECPs) that contain both estrogen and progestin are about 75 percent effective at keeping a woman from getting pregnant. In other words, if one hundred women had unprotected sex (sex without using birth control) in the fertile part of their cycle (when an egg is most likely to leave the ovary), about eight of those women would become pregnant. If all one hundred women took combined emergency contraceptive pills, only two would become pregnant. ECPs containing only progestin are about 89 percent effective. If those same one hundred women took progestin-only ECPs, only one would become pregnant. The IUD is 99.9 percent effective. If one thousand women had an IUD put in, only one would become pregnant.

The sooner you take emergency contraception after sex, the better your chances it will work.

My girlfriend took emergency contraceptive pills (ECPs) and they did not work. If she stays pregnant, will there be something wrong with her baby?

No. Studies have been done with women who did not know they were pregnant and kept taking birth control pills. These studies have found no greater risk for birth defects. Your girlfriend should see a doctor right away to talk about her options.

Is emergency contraception the same thing as the "abortion pill?"

No. Emergency contraception can keep a woman from becoming pregnant. It works one of three ways:

- By keeping the egg from leaving the ovary

- By keeping the sperm from meeting the egg
- By keeping the fertilized egg from attaching to the uterus (womb)

The abortion pill (Mifeprex®, also called RU-486) works after a woman becomes pregnant (after a fertilized egg has attached to the uterus). The abortion pill makes the uterus force out the egg, ending the pregnancy.

Chapter 25

Abortion

Chapter Contents

Section 25.1

Medical Abortion Procedures

"Medical Abortion Procedures," © 2004 American Pregnancy Association www.americanpregnancy.org), 866-942-6466. Reprinted with permission.

Medical abortion procedures are available to terminate a pregnancy during the early weeks of the first trimester. Before seeking a medical abortion procedure, it is recommended that you obtain a sonogram to determine if the pregnancy is viable (uterine, non-ectopic pregnancy) and for accurate pregnancy dating or gestation.

MTX: Methotrexate and Misoprostol

MTX is a medical abortion procedure used up to the first seven weeks of pregnancy.

Methotrexate is given orally or by injection during the first office visit. Misoprostol tablets are given orally or inserted vaginally during the second office visit, which occurs five to seven days later. You will return home, where the misoprostol will start contractions and expel the fetus. This may occur within a few hours or up to a few days. A physical exam is given seven days later to ensure that the abortion procedure is complete and that no complications are apparent. Methotrexate is primarily used in the treatment of cancer and rheumatoid arthritis because it attacks the most rapidly growing cells in the body. In the case of an abortion, it causes the fetus and placenta to separate from the lining of the uterus. The use of this drug for this purpose is not approved by the U.S. Food and Drug Administration.

The side effects and risks of methotrexate and misoprostol include the following:

- The procedure is unsuccessful approximately 10 percent of the time, thus requiring an additional surgical abortion procedure to complete the termination.
- Cramping, nausea, diarrhea, heavy bleeding, fever.

- Not advised for women who have anemia, bleeding disorders, liver or kidney disease, seizure disorder, acute inflammatory bowel disease, or use an intrauterine device (IUD).

RU-486: Mifepristone (Mifeprex®) and Misoprostol

Mifepristone (Mifeprex®) and misoprostol is a medical abortion procedure used up to the first seven to nine weeks of pregnancy. It is also referred to as RU-486 or the abortion pill.

A physical exam is given to determine if you are eligible for this medical abortion procedure. You are not eligible if you have any of the following: ectopic pregnancy, ovarian mass, IUD, corticosteroid use, adrenal failure, anemia, bleeding disorders or use of blood thinners, asthma, liver or kidney problems, heart disease, or high blood pressure.

Mifepristone is given orally during your first office visit. Mifepristone blocks progesterone from the uterine lining, causing the fetus to die. This alone may cause contractions to expel the fetus. Misoprostol tablets are given orally or inserted vaginally during the second office visit, which occurs thirty-six to forty-eight hours later. You will return home, where the misoprostol will start contractions and expel the fetus. This may occur within a few hours or in some cases up to two weeks after taking the misoprostol. A physical exam is given two weeks later to ensure the abortion was complete and that there are no immediate complications.

The side effects and risks of mifepristone and misoprostol include the following:

- The procedure is unsuccessful approximately 8 to 10 percent of the time, thus requiring an additional surgical abortion procedure to complete the termination.
- Cramping, nausea, vomiting, diarrhea, heavy bleeding, infection
- Not advised for women who have anemia, bleeding disorders, liver or kidney disease, seizure disorder, acute inflammatory bowel disease, or use an intrauterine device (IUD).

References

"Induced Abortion." The American College of Obstetricians and Gynecologists. 2001.

Pymar HC, Creinin MD (2000). Alternatives to mifepristone regimens for medical abortion. *American Journal of Obstetrics and Gynecology*, 183 (2): s54–s64.

Paul M, et al. (1999). *A Clinician's Guide to Medical and Surgical Abortion*. New York: Churchill Livingstone.

Creinin MD, et al. (2001). Medical management of abortion. *American Journal of Obstetrics and Gynecology Practice Bulletin*, no. 26, pg. 1–13.

Goldberg AB, et al. (2001). Misoprostol and pregnancy. *New England Journal of Medicine,* 344 (1): 3845.

Spitz IM, et al. (1998). Early pregnancy termination with mifepristone and misoprostol in the U.S. *New England Journal of Medicine*, 338 (18): 1241–47.

Section 25.2

Surgical Abortion Procedures

The type of surgical abortion procedure used is based on which stage of pregnancy a women is at. Before seeking a surgical abortion procedure, it is recommended that you obtain a sonogram to determine if the pregnancy is viable (uterine, non-ectopic pregnancy) and for accurate pregnancy dating or gestation.

Suction Aspiration

How is suction aspiration performed?

Suction aspiration is a surgical abortion procedure performed during the first six to twelve weeks gestation. It is also referred to as suction curettage or vacuum aspiration.

Your abortion provider may give you pain medication and misoprostol in preparation of the procedure. You will lie on your back with your feet in stirrups and a speculum is inserted to open the vagina. A local anesthetic is administered to your cervix. Then a tenaculum is used to hold the cervix in place for the cervix to be dilated by cone-shaped rods. When the cervix is wide enough, a cannula, which is a long plastic tube connected to a suction device, is inserted into the uterus to suction out the fetus and placenta. The procedure usually lasts ten to fifteen minutes, but recovery may require staying at the clinic for a few hours.

What are the side effects and risks of suction aspiration?

Common side effects that most women will experience following the procedure include cramping, nausea, sweating, and feeling faint.

Less frequent side effects include possible heavy or prolonged bleeding, blood clots, damage to the cervix, and perforation of the uterus. Infection due to retained products of conception or infection caused by an STD or bacteria being introduced to the uterus can cause fever, pain, abdominal tenderness, and possibly scar tissue.

Contact your healthcare provider immediately if your side effects persist or worsen.

Dilation and Curettage (D&C)

How is dilation and curettage performed?

Dilation and curettage is a surgical abortion procedure performed during the first twelve to fifteen weeks gestation. Dilation and curettage is similar to suction aspiration with the introduction of a curette. A curette is a long, looped shaped knife that scrapes the lining, placenta, and fetus away from the uterus. A cannula may be inserted for a final suctioning. This procedure usually lasts ten minutes with a possible stay of five hours.

What are the side effects and risks of dilation and curettage?

The side effects of dilation and curettage are the same as suction aspiration noted above with the exception that there is a slight increased chance for perforation of the uterus.

Contact your healthcare provider immediately if your symptoms persist or worsen.

Dilation and Evacuation (D&E)

How is dilation and evacuation performed?

Dilation and evacuation is a surgical abortion procedure performed between fifteen to twenty-one weeks gestation. In most cases, twenty-four hours prior to the actual procedure, your abortion provider will insert laminaria or a synthetic dilator inside your cervix. When the procedure begins the next day, your abortion provider will clamp a tenaculum to the cervix to keep the uterus in place and cone-shaped rods of increasing size are used to continue the dilation process.

The cannula is inserted to begin removing tissue away from the lining. Then using a curette, the lining is scraped to remove any residuals. If needed, forceps may be used to remove larger parts. The last step is usually a final suctioning to make sure the contents are completely removed.

The procedure normally takes about thirty minutes. Although some clinics may perform the procedure, it is usually performed in a hospital setting because of the greater risk for complications. The fetal remains are usually examined to ensure everything was removed and that the abortion was complete.

What are the side effects and risks of dilation and evacuation?

The common side effects for most women include nausea, bleeding. and cramping. which may occur for two weeks following the procedure. Although rare, the following are additional risks related to dilation and evacuation: damage to uterine lining or cervix, perforation of the uterus, infection, and blood clots.

Contact your healthcare provider immediately if your symptoms persist or worsen.

Induction Abortion

How is induction abortion performed?

Induction abortion is a procedure that uses saltwater, urea, or potassium chloride to terminate the viability of the pregnancy. Your abortion provider will insert prostaglandins into the vagina and Pitocin will be given intravenously. Laminaria is then usually inserted into your cervix to begin dilation. This procedure is rarely used, and normally only occurs when there is a medical problem or illness in the fetus or woman.

What are the side effects of induction abortion?

The side effects are similar to dilation and evacuation, although in rare cases it is possible for the mother's blood stream to be accidentally injected with saline or other medications. Excessive bleeding and cramping may also be experienced.

Contact your healthcare provider immediately if your symptoms persist or worsen.

Dilation and Extraction

How is dilation and extraction performed?

The dilation and extraction procedure is used after twenty-one weeks gestation. The procedure is also known as D & X, intact D & X, intrauterine cranial decompression, and partial birth abortion. Two days before the procedure, laminaria is inserted vaginally to dilate the cervix. Your water should break on the third day and you should return to the clinic. The fetus is rotated and forceps are used to grasp and pull the legs, shoulders, and arms through the birth canal. A small incision is made at the base of the skull to allow a suction catheter inside. The catheter removes the cerebral material until the skull collapses. Then the fetus is completely removed.

What are the side effects and risks related to dilation and extraction?

The side effects are the same as dilation and evacuation. However, there is an increased chance for additional emotional problems because of further fetal development.

Contact your healthcare provider immediately if your symptoms persist or worsen.

References

"Induced Abortion." The American College of Obstetricians and Gynecologists. 2001.

Paul M, et al. (1999). *A Clinician's Guide to Medical and Surgical Abortion*. New York: Churchill Livingstone.

Creinin MD, et al. (2001). Medical management of abortion. *American Journal of Obstetrics and Gynecology Practice Bulletin*, no. 26, pg. 1–13.

Chapter 26

Infertility

What is infertility?

Most experts define infertility as not being able to get pregnant after at least one year of trying. Women who are able to get pregnant but then have repeat miscarriages are also said to be infertile.

Pregnancy is the result of a complex chain of events. In order to get pregnant the following things must occur:

- A woman must release an egg from one of her ovaries (ovulation).
- The egg must go through a fallopian tube toward the uterus (womb).
- A man's sperm must join with (fertilize) the egg along the way.
- The fertilized egg must attach to the inside of the uterus (implantation).

Infertility can result from problems that interfere with any of these steps.

Is infertility a common problem?

About 12 percent of women (7.3 million) in the United States aged fifteen to forty-four had difficulty getting pregnant or carrying a baby

---

Reprinted from "Infertility," National Women's Health Information Center, May 2006.

to term in 2002, according to the National Center for Health Statistics of the Centers for Disease Control and Prevention.

Is infertility just a woman's problem?

No, infertility is not always a woman's problem. In only about one-third of cases is infertility due to the woman (female factors). In another one-third of cases, infertility is due to the man (male factors). The remaining cases are caused by a mixture of male and female factors or by unknown factors.

What causes infertility in men?

Infertility in men is most often caused by the following:

- **Problems making sperm:** Producing too few sperm or none at all
- **Problems with the sperm's ability to reach the egg and fertilize it:** Abnormal sperm shape or structure prevent it from moving correctly

Sometimes a man is born with the problems that affect his sperm. Other times problems start later in life due to illness or injury. For example, cystic fibrosis often causes infertility in men.

What increases a man's risk of infertility?

The number and quality of a man's sperm can be affected by his overall health and lifestyle. Some things that may reduce sperm number and/or quality include the following:

- Alcohol
- Drugs
- Environmental toxins, including pesticides and lead
- Smoking cigarettes
- Health problems
- Medicines
- Radiation treatment and chemotherapy for cancer
- Age

What causes infertility in women?

Problems with ovulation account for most cases of infertility in women. Without ovulation, there are no eggs to be fertilized. Some signs that a woman is not ovulating normally include irregular or absent menstrual periods.

Less common causes of fertility problems in women include the following:

- Blocked fallopian tubes due to pelvic inflammatory disease, endometriosis, or surgery for an ectopic pregnancy
- Physical problems with the uterus
- Uterine fibroids

What things increase a woman's risk of infertility?

Many things can affect a woman's ability to have a baby. These include the following:

- Age
- Stress
- Poor diet
- Athletic training
- Being overweight or underweight
- Tobacco smoking
- Alcohol
- Sexually transmitted diseases (STDs)
- Health problems that cause hormonal changes

How does age affect a woman's ability to have children?

More and more women are waiting until their thirties and forties to have children. Actually, about 20 percent of women in the United States now have their first child after age thirty-five. So age is an increasingly common cause of fertility problems. About one-third of couples in which the woman is over thirty-five have fertility problems.

Aging decreases a woman's chances of having a baby in the following ways:

- The ability of a woman's ovaries to release eggs ready for fertilization declines with age.
- The health of a woman's eggs declines with age.
- As a woman ages she is more likely to have health problems that can interfere with fertility.
- As a women ages, her risk of having a miscarriage increases.

How long should women try to get pregnant before calling their doctors?

Most healthy women under the age of thirty shouldn't worry about infertility unless they've been trying to get pregnant for at least a year. At this point, women should talk to their doctors about a fertility evaluation. Men should also talk to their doctors if this much time has passed.

In some cases, women should talk to their doctors sooner. Women in their thirties who've been trying to get pregnant for six months should speak to their doctors as soon as possible. A woman's chances of having a baby decrease rapidly every year after the age of thirty. So getting a complete and timely fertility evaluation is especially important.

Some health issues also increase the risk of fertility problems. So women with the following issues should speak to their doctors as soon as possible:

- Irregular periods or no menstrual periods
- Very painful periods
- Endometriosis
- Pelvic inflammatory disease
- More than one miscarriage

No matter how old you are, it's always a good idea to talk to a doctor before you start trying to get pregnant. Doctors can help you prepare your body for a healthy baby. They can also answer questions on fertility and give tips on conceiving.

How will doctors find out if a woman and her partner have fertility problems?

Sometimes doctors can find the cause of a couple's infertility by doing a complete fertility evaluation. This process usually begins with physical exams and health and sexual histories. If there are no obvious problems, like poorly timed intercourse or absence of ovulation, tests will be needed.

Finding the cause of infertility is often a long, complex, and emotional process. It can take months for you and your doctor to complete all the needed exams and tests. So don't be alarmed if the problem is not found right away.

For a man, doctors usually begin by testing his semen. They look at the number, shape, and movement of the sperm. Sometimes doctors also suggest testing the level of a man's hormones.

For a woman, the first step in testing is to find out if she is ovulating each month. There are several ways to do this. A woman can track her ovulation at home by the following methods:

- Recording changes in her morning body temperature (basal body temperature) for several months
- Recording the texture of her cervical mucus for several months
- Using a home ovulation test kit (available at drug or grocery stores)

Doctors can also check if a woman is ovulating by doing blood tests and an ultrasound of the ovaries. If the woman is ovulating normally, more tests are needed.

Some common tests of fertility in women include the following:

- **Hysterosalpingography:** In this test, doctors use x-rays to check for physical problems of the uterus and fallopian tubes. They start by injecting a special dye through the vagina into the uterus. This dye shows up on the x-ray. This allows the doctor to see if the dye moves normally through the uterus into the fallopian tubes. With these x-rays doctors can find blockages that may be causing infertility. Blockages can prevent the egg from moving from the fallopian tube to the uterus. Blockages can also keep the sperm from reaching the egg.
- **Laparoscopy:** During this surgery doctors use a tool called a laparoscope to see inside the abdomen. The doctor makes a small cut in the lower abdomen and inserts the laparoscope. Using the laparoscope, doctors check the ovaries, fallopian tubes, and uterus for disease and physical problems. Doctors can usually find scarring and endometriosis by laparoscopy.

How do doctors treat infertility?

Infertility can be treated with medicine, surgery, artificial insemination, or assisted reproductive technology. Many times these treatments are combined. About two-thirds of couples who are treated for infertility are able to have a baby. In most cases infertility is treated with drugs or surgery.

Doctors recommend specific treatments for infertility based on the following:

- Test results
- How long the couple has been trying to get pregnant
- The age of both the man and woman
- The overall health of the partners
- Preference of the partners

Doctors often treat infertility in men in the following ways:

- **Sexual problems:** If the man is impotent or has problems with premature ejaculation, doctors can help him address these issues. Behavioral therapy and/or medicines can be used in these cases.
- **Too few sperm:** If the man produces too few sperm, sometimes surgery can correct this problem. In other cases, doctors can surgically remove sperm from the male reproductive tract. Antibiotics can also be used to clear up infections affecting sperm count.

Various fertility medicines are often used to treat women with ovulation problems. It is important to talk with your doctor about the pros and cons of these medicines. You should understand the risks, benefits, and side effects.

Doctors also use surgery to treat some causes of infertility. Problems with a woman's ovaries, fallopian tubes, or uterus can sometimes be corrected with surgery.

Intrauterine insemination (IUI) is another type of treatment for infertility. IUI is known by most people as artificial insemination. In this procedure, the woman is injected with specially prepared sperm. Sometimes the woman is also treated with medicines that stimulate ovulation before IUI.

IUI is often used to treat the following:

- Mild male factor infertility
- Women who have problems with their cervical mucus
- Couples with unexplained infertility

What medicines are used to treat infertility in women?

Some common medicines used to treat infertility in women include the following:

- **Clomiphene citrate (Clomid®):** This medicine causes ovulation by acting on the pituitary gland. It is often used in women who have polycystic ovarian syndrome (PCOS) or other problems with ovulation. This medicine is taken by mouth.
- **Human menopausal gonadotropin or hMG (Repronex®, Pergonal®):** This medicine is often used for women who don't ovulate due to problems with their pituitary gland. hMG acts directly on the ovaries to stimulate ovulation. It is an injected medicine.
- **Follicle-stimulating hormone or FSH (Gonal-F®, Follistim®):** FSH works much like hMG. It causes the ovaries to begin the process of ovulation. These medicines are usually injected.
- **Gonadotropin-releasing hormone (Gn-RH) analog:** These medicines are often used for women who don't ovulate regularly each month. Women who ovulate before the egg is ready can also use these medicines. Gn-RH analogs act on the pituitary gland to change when the body ovulates. These medicines are usually injected or given with a nasal spray.
- **Metformin (Glucophage®):** Doctors use this medicine for women who have insulin resistance and/or polycystic ovarian syndrome (PCOS). This drug helps lower the high levels of male hormones in women with these conditions. This helps the body to ovulate. Sometimes clomiphene citrate or FSH is combined with metformin. This medicine is usually taken by mouth.
- **Bromocriptine (Parlodel®):** This medicine is used for women with ovulation problems due to high levels of prolactin. Prolactin is a hormone that causes milk production.

Many fertility drugs increase a woman's chance of having twins, triplets, or other multiples. Women who are pregnant with multiple fetuses have more problems during pregnancy. Multiple fetuses have a high risk of being born too early (prematurely). Premature babies are at a higher risk of health and developmental problems.

What is assisted reproductive technology (ART)?

Assisted reproductive technology (ART) is a term that describes several different methods used to help infertile couples. ART involves removing eggs from a woman's body, mixing them with sperm in the laboratory, and putting the embryos back into a woman's body.

How often is assisted reproductive technology (ART) successful?

Success rates vary and depend on many factors. Some things that affect the success rate of ART include the following:

- Age of the partners
- Reason for infertility
- Clinic
- Type of ART
- If the egg is fresh or frozen
- If the embryo is fresh or frozen

The U.S. Centers for Disease Prevention (CDC) collects success rates on ART for some fertility clinics. According to the 2003 CDC report on ART, the average percentage of ART cycles that led to a healthy baby were as follows:

- 37.3 percent in women under the age of thirty-five
- 30.2 percent in women aged thirty-five to thirty-seven
- 20.2 percent in women aged thirty-seven to forty
- 11.0 percent in women aged forty-one to forty-two

ART can be expensive and time-consuming. But it has allowed many couples to have children that otherwise would not have been conceived. The most common complication of ART is multiple fetuses. But this is a problem that can be prevented or minimized in several different ways.

What are the different types of assisted reproductive technology (ART)?

Common methods of ART include the following:

- **In vitro fertilization (IVF):** This means fertilization outside of the body. IVF is the most effective ART. It is often used when a woman's fallopian tubes are blocked or when a man produces too few sperm. Doctors treat the woman with a drug that causes the ovaries to produce multiple eggs. Once mature, the eggs are removed from the woman. They are put in a dish in the lab along with the man's sperm for fertilization. After three to five days, healthy embryos are implanted in the woman's uterus.
- **Zygote intrafallopian transfer (ZIFT) or tubal embryo transfer:** This is similar to IVF. Fertilization occurs in the laboratory. Then the very young embryo is transferred to the fallopian tube instead of the uterus.
- **Gamete intrafallopian transfer (GIFT):** This involves transferring eggs and sperm into the woman's fallopian tube, so fertilization occurs in the woman's body. Few practices offer GIFT as an option.
- **Intracytoplasmic sperm injection (ICSI):** This is often used for couples in which there are serious problems with the sperm. Sometimes it is also used for older couples or for those with failed IVF attempts. In ICSI, a single sperm is injected into a mature egg. Then the embryo is transferred to the uterus or fallopian tube.

ART procedures sometimes involve the use of donor eggs (eggs from another woman), donor sperm, or previously frozen embryos. Donor eggs are sometimes used for women who cannot produce eggs. Also, donor eggs or donor sperm are sometimes used when the woman or man has a genetic disease that can be passed on to the baby.

Chapter 27

Beginning a Pregnancy

Chapter Contents

Section 27.1

Preconception Care

Reprinted from "Preconception Care Questions and Answers," Centers for Disease Control and Prevention, April 16, 2006.

What is preconception health?

Preconception health is a woman's health before she becomes pregnant. It focuses on the conditions and risk factors that could affect a woman if she becomes pregnant. Preconception health applies to women who have never been pregnant, and also to women who could become pregnant again. Preconception health looks at factors that can affect a fetus or infant. These include factors such as taking prescription drugs or drinking alcohol. The key to promoting preconception health is to combine the best medical care, healthy behaviors, strong support, and safe environments at home and at work.

What is preconception health care?

Preconception health care is care given to a woman before pregnancy to manage conditions and behaviors which could be a risk to her or her baby. There are many topics covered under preconception care:

- Folic acid supplements to prevent neural tube defects.
- Rubella vaccinations to prevent congenital rubella syndrome.
- Detecting and treating existing health conditions to prevent complications in the mother, and reduce the risk of birth defects, such as diabetes, hypothyroidism, human immunodeficiency virus/acquired immunodeficiency syndrome (HIV/AIDS), hepatitis B, phenylketonuria (PKU), hypertension, blood diseases, and eating disorders.
- Reviewing medications that can affect the fetus or the mother, such as epilepsy medicine, blood thinners, and some medicines used to treat acne, such as Accutane®.
- Reviewing a woman's pregnancy history—has she lost a baby before?

- Stopping smoking to reduce the risk of low birth weight.
- Eliminating alcohol consumption to prevent fetal alcohol syndrome and other complications.
- Family planning counseling to avoid unplanned pregnancies.
- Counseling to promote healthy behaviors such as appropriate weight, nutrition, exercise, and oral health. Counseling can help a woman avoid substance abuse and toxic substances. It can help women and couples understand genetic risks, mental health issues (such as depression), and intimate partner domestic violence.

Good preconception health care is about managing current health conditions. By taking action on health issues *before* pregnancy, future problems for the mother and baby can be prevented. Preconception health care must be tailored to each individual woman. It means helping women and their partners reduce risks and get ongoing care. Men and other family members are also very important in supporting the goals of preconception health.

Why are there new recommendations on preconception health and health care now?

There have been important advances in medicine and prenatal care in recent years. Despite these advances, birth outcomes are worse in the United States than in other developed countries. Many babies are born prematurely or have low birth weight. In some groups of people, the problems are actually getting worse.

Experts agree that women need to be healthier before becoming pregnant. While this is not a new idea, there has not been an organized effort to promote preconception health and health care until now. The recommendations shown here have been developed by local, state, and federal government agencies, with help from national medical organizations and groups such as the March of Dimes. They offer guidance to individuals and their families, health care providers, planners, and policymakers. The goal is to improve the health of women so that babies can be born healthier in the future.

Does preconception health apply to women who do not plan to get pregnant?

Absolutely. Every woman should be thinking about her health, whether or not she wants to get pregnant. Some of the basic recommendations for preconception health include healthy weight and nutrition, and identifying and managing existing conditions and infections. All women should quit smoking and avoid other harmful substances. These are important health goals for everyone, not just women planning to get pregnant.

Since over half of all pregnancies in the United States are unplanned, women who might be sexually active with male partners should consider their health. As they might not know they are pregnant, women need to avoid risks, such as using medications that could harm a fetus, whenever possible.

The Centers for Disease Control and Prevention (CDC) recommends that men and women think about a reproductive life plan. This means deciding the ideal time and conditions for having children and learning how to achieve these goals. This can include effective contraception. Women's lives are rich and complex, and the possibility of pregnancy is only one factor affecting women's health choices. The more that women know about the health care relevant to their own circumstances, the more empowered they are to make the right choices for their lives.

How long before becoming pregnant should a woman start preparing for pregnancy? What are the five most important things she should do before pregnancy for her and her baby's health?

Every man and woman should prepare for pregnancy before becoming sexually active, or at least three months before conception. Women should begin some of the recommendations even sooner—such as quitting smoking, reaching healthy weight, and adjusting medications. Planning for pregnancy is also a good time to talk about other concerns. Issues such as intimate partner domestic violence, mental health, and previous pregnancy problems need to be discussed. Although men and women can do much on their own, a health care provider is necessary for finding and treating existing health problems. They can also help a woman improve her health before pregnancy.

The five most important things a woman can do for preconception health are as follows:

- Take 400 micrograms of folic acid a day for at least three months before becoming pregnancy to reduce the risk of birth defects.
- Stop smoking and drinking alcohol.
- If you currently have a medical condition, be sure these conditions are under control. Conditions include but are not limited

to asthma, diabetes, oral health, obesity, or epilepsy. Be sure that your vaccinations are up to date.

- Talk to your doctor and pharmacist about any over-the-counter and prescription medicines you are taking, including vitamins, and any dietary or herbal supplements you are taking.
- Avoid exposures to toxic substances or potentially infectious materials at work or at home, such as chemicals, or cat and rodent feces.

The new recommendations say that everyone should have a reproductive life plan. What does this really mean?

A reproductive life plan is a set of personal goals about having (or not having) children. It also states how to achieve those goals. Everyone needs to make a reproductive plan based on personal values and resources. Here are some examples:

- "I'm not ready to have children now. I'll make sure I don't get pregnant. Either I won't have heterosexual sex, or I'll correctly use effective contraception."
- "I'll want to have children when my relationship feels secure and I've saved enough money. I won't become pregnant until then. After that, I'll visit my doctor to discuss preconception health. I'll try to get pregnant when I'm in good health."
- "I'd like to be a father after I finish school and have a job to support a family. While I work toward those goals, I'll talk to my wife about her goals for starting a family. I'll make sure we correctly use an effective method of contraception every time we have sex until we're ready to have a baby."
- "I'd like to have two children, and space my pregnancies by at least two years. I'll visit my certified nurse midwife to discuss preconception health now. I'll start trying to get pregnant as soon as I'm healthy. Once I have a baby, I'll get advice from a health professional on birth control. I don't want to have a second baby before I'm ready."
- "I will let pregnancy happen whenever it happens. Because I don't know when that will be, I'll make sure I'm in optimal health for pregnancy at all times."

There are many kinds of reproductive life plans. What's important is that you think about when and under what conditions you want to become pregnant. Then make sure your actions support these goals. Health care providers and counselors can help you understand the clinical and lifestyle options that are best for you.

What can men do to support the preconception health of their female partners and their future babies?

Men can make a big difference in promoting good preconception health. As boyfriends, husbands, fathers-to-be, partners, and family members, they can learn how their loved ones can achieve optimal preconception health. They can encourage and support women in every aspect of preparing for pregnancy.

There are other ways men can help. Men who work with chemicals or other toxins need to be careful that they don't expose women to them. For example, men who use fertilizers or pesticides in agricultural jobs should change out of dirty work clothes before coming near their female partners. They should handle and wash soiled clothes separately.

The family health histories of men are also important when planning a pregnancy. Understanding genetic risks from both sides enables providers to give more accurate advice. Screening for and treating sexually transmitted infections (STIs) in men can help make sure that the infections are not passed to female partners. Men can improve their own reproductive health by reducing stress, eating right, avoiding excessive alcohol use, not smoking, and talking to their health care providers about their own medications. It is also important for men who smoke to stop smoking around their partners, to avoid the harmful effects of secondhand smoke.

What is the role of community groups in promoting preconception health?

Since preconception health affects so many women, community groups can help ensure that no one gets left out. They can learn about preconception health and make sure their members know. Also, because community groups are often trusted sources of support, they can be effective in encouraging healthy choices.

What should my health care provider be doing about preconception care at my regular visits?

Health care providers have a lot to cover during an appointment, so it's always a good idea to make a list and bring up any issues on your mind. Do this even if the health care provider doesn't ask about them. The first thing to discuss is your plan for pregnancy. If you tell your provider that you might become pregnant in the near future, there will be a number of things to discuss. You may need to schedule another visit to make sure everything gets covered.

Your health care provider should do the following things:

- Review your family's medical history. This includes your previous experiences with pregnancy, fertility, birth, and use of birth control methods.
- Ask about your lifestyle, behaviors, and social support concerns that affect your health. Do you smoke, drink alcohol, use drugs, or have psychological problems, including depression? Do you have nutrition and diet issues? Concerns about health conditions in your or your partner's family? Are there issues around intimate partner domestic violence? What are the medications you are taking? Are there chemicals, solvents, radiation, or other potential risks at your workplace or home that could harm you or your baby?
- Schedule health screening tests—Pap smear, urinalysis, blood tests. Your provider needs to know your blood type, Rh factor, and whether you have diabetes, hypertension, sexually transmitted infections, or other conditions.
- Review your immunization status and update them if needed.
- Perform a physical exam, including a pelvic exam and a blood pressure check.

Based on your individual health, your health care provider will suggest a course of treatment or follow-up care as needed.

Section 27.2

Doctor's Visits and Prenatal Tests

Reprinted from "Healthy Pregnancy: Doctor's Visits and Tests," National Women's Health Information Center, March 2007.

Doctor Visits

During pregnancy visiting your doctor regularly is very important. Regular check-ups throughout the nine months of pregnancy is called prenatal care. This consistent care will keep you and your baby healthy, spot problems if they occur, and prevent difficulties during delivery.

Become a partner with your doctor to manage your care. Keep all of your appointments—every one is important! Ask questions and read to educate yourself about this exciting time.

Regular Check-Ups

Your doctor or midwife will give you a schedule for your prenatal visits. An average pregnancy lasts about forty weeks. You can expect to see your doctor more often as you approach the end of your pregnancy. A typical schedule includes visiting your doctor or midwife:

- about once each month during your first six months of pregnancy;
- every two weeks during the seventh and eighth month of pregnancy;
- weekly in the ninth month of pregnancy.

If you are over thirty-five years old or your pregnancy is high risk because you have certain health problems (like diabetes or high blood pressure), your doctor or midwife will probably want to see you more often.

The first time you see your doctor you'll probably have a pelvic exam to check your uterus (womb) and to have a Pap test. After the first visit, most prenatal visits will include the following:

- Checking the baby's heart rate
- Checking your blood pressure
- Checking your urine for signs of diabetes
- Measuring your weight gain

Prenatal Tests and Procedures

While you are pregnant your doctor or midwife may suggest a number of laboratory tests, ultrasound exams, or other screening tests. Read on to find out the basics of the most common tests done during pregnancy.

Screening Tests

Screening tests measure the risk of having a baby with some genetic birth defects. Birth defects are caused by problems with a baby's genes, inherited factors passed down from the mother and the father. Birth defects can also occur randomly in people with no family history of that disorder. Women over the age of thirty-five have the greatest risk of having babies with birth defects.

The benefit of screening tests is that they do not pose any risk to the fetus or mother. But screening tests cannot tell for sure if the baby has a birth defect. So, they do not give a "yes" or "no" answer. Instead, screening tests give the odds of your baby having a birth defect based on your age. Women under the age of thirty-five will find out if their risk is as high as that of a thirty-five-year-old woman. For women over age thirty-five, screening tests will help them find out if their risk for their age is higher or lower than average.

Some common screening tests used during pregnancy include the following.

Targeted ultrasound: The best time to receive this test is between eighteen and twenty weeks of pregnancy. Most major problems with the way your baby might be formed can be seen at this time. But some problems like clubbed feet and heart defects can be missed on ultrasound. Your doctor also will be able to see if your baby has any neural tube defects, such as spina bifida. This test is not the most accurate for finding out whether your baby has Down syndrome. Only one in three babies with Down syndrome have an abnormal second-trimester ultrasound. In most cases, your doctor can find out the sex of your baby by using ultrasound.

Maternal serum marker screening test: This blood test can be called by many different names including multiple marker screening test, triple test, quad screen, and others. This test is usually given between fifteen and twenty weeks of pregnancy. It checks for birth defects such as Down syndrome, trisomy 18, or open neural tube defects. Doctors take a sample of your blood. They check the blood for three chemicals: alpha-fetoprotein (AFP) (made by the liver of the fetus), and two pregnancy hormones, estriol and human chorionic gonadotropin (hCG). Sometimes, doctors test for a fourth substance in the blood called inhibin-A. Testing for inhibin-A may improve the ability to detect fetuses with a high risk of Down syndrome.

Higher levels of AFP are linked with open neural tube defects. In women age thirty-five and over, this test finds about 80 percent of fetuses with Down syndrome, trisomy 18, or an open neural tube defect. In this age group, there is a false positive rate (having a positive result without actually having a fetus with one of these health problems) of 22 percent. In women under age thirty-five, this test finds about 65 percent of fetuses with Down syndrome, and there is a false positive rate of about 5 percent.

Nuchal translucency screening (NTS): This new type of screening can be done between eleven and fourteen weeks of pregnancy. It uses an ultrasound and blood test to calculate the risk of some birth defects. Doctors use the ultrasound exam to check the thickness of the back of the fetus's neck. They also test your blood for levels of a protein called pregnancy-associated plasma protein and a hormone called human chorionic gonadotropin (hCG). Doctors use this information to tell if the fetus has a normal or greater than normal chance of having some birth defects.

In an important recent study, NTS found 87 percent of cases of Down syndrome when done at eleven weeks of pregnancy. When NTS was followed by another blood test done in the second trimester (maternal serum screening test), 95 percent of fetuses with Down syndrome were identified.

Like all screening tests, the results are sometimes misleading. In 5 percent of women who have NTS, results show that their babies have a high risk of having a birth defect when they are actually healthy. This is called a false positive. To find out for sure if the fetus has a birth defect, NTS must be followed by a diagnostic test like chorionic villus sampling or amniocentesis.

NTS is not yet widely used. If you are interested in NTS, talk to your doctor. If he or she is unable to do the test, he or she can refer you to someone who can. You should also call your insurance company to find out if they cover the cost of this procedure. NTS allows women to find out early if there are potential health problems with the fetus. This may help them decide whether to have follow-up tests.

Diagnostic Tests

Diagnostic tests can give definite "yes" or "no" answers about whether your baby has a birth defect. But, unlike screening tests, they are invasive or come with a risk of miscarriage. Amniocentesis and chorionic villus sampling (CVS) are the two most commonly used. Both tests are more than 99 percent accurate for finding these problems. These tests also can tell you your baby's sex. In most cases, results take about two weeks.

Amniocentesis: This test is performed in pregnancies of at least sixteen weeks. It involves your doctor inserting a thin needle through your abdomen, into your uterus, and into the amniotic sac to take out a small amount of amniotic fluid for testing. The cells from the fluid are grown in a lab to look for problems with chromosomes. The fluid also can be tested for AFP. About one in two hundred women have a miscarriage as a result of this test.

Chorionic villus sampling (CVS): This test is performed between ten and twelve weeks of pregnancy. The doctor inserts a needle through your abdomen or inserts a catheter through your cervix in order to reach the placenta. Your doctor then takes a sample of cells from the placenta. These cells are used in a lab to look for problems with chromosomes. This test cannot find out whether your baby has open neural tube defects. About one in two hundred women have a miscarriage as a result of this test.

Chapter 28

Staying Healthy during Pregnancy

Now that you're pregnant, taking care of yourself has never been more important. Of course, you'll probably get advice from everyone—your doctor, family members, friends, co-workers, and even complete strangers—about what you should and shouldn't be doing. But staying healthy during pregnancy depends on you, so it's crucial to arm yourself with information about the many ways to keep you and your baby as healthy as possible.

Prenatal Health Care

Key to protecting the health of your child is to get regular prenatal care. If you think you're pregnant, call your health care provider to schedule an appointment.

You should have your first examination during the first six to eight weeks of your pregnancy, which is when your menstrual period is two to four weeks late.

At this first visit, your health care provider will figure out how many weeks pregnant you are based on a physical examination and the date of your last period. He or she will also use this information to predict your delivery date (however, an ultrasound performed sometime during your pregnancy will help to verify that date).

"Staying Healthy during Pregnancy," July 2005, reprinted with permission from www.kidshealth.org. Copyright © 2005 The Nemours Foundation. This information was provided by KidsHealth, one of the largest resources online for medically reviewed health information written for parents, kids, and teens. For more articles like this one, visit www.KidsHealth.org, or www.TeensHealth.org.

If you're healthy and there are no complicating risk factors, you can expect to see your health care provider:

- every four weeks until the twenty-eighth week of pregnancy;
- then every two weeks until thirty-six weeks;
- then once a week until delivery.

Throughout your pregnancy, your health care provider will check your weight and blood pressure while also checking the growth and development of your baby (by doing things like feeling your abdomen, listening for the fetal heartbeat starting during the second trimester, and measuring your belly). During the span of your pregnancy, you'll also have prenatal tests, including blood, urine, and cervical tests, and probably at least one ultrasound.

If you still need to choose a health care provider to counsel and treat you during your pregnancy, there are several options:

- Obstetricians/gynecologists (also known as OB/GYNs—doctors who specialize in pregnancy and childbirth, as well as women's health care)
- family practitioners (doctors who provide a range of services for patients of all ages—in some cases, this includes obstetrical care)
- certified nurse-midwives (advanced practice nurses specializing in women's health care needs, including prenatal care, labor and delivery, and postpartum care for "normal" pregnancies; there are also other kinds of midwives, but you should look for one with formal training who's been certified in the field)

Any of these is a good choice if you're healthy and there's no reason to anticipate complications with your pregnancy and delivery. However, nurse-midwives do need to have a doctor available for the delivery in case an unexpected problem arises or a cesarean section (C-section) has to be performed.

Nutrition and Supplements

Now that you're eating for two (or more!), this is not the time to cut calories or go on a diet. In fact, it's just the opposite—you need about three hundred extra calories a day, especially later in your pregnancy when your baby grows quickly. If you're very thin or carrying twins, you'll need even more. But if you're overweight, your health care provider may advise that you consume fewer extra calories.

Healthy eating is always important, but especially when you're pregnant. So, it's important to make sure your calories come from nutritious foods so they can contribute to your baby's growth and development.

Try to maintain a well-balanced diet that incorporates the dietary guidelines including:

- lean meats;
- fruits;
- vegetables;
- whole-grain breads;
- low-fat dairy products.

By eating a healthy, balanced diet you're more likely to get the nutrients you need. But you will need more of the essential nutrients (especially calcium, iron, and folic acid) than you did before you became pregnant. Your health care provider will prescribe prenatal vitamins to be sure both you and your growing baby are getting enough.

But taking prenatal vitamins doesn't mean you can eat a diet that's completely lacking in nutrients. It's important to remember that you still need to eat well while pregnant. Prenatal vitamins are meant to supplement your diet not be your only source of much-needed nutrients.

Calcium

Most women nineteen and older—including those who are pregnant—don't often get the daily 1,000 mg of calcium that's recommended. Because your growing baby's calcium demands are high, you should increase your calcium consumption to prevent a loss of calcium from your own bones. Your doctor will also likely prescribe prenatal vitamins for you, which may contain some extra calcium.

Good sources of calcium include:

- low-fat dairy products including milk, cheese, and yogurt;
- calcium-fortified products, including orange juice, soy milk, and cereals;
- dark green vegetables including spinach, kale, and broccoli;
- tofu;
- dried beans;
- almonds.

Iron

Pregnant women need 27 to 30 mg of iron every day. Why? Because iron is needed to make hemoglobin, the oxygen-carrying component of red blood cells. Red blood cells circulate throughout the body to deliver oxygen to all its cells.

Without enough iron, the body can't make enough red blood cells and the body's tissues and organs won't get the oxygen they need to function well. So it's especially important for pregnant women to get enough iron in their daily diets—for themselves and their growing babies.

Although the nutrient can be found in various kinds of foods, iron from meat sources is more easily absorbed by the body than iron found in plant foods. Some examples of iron-rich foods include:

- red meat;
- dark poultry;
- salmon;
- eggs;
- tofu;
- enriched grains;
- dried beans and peas;
- dried fruits;
- leafy green vegetables;
- blackstrap molasses;
- iron-fortified breakfast cereals.

Folate (Folic Acid)

The U.S. Centers for Disease Control and Prevention (CDC) recommends that all women of childbearing age—and especially those who are planning a pregnancy—get about 400 micrograms (0.4 milligrams) of folic acid supplements every day. That can be from a multivitamin or folic acid supplement in addition to the folic acid found in food.

So, why is folic acid so important? Studies have shown that taking folic acid supplements one month prior to and throughout the first three months of pregnancy decrease the risk of neural tube defects by up to 70 percent.

The neural tube—formed during the first twenty-eight days of the pregnancy, usually before a woman even knows she's pregnant—goes on to become the baby's developing brain and spinal cord. When the neural tube doesn't form properly, the result is a neural tube defect such as spina bifida.

Again, your health care provider can prescribe a prenatal vitamin that contains the right amount of folic acid. Some pregnancy health care providers even recommend taking an additional folic acid supplement, especially if a woman has previously had a child with a neural tube defect.

If you're buying an over-the-counter supplement, keep in mind that most multivitamins contain folic acid, but not all of them have enough folic acid to meet the nutritional needs of a pregnant woman. So, be sure to check labels carefully before choosing one and check with your health care provider.

Fluids

It's also important to drink plenty of fluids, especially water, during pregnancy. A woman's blood volume increases dramatically during pregnancy, and drinking enough water each day can help prevent common problems such as dehydration and constipation.

Exercise

The 2005 dietary guidelines recommend that healthy pregnant women get thirty minutes or more of moderate-intensity physical activity every day. Exercising during pregnancy has been shown to be extremely beneficial.

Regular exercise can help:

- prevent excess weight gain;
- reduce pregnancy-related problems, like back pain, swelling, and constipation;
- improve sleep;
- increase energy;
- improve outlook;
- prepare for labor;
- lessen recovery time.

If you've been involved in an exercise program before becoming pregnant, talk to your health care provider about whether it's safe to continue. If you haven't been active and/or you have a high-risk pregnancy, ask your health care provider how you can safely start.

Low-impact, moderate-intensity exercise activities (such as walking and swimming) are great choices. You can also opt for yoga or Pilates classes, DVDs, or videos that are tailored for pregnancy. These are both low-impact and work on strength, flexibility, and relaxation.

But you should limit high-impact aerobics and avoid certain sports and activities that pose a risk of falling or abdominal injury. Typical limitations include contact sports, downhill skiing, and horseback riding.

It's also important to be aware of how your body changes. During pregnancy, your body produces a hormone known as relaxin, which is believed to help prepare the pubic area and the cervix for the birth. The relaxin loosens the ligaments in your body, making you less stable and more prone to injury.

So, it's easy to overstretch or strain yourself, especially the joints in your pelvis, lower back, and knees. In addition, your center of gravity shifts as your pregnancy progresses, so you may feel off-balance and at risk of falling. Keep these in mind when you choose an activity, and don't overdo it.

Whatever type of exercise you choose, make sure to take frequent breaks and remember to drink plenty of fluids. And use common sense—slow down or stop if you get short of breath or feel uncomfortable. If you have any questions about doing a certain sport or activity during your pregnancy, talk to your health care provider for specific guidelines.

Sleep

It's important to get enough sleep during your pregnancy. Your body is working hard to accommodate a new life, so you'll probably feel more tired than usual. And as your baby gets bigger, it will be harder to find a comfortable position when you're trying to sleep.

Lying on your side with your knees bent is likely to be the most comfortable position as your pregnancy progresses. It also makes your heart's job easier because it keeps the baby's weight from applying pressure to the large blood vessels that carry blood to and from your heart and your feet and legs. Lying on your side can also help prevent or reduce varicose veins, constipation, hemorrhoids, and swelling in your legs.

Some doctors specifically recommend that pregnant women sleep on the left side. Because your liver is on the right side of your abdomen, lying on your left side helps keep the uterus off that large organ.

Lying on your left side also optimizes blood flow to the placenta and, therefore, your baby.

Ask what your health care provider recommends. In most cases, lying on either side should do the trick and help take some pressure off your back. To create a more comfortable resting position, either way, prop pillows between your legs, behind your back, and underneath your belly.

Some Things to Avoid

When you're pregnant, what you don't put into your body (or expose your body to) is almost as important as what you do. Here are some things to avoid.

Alcohol

Although it may seem harmless to have a glass of wine at dinner or a mug of beer out with friends, no one has determined what's a "safe amount" of alcohol to consume during pregnancy. One of the most common known causes of mental and physical birth defects, alcohol produces more severe abnormalities in a developing fetus than heroin, cocaine, or marijuana.

Alcohol is easily passed along to the baby, who is less equipped to eliminate alcohol than the mother. That means an unborn baby tends to develop a high concentration of alcohol, which stays in the baby's system for longer periods than it would in the mother's. And moderate alcohol intake, as well as periodic binge drinking, can damage a baby's developing nervous system.

If you had a drink or two before you even knew you were pregnant (as many women do), don't worry too much about it. But your best bet is to not drink any alcohol at all for the rest of your pregnancy.

Recreational Drugs

Pregnant women who use drugs may be placing their unborn babies at risk for premature birth, poor growth, birth defects, and behavior and learning problems. And their babies could also be born addicted to those drugs themselves.

If you're pregnant and using drugs, a health clinic such as Planned Parenthood can recommend health care providers, at little or no cost, who can help you quit your habit and have a healthier pregnancy.

If you've used any drugs at any time during your pregnancy, it's important to inform your health care provider. Even if you've quit, your unborn child could still be at risk for health problems.

Nicotine

You wouldn't light a cigarette, put it in your baby's mouth, and encourage your little one to puff away. As ridiculous as this scenario seems, pregnant women who continue to smoke are allowing their fetus to smoke, too. The smoking mother passes nicotine and carbon monoxide to her growing baby.

The risks of smoking to the fetus include:

- stillbirth;
- prematurity;
- low birth weight;
- sudden infant death syndrome (SIDS);
- asthma and other respiratory problems.

If you smoke, having a baby may be the motivation you need to quit. Talk to your health care provider about options for stopping your smoking habit.

Caffeine

High caffeine consumption has been linked to an increased risk of miscarriage, so it's probably wise to limit or avoid caffeine altogether if you can.

If you're having a hard time cutting out coffee cold turkey, here's how you can start:

- Cut your consumption down to one or two cups a day.
- Gradually reduce the amount by combining decaffeinated coffee with regular coffee.
- Eventually cut out the regular coffee altogether.

And remember that caffeine is not limited to coffee. Green and black tea, cola, and other soft drinks contain caffeine. Try switching to decaffeinated products (which may still have some caffeine, but in much smaller amounts) or caffeine-free alternatives.

If you're wondering whether chocolate, which also contains caffeine, is a concern, the good news is that you can have it in moderation. Whereas the average chocolate bar has anywhere from 5 to 30 milligrams of caffeine, there's 95 to 135 milligrams in a cup of brewed coffee. So, small amounts of chocolate are fine.

Certain Foods

Although you need to eat plenty of healthy foods during pregnancy, you also need to avoid food-borne illnesses, such as listeriosis and toxoplasmosis, which can be life-threatening to an unborn baby and may cause birth defects or miscarriage.

Foods you'll want to steer clear of include:

- soft, unpasteurized cheeses (often advertised as "fresh") such as feta, goat, Brie, Camembert, and blue cheese;
- unpasteurized milk, juices, and apple cider;
- raw eggs or foods containing raw eggs, including mousse, tiramisu, raw cookie dough, homemade ice cream, and Caesar dressing (although some store-bought brands of the dressing may not contain raw eggs);
- raw or undercooked meats, fish (sushi), or shellfish;
- processed meats such as hot dogs and deli meats (these should be well cooked).

Also, although fish and shellfish can be an extremely healthy part of your pregnancy diet (they contain beneficial omega-3 fatty acids and are high in protein and low in saturated fat), you should avoid eating:

- shark;
- swordfish;
- king mackerel;
- tilefish.

These types of fish may contain high levels of mercury, which can cause damage to the developing brain of a fetus. When you choose seafood, eat a variety of fish and shellfish and limit the amount to about twelve ounces per week—that's about two meals. Also, when you're eating canned tuna, you may want to choose light tuna, which has less mercury than canned white tuna. You should eat no more than six ounces per week of canned albacore or white tuna. Also, it's a good idea to check any local advisories before consuming any recreationally caught fish.

Changing the Litter Box

Pregnancy is the prime time to get out of cleaning kitty's litter box. Why? Because an infection called toxoplasmosis can be spread through soiled cat litter boxes and can cause serious problems, including prematurity, poor growth, and severe eye and brain damage. A pregnant woman who becomes infected often has no symptoms but can still pass the infection on to her developing baby.

Over-the-Counter and Prescription Medications

Even common over-the-counter medications that are generally safe may be considered off-limits during pregnancy because of their potential effects on the baby. And certain prescription medications may also cause harm to the developing fetus.

To make sure you don't take anything that could be harmful to your baby:

- Ask your health care provider which medicines—both over-the-counter and prescription—are safe to take during pregnancy.
- Talk to your health care provider about any prescription drugs you're taking.
- Let all of your health care providers know that you're pregnant so that they'll keep that in mind when recommending or prescribing any medications.
- Discuss any questions about natural remedies, supplements, and vitamins.

If you were prescribed a medication before you became pregnant for an illness, disease, or condition you still have, consult with your health care provider, who can help you weigh potential benefits and risks of continuing your prescription.

If you become sick (i.e., with a cold) or have symptoms that are causing you discomfort or pain (i.e., a headache or backache), talk to your health care provider about medications you can take and alternative ways to help you feel better without medication.

Healthy Pregnancy Habits: From Start to Finish

During pregnancy, from the first week to the fortieth, it's important to take care of yourself in order to take care of your baby. Even though you have to take some precautions and be ever-aware of how what you what you do—and don't do—may affect your baby, many women say they've never felt healthier than when they carried their children.

Chapter 29

Pregnancy and Medicines

Is it safe to use medicine while I am pregnant?

There is no clear-cut answer to this question. Before you start or stop any medicine, it is always best to speak with the doctor who is caring for you while you are pregnant. Read on to learn about deciding to use medicine while pregnant.

How should I decide whether to use a medicine while I am pregnant?

When deciding whether or not to use a medicine in pregnancy, you and your doctor need to talk about the medicine's benefits and risks:

- **Benefits:** What are the good things the medicine can do for me and my growing baby (fetus)?
- **Risks:** What are the ways the medicine might harm me or my growing baby (fetus)?

There may be times during pregnancy when using medicine is a choice. Some of the medicine choices you and your doctor make while you are pregnant may differ from the choices you make when you are not pregnant. For example, if you get a cold, you may decide to "live

---

Reprinted from "Pregnancy and Medicines," National Women's Health Information Center, April 2007.

with" your stuffy nose instead of using the "stuffy nose" medicine you use when you are not pregnant.

Other times, using medicine is not a choice—it is needed. Some women need to use medicines while they are pregnant. Sometimes, women need medicine for a few days or a couple of weeks to treat a problem like a bladder infection or strep throat. Other women need to use medicine every day to control long-term health problems like asthma, diabetes, depression, or seizures. Also, some women have a pregnancy problem that needs medicine treatment. These problems include severe nausea and vomiting, earlier pregnancy losses, or preterm labor.

Where do doctors and nurses find out about using medicines during pregnancy?

Doctors and nurses get information from medicine labels and packages, textbooks, and research journals. They also share knowledge with other doctors and nurses and talk to the people who make and sell medicines.

The Food and Drug Administration (FDA) is the part of our country's government that controls the medicines that can and can't be sold in the United States. The FDA lets a company sell a medicine in the United States if it is safe to use and works for a certain problem. Companies that make medicines usually have to show FDA doctors and scientists whether birth defects or other problems occur in baby animals when the medicine is given to pregnant animals. Most of the time, drugs are not studied in pregnant women.

The FDA works with the drug companies to make clear and complete labels. But in most cases, there is not much information about how a medicine affects pregnant women and their growing babies. Many prescription medicine labels include the results of studies done in pregnant animals. But a medicine does not always affect growing humans and animals in the same way. Here is an example: A medicine is given to pregnant rats. If the medicine causes problems in some of the rat babies, it may or may not cause problems in human babies. If there are no problems in the rat babies, it does not prove that the medicine will not cause problems in human babies.

The FDA asks for studies in two different kinds of animals. This improves the chance that the studies can predict what may happen in pregnant women and their babies.

There is a lot that FDA doctors and scientists do not know about using medicine during pregnancy. In a perfect world, every medicine label would include helpful information about the medicine's effects on pregnant women and their growing babies. Unfortunately, this is not the case.

How do prescription and over-the-counter (OTC) medicine labels help my doctor choose the right medicine for me when I am pregnant?

Doctors use information from many sources when they choose medicine for a patient, including medicine labels. To help doctors, the FDA created pregnancy letter categories to help explain what is known about using medicine during pregnancy. This system assigns letter categories to all prescription medicines. The letter category is listed in the label of a prescription medicine. The label states whether studies were done in pregnant women or pregnant animals and if so, what happened. Over-the-counter (OTC) medicines do not have a pregnancy letter category. Some OTC medicines were prescription medicines first and used to have a letter category. Talk to your doctor and follow the instructions on the label before taking OTC medicines.

Prescription medicines: The FDA chooses a medicine's letter category based on what is known about the medicine when used in pregnant women and animals (see Table 29.1).

The FDA is working hard to gather more knowledge about using medicine during pregnancy. The FDA is also trying to make medicine labels more helpful to doctors. Medicine label information for prescription medicines is now changing, and the pregnancy part of the label will change over the next few years.

OTC medicines: All OTC medicines have a Drug Facts label. The Drug Facts label is arranged the same way on all OTC medicines. This makes information about using the medicine easier to find. One section of the Drug Facts label is for pregnant women. With OTC medicines, the label usually tells a pregnant woman to speak with her doctor before using the medicine. Some OTC medicines are known to cause certain problems in pregnancy. The labels for these medicines give pregnant women facts about why and when they should not use the medicine. Here are some examples:

- Nonsteroidal anti-inflammatory drugs (NSAIDs) like ibuprofen (Advil®, Motrin®), naproxen (Aleve®), and aspirin (acetylsalicylate), can cause serious blood flow problems in the baby if used

Table 29.1. Pregnancy Letter Categories for Prescription Medicines

Pregnancy Category	Definition	Examples of Drugs
A	In human studies, pregnant women used the medicine and their babies did not have any problems related to using the medicine.	• Folic acid • Levothyroxine (thyroid hormone medicine)
B	In humans, there are no good studies. But in animal studies, pregnant animals received the medicine, and the babies did not show any problems related to the medicine. ***Or*** In animal studies, pregnant animals received the medicine, and some babies had problems. But in human studies, pregnant women used the medicine and their babies did not have any problems related to using the medicine.	• Some antibiotics like amoxicillin • Zofran® (ondansetron) for nausea • Glucophage® (metformin) for diabetes • Some insulins used to treat diabetes such as regular and neutral protamine Hagedorn (NPH) insulin
C	In humans, there are no good studies. In animals, pregnant animals treated with the medicine had some babies with problems. However, sometimes the medicine may still help the human mothers and babies more than it might harm. ***Or*** No animal studies have been done, and there are no good studies in pregnant women.	• Diflucan® (fluconazole) for yeast infections • Ventolin® (albuterol) for asthma • Zoloft® (sertraline) and Prozac® (fluoxetine) for depression
D	Studies in humans and other reports show that when pregnant women use the medicine, some babies are born with problems related to the medicine. However, in some serious situations, the medicine may still help the mother and the baby more than it might harm.	• Paxil® (paroxetine) for depression • Lithium for bipolar disorder • Dilantin® (phenytoin) for epileptic seizures • Some cancer chemotherapy
X	Studies or reports in humans or animals show that mothers using the medicine during pregnancy may have babies with problems related to the medicine. There are no situations where the medicine can help the mother or baby enough to make the risk of problems worth it. These medicines should never be used by pregnant women.	• Accutane® (isotretinoin) for cystic acne • Thalomid® (thalidomide) for a type of skin disease

during the last third of pregnancy (after twenty-eight weeks). Also, aspirin may increase the chance for bleeding problems in the mother and the baby during pregnancy or at delivery.

- The labels for nicotine therapy drugs, like the nicotine patch and lozenge, remind women that smoking can harm an unborn child. While the medicine is thought to be safer than smoking, the risks of the medicine are not fully known. Pregnant smokers are told to try quitting without the medicine first.

What if I'm thinking about getting pregnant?

If you are not pregnant yet, you can help your chances for having a healthy baby by planning ahead. Schedule a pre-pregnancy checkup. At this visit, you can talk to your doctor about the medicines, vitamins, and herbs you use. It is very important that you keep treating your health problems while you are pregnant. Your doctor can tell you if you need to switch your medicine. Ask about vitamins for women who are trying to get pregnant. All women who can get pregnant should take a daily vitamin with folic acid (a B vitamin) to prevent birth defects of the brain and spinal cord. You should begin taking these vitamins before you become pregnant or if you could become pregnant. It is also a good idea to discuss caffeine, alcohol, and smoking with your doctor at this time.

Is it safe to use medicine while I am trying to become pregnant?

It is hard to know exactly when you will get pregnant. Once you do get pregnant, you may not know you are pregnant for ten to fourteen days or longer. Before you start trying to get pregnant, it is wise to schedule a meeting with your doctor to discuss medicines that you use daily or every now and then. Sometimes, medicines should be changed, and sometimes they can be stopped before a woman gets pregnant. Each woman is different. So you should discuss your medicines with your doctor rather than making medicine changes on your own.

What if I get sick and need to use medicine while I am pregnant?

Whether or not you should use medicine during pregnancy is a serious question to discuss with your doctor. Some health problems need treatment. Not using a medicine that you need could harm you and your baby. For example, a urinary tract infection (UTI) that is not treated may become a kidney infection. Kidney infections can cause preterm labor and low birth weight. An antibiotic is needed to get rid of a UTI. Ask your doctor whether the benefits of taking a certain medicine outweigh the risks for you and your baby.

I have a health problem. Should I stop using my medicine while I am pregnant?

If you are pregnant or thinking about becoming pregnant, you should talk to your doctor about your medicines. Do not stop or change them on your own. This includes medicines for depression, asthma, diabetes, seizures (epilepsy), and other health problems. Not using medicine that you need may be more harmful to you and your baby than using the medicine.

For women living with human immunodeficiency virus (HIV), the Centers for Disease Control and Prevention (CDC) recommends using zidovudine (AZT) during pregnancy. Studies show that HIV-positive women who use AZT during pregnancy greatly lower the risk of passing HIV to their babies. If a diabetic woman does not use her medicine during pregnancy, she raises her risk for miscarriage, stillbirth, and some birth defects. If asthma and high blood pressure are not controlled during pregnancy, problems with the fetus may result.

Are vitamins safe for me while I am pregnant?

Regular multivitamins and prenatal vitamins are safe to take during pregnancy and can be helpful. Women who are pregnant or trying to get pregnant should take a daily multivitamin or prenatal vitamin that contains at least 400 micrograms (µg) of folic acid. It is best to start taking these vitamins before you become pregnant or if you could become pregnant. Folic acid reduces the chance of a baby having a neural tube defect, like spina bifida, where the spine or brain does not form the right way. It's important to take the vitamin dose prescribed by your doctor. Too many vitamins can harm your baby. For example, very high levels of vitamin A have been linked with severe birth defects.

What should I know about vaccines and pregnancy?

Vaccines protect your body against dangerous diseases. Some vaccines are not safe to receive during pregnancy. For some vaccines, the decision to give a vaccine during pregnancy depends on a pregnant woman's own situation. Her doctor may consider these questions before giving a vaccine:

- Is there is a high chance she will be exposed to the disease?
- Would the infection pose a risk to the mother or fetus?
- Is the vaccine unlikely to cause harm?

The Advisory Committee on Immunization Practices recommends that Hepatitis B vaccination should be considered when women are at risk for developing Hepatitis B during pregnancy, and inactivated influenza vaccine should be considered for women who are pregnant during flu season. On the other hand, a pregnant woman who is not immune to rubella (German measles) is not given a rubella vaccine until after pregnancy. Talk with your doctor to make sure you are fully protected. The Centers for Disease Control and Prevention (CDC) provides vaccine guidelines for pregnant women.

Are herbal remedies, "natural" products, or dietary supplements safe for me while I am pregnant?

Except for some vitamins, little is known about using dietary supplements while pregnant. Some herbal remedy labels claim they will help with pregnancy. But, most often there are no good studies to show if these claims are true or if the herb can cause harm to or your baby. Talk with your doctor before using any herbal product or dietary supplement. These products may contain things that could harm you or your growing baby during your pregnancy.

In the United States, there are different laws for medicines and for dietary supplements. The part of the FDA that controls dietary supplements is the same part that controls foods sold in the United States. Only dietary supplements containing new dietary ingredients that were not marketed before October 15, 1994, submit safety information for review by the FDA. However, unlike medicines, herbal remedies and "natural products" are not approved by the FDA for safety or for what they say they will do. Most have not even been evaluated for their potential to cause harm to you or the growing fetus, let alone shown to be safe for use in pregnancy. Before a company can sell a medicine, the company must complete many studies and send the results to the FDA. Many scientists and doctors at the FDA check the study results. The FDA allows the medicine to be sold only if the studies show that the medicine works and is safe to use.

In the future, will there be better ways to know if medicines are safe to use during pregnancy?

At this time, drugs are rarely tested for safety in pregnant women for fear of harming the unborn baby. Until this changes, pregnancy exposure registries help doctors and researchers learn how medicines affect pregnant mothers and their growing baby. A pregnancy exposure registry is a study that enrolls pregnant women who are using a certain medicine. The women sign up for the study while pregnant and are followed for a certain length of time after the baby is born. Researchers compare babies with mothers who used the medicine while pregnant to babies with mothers who did not use the medicine. This type of study compares large groups of pregnant mothers and babies to look for medicine effects. A woman and her doctor can use registry results to make more informed choices about using medicine while pregnant.

If you are pregnant and are using a medicine or were using one when you got pregnant, check to see if there is a pregnancy exposure registry for that medicine. The Food and Drug Administration has a list of pregnancy exposure registries that pregnant women can join.

Chapter 30

The Birth of Your Baby

Chapter Contents

Section 30.1

Frequently Asked Questions about Labor and Delivery

How will I know when I'm in labor?

It is often difficult to know when you are in true labor. Your body will give you signals, but there is no guarantee that you will experience them. Here are some signs to watch for:

- **Contractions:** Braxton Hicks are contractions that prepare your body for true labor and they are felt more in your abdomen. When you start feeling contractions in your back that is a sign that true labor is beginning. True labor contractions are usually painful and you may not be able to talk or move much during them. You need to time your true labor contractions from the start of one to the start of the next one. Also, time how long each one lasts.
- **Lightening:** When your baby moves into position for birth, you may feel like your baby has "dropped" slightly. This relieves pressure on your diaphragm, makes it easier to breathe, and may make you feel lighter.
- **Mucous plug:** As your cervix begins to dilate you may pass a small clot-like plug. Although this does not signify that you will go into labor immediately, it does mean that you will probably go into labor within the next couple days or weeks, if not sooner.
- **Nesting:** Some women experience a sudden urge to clean or a burst of energy.
- **Effacement (thinning of the cervix) and dilation (opening of the cervix):** These signs will need to be measured by your health care provider and will give a more accurate indication of what stage of labor you are in.

Do not wait for your water to break before calling your doctor—for most women this does not happen until the labor has progressed.

If you notice any bright red discharge call your health care provider immediately! Pinkish spotting (bloody show) is normal after thirty-seven weeks, particularly after you have had a vaginal exam, have had sex, or are in early labor. Call your health care provider if you experience any bleeding that occurs before thirty-seven weeks. This is not normal.

What should I expect when I get to the hospital?

When you first get to the hospital, you will go to the birth center or labor and delivery area, based on your birthing choices, room availability, and instructions from your health care provider. You either may walk or need to take a wheelchair, depending on how you feel. When you arrive on the unit, you will need to change into a hospital gown and give a urine sample. The nurse will help you into bed, ask questions about your health history, and take your temperature, pulse, and blood pressure. A fetal monitor may be used to listen to your baby's heart rate and to record any contractions which you may be having. The monitor is attached to a computer screen, so you can also see the tracing or recording of your baby's heartbeat. You may have a sterile exam with a speculum placed into the vagina to see if your water has broken. An exam can tell if your cervix (the opening to your uterus where the baby will come out) is dilating (opening).

What will happen during labor?

During labor, your uterus (which is made up of muscles) will tighten and relax. This causes your cervix to open. Once the cervix is fully open (dilated), you will start to push the baby down through the birth canal. Labor is hard work and can be uncomfortable.

Every labor is different, but labor usually starts out slowly, with cramps. The cramps become stronger and closer together. As you become more uncomfortable, you can try different ways to help make labor go smoothly.

Your amniotic sac (bag of water) may break on its own before or during labor. Sometimes, your health care provider may decide to break the bag of water if it has not broken on its own. This is not any more uncomfortable than a vaginal exam. The amniotic fluid may feel warm as it leaks out. The fluid will continue to leak during labor. Your contractions may or may not feel stronger to you after your water has broken. You may need to wear a sanitary pad if you are out of bed or walking.

First stage: During the first stage of labor uterine contractions begin. They will be relatively mild at first and they will increase in intensity and duration as labor progresses. Usually contractions will become more frequent after your water breaks. Throughout this stage your cervix thins (effaces) and opens (dilation) and by the time you are ready to deliver your baby your cervix will be dilated to 10 centimeters. The typical duration of this stage is thirteen hours—if it's your first child.

Second stage: During the second stage of labor your cervix will open sufficiently and your baby begins to move down the birth canal. At this time you will push the baby through the birth canal and you'll finally be able to meet your new baby. The typical duration of this stage is ninety minutes.

Third stage: In the third stage you will deliver the placenta or afterbirth. This usually happens within thirty minutes after the birth.

How long will my labor last?

If it's your first child, labor will typically last between twelve and twenty-four hours, with an average of fourteen hours. However, if you've given birth before, labor usually averages between six and eight hours.

Is there anything I can do to lessen the pain of the contractions?

- Change positions often
- Use relaxation techniques from your childbirth class, or ask your nurse to help you
- Have your support person massage your feet. This does help and feels great
- Go to the bathroom every hour or so. A full bladder hurts and keeps the baby from moving into the birth canal
- Turn the lights down and listen to quiet music
- Have your support person give you a back rub
- Use a cool, moist washcloth on your face or forehead
- Take a warm shower or whirlpool bath, to help you relax

What if something doesn't go as planned?

Be assured, many women give birth to healthy babies with no complications at all. If complications do occur, they are many times related to timing and your doctor or other health care provider know exactly how to handle them. Serious problems are relatively rare and often can be anticipated:

- Premature rupture of the membranes (water breaking)
- Pre-term labor (labor that begins before the thirty-seventh week of pregnancy)
- Post-term pregnancy (pregnancy that continues beyond forty-two weeks)
- Excessive vaginal bleeding
- An abnormal heart rate in the fetus
- Labor that progresses too slowly
- Abnormal position of the fetus including breech presentation

Section 30.2

Risks and Warning Signs of Premature Labor

Pregnancy is normally a time of happiness and anticipation, but it can also be a time of unknowns. Many women have concerns about what is happening with their baby. Is everything okay? Some women wonder about going into labor early. Premature labor occurs in about 12 percent of all pregnancies. However, knowing the symptoms and avoiding particular risk factors can lower a woman's chance of premature labor.

What is premature labor?

A normal pregnancy should last about forty weeks. Occasionally, labor may begin prematurely before the thirty-seventh week of pregnancy because uterine contractions cause the cervix to open earlier than normal. When this happens, the baby is born premature and can be at risk for health problems. Fortunately, due to research, technology, and medicine, the health of premature babies is improving.

What risk factors place me at a high risk for premature labor?

Certain factors may increase a woman's risk of having premature labor, although the specific causes of premature labor are not known. However, having a specific risk factor does not mean a woman is predetermined to have premature labor. A woman may have premature labor for no apparent reason. If you have any of these risk factors, it's important to know the symptoms of premature labor and what you should do if they occur.

Women are at greatest risk for premature labor if:

- they are pregnant with multiples;
- they have had a previous premature birth;
- they have certain uterine or cervical abnormalities.

Medical risk factors include:

- recurring bladder and/or kidney infections;
- urinary tract infections, vaginal infections, and sexually transmitted infections;
- infection with fever (greater than 101 degrees Fahrenheit) during pregnancy;
- unexplained vaginal bleeding after twenty weeks of pregnancy;
- chronic illness such as high blood pressure, kidney disease, or diabetes;
- multiple first trimester abortions or one or more second trimester abortions;
- underweight or overweight before pregnancy;
- clotting disorder (thrombophilia);
- being pregnant with a single fetus after in vitro fertilization (IVF);
- short time between pregnancies (less than six to nine months between birth and beginning of the next pregnancy).

Lifestyle risks for premature labor include:

- little or no prenatal care;
- smoking;
- drinking alcohol;
- using illegal drugs;
- domestic violence, including physical, sexual or emotional abuse;
- lack of social support;
- high levels of stress;
- low income;
- long working hours with long periods of standing.

What are warning signs of premature labor?

It may be possible to prevent a premature birth by knowing the warning signs and calling your health care provider if you suspect you are having premature labor. Warning signs and symptoms of premature labor include:

- A contraction every ten minutes, or more frequently within one hour (five or more uterine contractions in an hour);
- watery fluid leaking from your vagina (this could indicate that your bag of water is broken);
- menstrual-like cramps felt in the lower abdomen that may come and go or be constant;
- low, dull backache felt below the waistline that may come and go or be constant;
- pelvic pressure that feels like your baby is pushing down;
- abdominal cramps that may occur with or without diarrhea;
- increase or change in vaginal discharge.

What does a contraction feel like?

As the muscles of your uterus contract, you will feel your abdomen harden. As the contraction goes away, your uterus becomes soft. Throughout pregnancy, the layers of your uterus will tighten irregularly which are usually not painful. These are known as Braxton-Hicks contractions and are usually irregular and do not open the cervix. If these contractions become regular or more frequent (one every ten to twelve minutes for at least an hour) they may be premature labor contractions which can cause the cervix to open. It is important to contact your health care provider immediately.

How can I check for contractions?

While lying down, use your fingertips to feel your uterus tighten and soften. This is called "palpation." During a contraction your abdomen will feel hard all over, not just in one area. However, as your baby grows you may feel your abdomen become firmer in one area and then become soft again.

What should I do if I think I am experiencing premature labor?

If you suspect you are having signs and symptoms of premature labor call your health care provider immediately. This can be a scary time for you but there are some ways you can help to prevent premature labor by becoming aware of the symptoms and following these directions:

- Empty your bladder.
- Lie down tilted towards your left side; this may slow down or stop signs and symptoms.
- Avoid lying flat on your back; this may cause the contractions to increase.
- Drink several glasses of water because dehydration can cause contractions.
- Monitor contractions for one hour by counting the minutes that elapse from the beginning of one contraction to the beginning of the next.

If symptoms get worse, or don't go away after one hour, call your health care provider again or go to the hospital. When you call your health care provider, be sure to mention that you are worried about premature labor. The only sure way to know if you are in premature labor is by examination of your cervix. If your cervix is opening up, premature labor could be starting.

What is the treatment to prevent premature labor from starting or continuing?

- Magnesium sulfate is a medication given through an intravenous (IV) line, which may cause nausea temporarily. A large dose is given initially and then a smaller continuous dose is given for twelve to twenty-four hours or more.
- Corticosteroid is a medication given twenty-four hours before birth to help accelerate the baby's lung and brain maturity.
- Oral medications are sometimes used to decrease the frequency of contractions, and may make women feel better.

What impact does premature labor have on my pregnancy?

The longer your baby is in the womb, the better the chance he or she will be healthy. Babies who are born prematurely are at higher risks for brain and other neurological complications, as well as breathing and digestive problems. Some premature babies grow up with a developmental delay, and/or have learning difficulties in school. The earlier in pregnancy a baby is born, the more health problems are likely to develop.

Premature labor does not always result in premature delivery. Some women with premature labor and early dilation of the cervix are sometimes put on bed rest until the pregnancy progresses further.

Most babies born prior to twenty-four weeks have little chance of survival. Only about 50 percent will survive and the other 50 percent may die or have permanent problems. However, babies born after thirty-two weeks have a very high survival rate, and usually do not have long-term complications.

Babies born at hospitals with neonatal intensive care units (NICU) do best. If you deliver at a hospital that does not have a NICU, you may be transferred to a nearby hospital.

Chapter 31

Questions about Pregnancy Loss

Chapter Contents

Section 31.1

Ectopic Pregnancy

"Ectopic Pregnancy," © 2007 American Pregnancy Association (www.americanpregnancy.org). Reprinted with permission.

An ectopic pregnancy occurs when the fertilized egg attaches itself in a place other than inside the uterus. Almost all ectopic pregnancies occur in a fallopian tube, and are thus sometimes called tubal pregnancies. The fallopian tubes are not designed to hold a growing embryo; the fertilized egg in a tubal pregnancy cannot develop normally and must be treated. An ectopic pregnancy happens in one out of sixty pregnancies.

What causes an ectopic pregnancy?

Ectopic pregnancies are caused by one or more of the following:

- An infection or inflammation of the fallopian tube can cause it to become partially or entirely blocked.
- Scar tissue left behind from a previous infection or an operation on the tube may also impede the egg's movement.
- Previous surgery in the pelvic area or on the tubes can cause adhesions.
- An abnormality in the tube's shape can be caused by abnormal growths or a birth defect.

Who is at risk for having an ectopic pregnancy?

Women who are more at risk for having an ectopic pregnancy include the following:

- Are thirty-five to forty-four years of age
- Have had a previous ectopic pregnancy
- Have had pelvic or abdominal surgery

- Have pelvic inflammatory disease (PID)
- Have had several induced abortions
- Women who get pregnant after having a tubal ligation or while an intrauterine device (IUD) is in place

What are the symptoms of an ectopic pregnancy?

Although you may experience typical signs and symptoms of pregnancy, the following symptoms may be used to help recognize a potential ectopic pregnancy:

- Sharp or stabbing pain that may come and go and vary in intensity. The pain may be in the pelvis, abdomen, or even the shoulder and neck (due to blood from a ruptured ectopic pregnancy gathering up under the diaphragm).
- Vaginal bleeding, heavier or lighter than your normal period.
- Gastrointestinal symptoms.
- Weakness, dizziness, or fainting.

It is important for you to seek emergency care if you are experiencing sharp pain or have bleeding.

How is an ectopic pregnancy diagnosed?

Ectopic pregnancies are diagnosed by your physician, who will probably first perform a pelvic exam to locate pain, tenderness, or a mass in the abdomen. Your physician will also use an ultrasound to determine whether the uterus contains a developing fetus.

The measurement of human chorionic gonadotropin (hCG) levels is also important. An hCG level that is lower than what would be expected is one reason to suspect an ectopic pregnancy. Low levels of progesterone may also indicate that a pregnancy is abnormal.

Your physician may do a culdocentesis, which is a procedure that involves inserting a needle into the space at the very top of the vagina, behind the uterus and in front of the rectum. The presence of blood in this area may indicate bleeding from a ruptured fallopian tube.

How is an ectopic pregnancy treated?

An ectopic pregnancy may be treated in any of the following ways:

- Methotrexate may be given, which allows the body to absorb the pregnancy tissue and may save the fallopian tube, depending on how far the pregnancy has developed.
- If the tube has become stretched or it has ruptured and started bleeding, all or part of the fallopian tube may have to be removed. Bleeding needs to be stopped promptly, and emergency surgery is needed.
- Laparoscopic surgery under general anesthesia may be performed. This procedure involves a surgeon using a laparoscope to remove the ectopic pregnancy and repair or remove the affected fallopian tube. If the ectopic pregnancy cannot be removed by a laparoscope procedure, then another surgical procedure called a laparotomy may be done.

What about my future?

Your hCG level will need to be rechecked on a regular basis until it reaches zero if you did not have your entire fallopian tube removed. An hCG level that remains high could indicate that the ectopic tissue was not entirely removed, which would require surgery or medical management with methotrexate.

The chances of having a successful pregnancy after an ectopic pregnancy may be lower than normal, but this will depend on why the pregnancy was ectopic and your medical history. If the fallopian tubes have been left in place, you have approximately a 60 percent chance of having a successful pregnancy in the future.

Section 31.2

Miscarriage

Reprinted from "Miscarriage," National Institute of Child Health and Human Development, May 24, 2007.

What is a miscarriage?

A miscarriage, sometimes called pregnancy loss, is the loss of pregnancy from natural causes before the twentieth week of pregnancy. Most miscarriages occur very early in the pregnancy, often before a woman even knows she is pregnant.

What causes a miscarriage?

There are many different causes for a miscarriage, some known and others unknown. In most cases, there is nothing a woman can do to prevent a miscarriage.

There are some factors that may contribute to miscarriage:

- The most common cause of miscarriage in the first trimester is a chromosomal abnormality in the fetus. This usually results from a problem with the sperm or egg that prevents the fetus from developing properly.
- During the second trimester, problems with the uterus or cervix can contribute to miscarriage.
- Women with a disorder called polycystic ovary syndrome are three times more likely to miscarry during the early months of pregnancy than women who don't have the syndrome.
- Women who have miscarriages can and often do become pregnant again, with normal pregnancy outcomes.

What are the symptoms of and treatments for miscarriage?

Signs of a miscarriage can include the following:

- Vaginal spotting or bleeding

- Cramping or abdominal pain
- Fluid or tissue passing from the vagina

Although vaginal bleeding is a common symptom when a woman has a miscarriage, many pregnant women have spotting early in their pregnancy but do not miscarry. But, pregnant women who have symptoms such as bleeding should contact their health care provider immediately.

Women who miscarry early in their pregnancy usually do not need any treatment. In some cases, a woman may need a procedure called a dilatation and curettage (D&C) to remove tissue remaining in the uterus. A D&C can be done in a health care provider's office, an outpatient clinic, or a hospital.

Section 31.3

Stillbirth

Reprinted from "Stillbirth," National Institute of Child Health and Human Development, September 10, 2006.

What is a stillbirth?

A stillbirth is the loss of pregnancy due to natural causes after the twentieth week of pregnancy. It can occur before delivery or during delivery.

What are the signs of a stillbirth?

In some cases of stillbirth, the mother may notice a decrease in the movement or kicking of the fetus. In these cases, the health care provider uses an ultrasound, a machine that uses sound waves to create a picture of the fetus, to learn more about its health.

If the fetus has died, an autopsy and placental examination is performed to get information on why the baby died. But it is not always possible to tell why the baby died.

If you are pregnant and have concerns about stillbirth, ask your health care provider if there are ways he or she wants you to track movement.

What are the causes of a stillbirth?

Causes of a stillbirth may include the following:

- Problems with the placenta, such an abruption in which the placenta peels away from the uterine wall
- Chromosomal abnormalities resulting from defects in the sperm or egg that make the fetus unable to develop properly
- Other physical problems in the fetus
- Fetuses that are small for their gestational age or not growing at an appropriate rate
- Bacterial infections that can cause complications and death to the fetus

In at least half of all cases, researchers can find no cause for the pregnancy loss.

What medical procedures are used when there is a stillbirth?

In some cases it is medically necessary for a woman to deliver the fetus immediately after the diagnosis of a stillbirth.

In other cases, the couple can decide when they want to deliver the fetus.

A healthcare provider can induce labor or perform a caesarean section to deliver the fetus. A woman will usually go into labor on her own within two weeks after the fetal death.

Part Four

Cancer in Women

Chapter 32

Self-Examination Can Lead to Early Cancer Detection

Chapter Contents

Section 32.1

How to Spot Skin Cancer

This section includes text from "Self-Examination" and "Warning Signs: The ABCDEs of Melanoma," and excerpts from "The Ugly Duckling Sign: An Early Melanoma Recognition Tool," © 2008 Skin Cancer Foundation (www.skincancer.org). Reprinted with permission.

Self-Examination

Coupled with a yearly skin exam by a doctor, self-examination of your skin once a month is the best way to detect the early warning signs of basal cell carcinoma, squamous cell carcinoma, and melanoma, the three main types of skin cancer. Look for a new growth or any skin change.

What you'll need: a bright light; a full-length mirror; a hand mirror; two chairs or stools; a blow dryer.

Examine head and face, using one or both mirrors. Use blow dryer to inspect scalp.

Check hands, including nails. In full-length mirror, examine elbows, arms, underarms.

Focus on neck, chest, torso. Women: Check under breasts.

With back to the mirror, use hand mirror to inspect back of neck, shoulders, upper arms, back, buttocks, legs.

Sitting down, check legs and feet, including soles, heels, and nails. Use hand mirror to examine genitals.

Melanoma, the deadliest form of skin cancer, is especially hard to stop once it has spread (metastasized) to other parts of the body. But it can be readily treated in its earliest stages.

Warning Signs: The ABCDEs of Melanoma

Moles, brown spots, and growths on the skin are usually harmless—but not always. Anyone who has more than one hundred moles is at greater risk for melanoma. The first signs can appear in one or more of these moles. That's why it's so important to get to know your skin very well, so you can recognize any changes in the moles on your body. Look for the ABCDEs of melanoma, and if you see one or more, make an appointment with a dermatologist immediately.

Asymmetry: If you draw a line through the mole, the two halves will not match, meaning it is asymmetrical, a warning sign for melanoma.

Border: The borders of an early melanoma tend to be uneven. The edges may be scalloped or notched.

Color: Having a variety of colors is another warning signal. A number of different shades of brown, tan, or black could appear. A melanoma may also become red, white, or blue.

Diameter: Melanomas usually are larger in diameter than the size of the eraser on your pencil (1/4 inch or 6 mm), but they may sometimes be smaller when first detected.

Evolving: Any change—in size, shape, color, elevation, or another trait, or any new symptom such as bleeding, itching, or crusting—points to danger.

Prompt action is your best protection. Common moles and melanomas do not look alike.

Table 32.1. Characteristics of Benign and Malignant Skin Growths

Benign	Malignant
Symmetrical	Asymmetrical
Borders are even	Borders are uneven
One shade	Two or more shades
Smaller than 1/4 inch	Larger than 1/4 inch

The Ugly Duckling Sign: An Early Melanoma Recognition Tool

A recently developed early detection tool can improve early diagnosis critical to the successful treatment of melanoma.

For many years, the early warning signs of melanoma have been identified by the acronym "ABCDE" (A stands for asymmetry, B stands for border, C for color, D for diameter, and E for evolving or changing was recently added.). While the ABCDE rule helps detect many melanomas, there are a group of melanomas that do not manifest the ABCDE features. Recently, several melanoma specialists developed a new method of sight detection for skin lesions which could be melanoma.

This new method of sight detection for skin lesions is based on the concept that these melanomas look different—i.e., "the ugly duckling"—compared to surrounding moles. Thus, during skin self examination, patients and physicians should be looking for lesions that manifest the ABCDEs *and* for lesions that look different compared to surrounding moles.

As reported in the December 2007 issue of *The Melanoma Letter*, a publication of the Skin Cancer Foundation, an approach combining the ABCDEs and the "Ugly Duckling" technique should improve the chances of early detection of all types of melanoma. In the article "The 'Ugly Duckling' Sign: An Early Melanoma Recognition Tool For Clinicians and the Public" by Dr. Alon Scope and Dr. Ashfaq A. Marghoob of Memorial Sloan Kettering Cancer Center (New York, N.Y.), the premise of the ugly duckling sign is that the patient's "normal" moles resemble each other, like siblings.

The doctors suggest thinking of "the ugly duckling" mole, a.k.a. "the outlier," as the lesion that, at a given moment in time, looks or feels different than the patient's other moles, or that over time, changes differently than the patient's other moles. The "ugly duckling" methodology may be especially useful in the detection of nodular melanoma, a dangerous type of melanoma, which notoriously lacks the classic ABCDE signs.

Section 32.2

How to Do a Breast Self-Examination

Excerpted from "Questions and Answers about Breast Health and Breast Cancer," © 2007. Reprinted with permission from the American Institute for Cancer Research.

Breast Self-Examination

Breast self-examination (BSE) should be done once a month so you become familiar with the usual appearance and feel of your breasts. Familiarity makes it easier to notice any changes. Early discovery of a change from what is normal for you is the main purpose of BSE.

The best time to do BSE is one week after your period ends, when your breasts are least likely to be tender and swollen. After menopause, or if you have had a hysterectomy, perform your BSE on the first day of each month.

How to Do a Breast Self-Examination

1. Stand before a mirror with your arms at your sides. Look at both breasts for anything unusual, such as puckering, dimpling, scaling of the skin, or fluid leaking from the nipples.

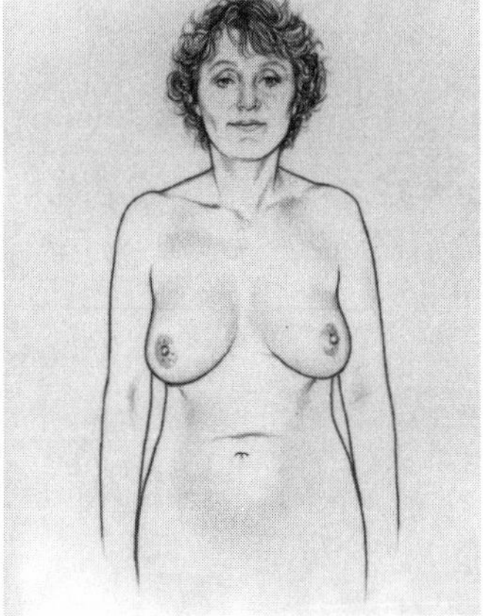

Figure 32.1. *Breast self-exam: Step one. (Source: National Cancer Institute)*

The next two steps are designed to emphasize any change in the shape or contour of your breasts. As you do them you should be able to feel your chest muscles tighten.

2. Clasp your hands behind your head and press your hands forward. Look closely at your breasts in the mirror.

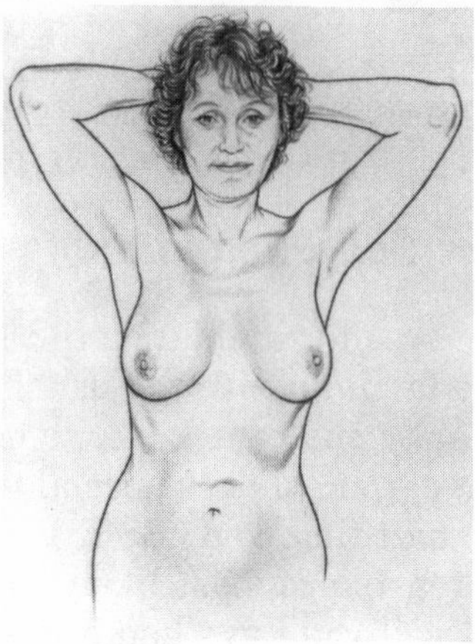

Figure 32.2. *Breast self-exam: Step two. (Source: National Cancer Institute)*

3. Press your hands firmly on your hips and bow slightly toward the mirror as you pull your shoulders and elbows forward. Once again, look closely at your breasts in the mirror. Some women do the next part of the exam in the shower. Fingers glide over soapy skin, making it easy to concentrate on the texture underneath.

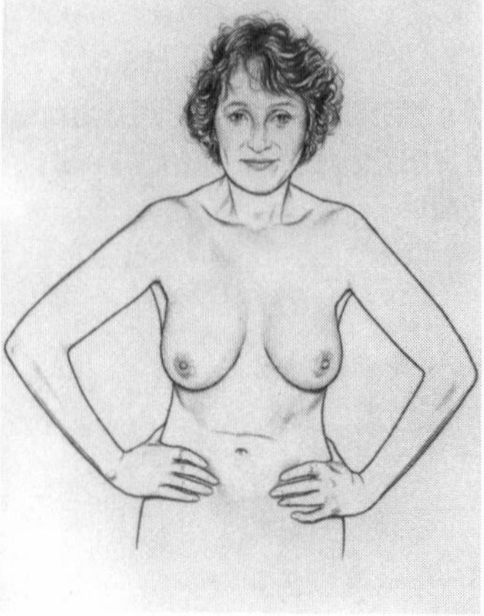

Figure 32.3. *Breast self-exam: Step three. (Source: National Cancer Institute)*

4. Raise your left arm. Use three or four fingers of your right hand to explore your left breast carefully. Beginning at the outer edge, firmly press the flat part of your fingers in small circles, moving the circles slowly around the breast. Gradually work toward the nipple. Be sure to cover the entire breast. Pay special attention to the area between the breast and armpit, including the armpit itself. Feel for any unusual lumps or masses under the skin.

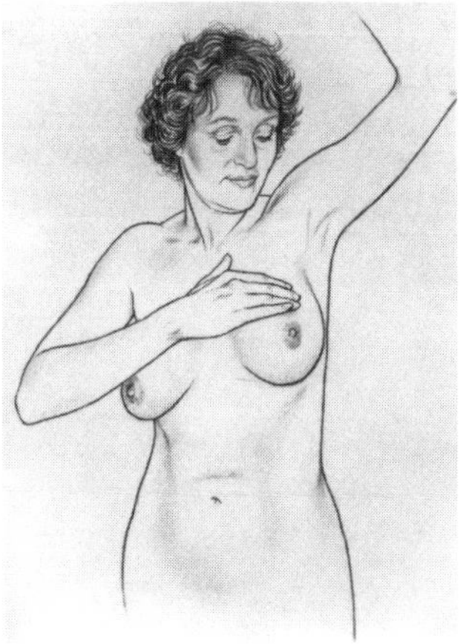

Figure 32.4. *Breast self-exam: Step four. (Source: National Cancer Institute)*

5. Gently squeeze the nipple and look for any fluid discharge. Repeat steps 4 and 5 on your right breast. The last part of the exam should be done while lying down.

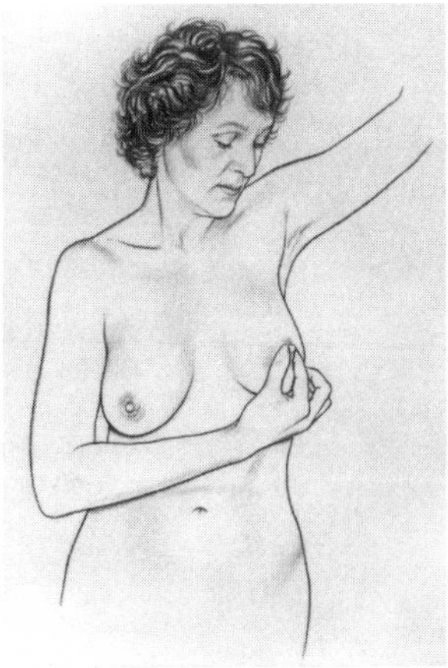

Figure 32.5. *Breast self-exam: Step five. (Source: National Cancer Institute)*

6. Lie flat on your back with your left arm over your head and a pillow or folded towel under your left shoulder. This position flattens the breast and makes it easier to examine. Using the same motions described in steps 4 and 5, examine your left breast, underarm area, and nipple. Repeat on your right side.

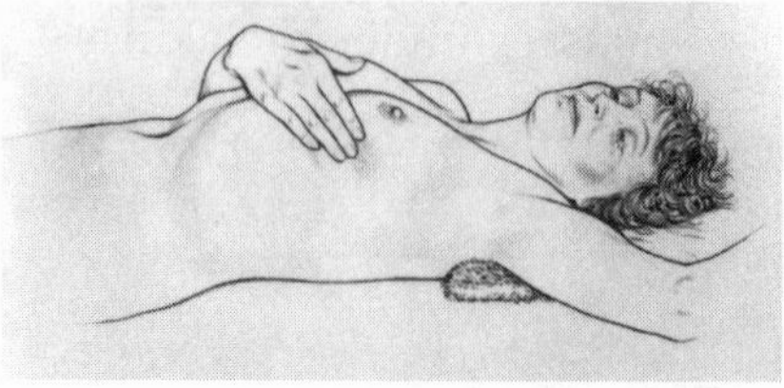

Figure 32.6. *Breast self-exam: Step six. (Source: National Cancer Institute)*

Chapter 33

Breast Cancer

Breast cancer is one of the most common cancers in American women. It is more common among older women than younger women. Men can get breast cancer too, although they account for only 1 percent of all reported cases.

When cancer grows in breast tissue and spreads outside the breast, cancer cells are often found in the lymph nodes under the arm. If the cancer has reached these nodes, it means that cancer cells may have spread, or metastasized, to other parts of the body.

Breast cancer is not contagious. A woman cannot "catch" breast cancer from other women who have the disease. Also, breast cancer is not caused by an injury to the breast. Most women who develop breast cancer do not have any known risk factors or a history of the disease in their families.

Today, more women are surviving breast cancer than ever before. Over two million women are breast cancer survivors.

There are several ways to treat breast cancer, but all treatments work best when the disease is found early.

Every day, researchers are working to find new and better ways to detect and treat cancer. Many studies of new approaches for women with breast cancer are under way. With early detection and prompt and appropriate treatment, the outlook for women with breast cancer can be positive.

Excerpted from "Breast Cancer," NIH Senior Health, October 26, 2006.

Causes and Risk Factors

No one knows why some women develop breast cancer and others do not. Although the disease may affect younger women, three-fourths of all breast cancer occurs in women age fifty or older.

Researchers often talk about breast cancer in two ways: *in situ* and invasive. *In situ* refers to cancer that has not spread beyond its site of origin. Invasive applies to cancer that has spread to the tissue around it.

Table 33.1 shows what the approximate chances are of a woman getting invasive breast cancer in her lifetime.

Older age and the following risk factors increase a woman's chance of getting breast cancer:

- Breast cancer among one or more of your close relatives, such as a sister, mother, or daughter, increases the risk.
- Having no children or having your first child in your mid-thirties or later increases the risk.
- Having your first menstrual period before age twelve increases the risk
- Gaining weight after menopause, especially after natural menopause or after age sixty increases the risk.
- Race can be a factor. White women are at greater risk than black women. However, black women diagnosed with breast cancer are more likely to die of the disease.
- Five to 10 percent of all breast cancers are thought to be inherited.

When breast cancer first develops, there may be no symptoms at all. But as the cancer grows, it can cause changes that women should

Table 33.1. Age-Adjusted Likelihood of Developing Breast Cancer

Ages	Chances
30 to 40	1 out of 257
40 to 50	1 out of 67
50 to 60	1 out of 36
60 to 70	1 out of 28
70 to 80	1 out of 24

watch for. You can help safeguard your health by learning the following warning signs of breast cancer:

- A lump or thickening in or near the breast or in the underarm area
- A change in the size or shape of the breast
- Nipple discharge or tenderness, or the nipple is pulled back or inverted into the breast
- Ridges or pitting of the breast—the skin looks like the skin of an orange
- A change in the way the skin of the breast, areola, or nipple looks or feels (for example, the skin may be warm, swollen, red, or scaly)

You should see your doctor about any symptoms like these. Most often, they are not cancer, but it's important to check with the doctor so that any problems can be diagnosed and treated as early as possible.

Testing and Diagnosis

Most cancers in their early, most treatable stages do not cause any symptoms. That is why it's important to have regular tests to check for cancer long before you might notice anything wrong.

When breast cancer is found early, it is more likely to be treated successfully. Checking for cancer in a person who does not have any symptoms is called screening. Screening tests for breast cancer include, among others, clinical breast exams and mammograms.

During a clinical breast exam, the doctor or other health care professional checks the breasts and underarms for lumps or other changes that could be a sign of breast cancer. A mammogram is a special x-ray of the breast that often can detect cancers that are too small for a woman or her doctor to feel.

Several studies show that mammography screening has reduced the number of deaths from breast cancer. However, some other studies have not shown a clear benefit from mammography.

Scientists are continuing to examine the level of benefit that mammography can produce. For the time being, the National Cancer Institute recommends the following:

- If you are a woman in your forties, you should have mammography screening every one to two years.

- If you are a woman age fifty and older, you should have mammography screening every one to two years.
- If you are a woman who is at higher than average risk for breast cancer, you should seek expert medical advice about whether to begin screening before age forty and how often to have screening mammography.

Between 5 and 10 percent of mammogram results are abnormal and require more testing. Most of these follow-up tests confirm that no cancer was present.

If needed, the most common follow-up test a doctor will recommend is called a biopsy. This is a procedure where a small amount of fluid or tissue is removed from the breast to make a diagnosis. A doctor might perform fine needle aspiration, a needle or core biopsy, or a surgical biopsy.

With fine needle aspiration, doctors numb the area and use a thin needle to remove fluid and/or cells from a breast lump. If the fluid is clear, it may not need to be checked out by a lab.

For a needle biopsy, sometimes called a core biopsy, doctors use a needle to remove tissue from an area that looks suspicious on a mammogram but cannot be felt. This tissue goes to a lab where a pathologist examines it to see if any of the cells are cancerous.

In a surgical biopsy, a surgeon removes a sample of a lump or suspicious area. Sometimes it is necessary to remove the entire lump or suspicious area, plus an area of healthy tissue around the edges. The tissue then goes to a lab where a pathologist examines it under a microscope to check for cancer cells.

Doctors are studying another type of surgical biopsy that removes less breast tissue. It is called an image-guided needle breast biopsy, or stereotactic biopsy. If approved for general use, it would become an important surgical tool.

Other techniques used to find cancer include a new way of reading mammograms called digital mammography. Magnetic resonance imaging, or MRI, and ultrasound are two other techniques which researchers think might detect breast cancer with greater accuracy.

Treatment and Research

There are many treatment options for women with breast cancer. The choice of treatment depends on your age and general health, the stage of the cancer, whether or not it has spread beyond the breast, and other factors.

Planning Treatment

If tests show that you have cancer, you should talk with your doctor and make treatment decisions as soon as possible. Studies show that early treatment leads to better outcomes.

Before starting treatment, you may want another doctor to review the diagnosis and treatment plan. Some insurance companies require a second opinion. Others may pay for a second opinion if you request it.

Some breast cancer patients take part in studies of new treatments. These studies, called clinical trials, are designed to find out whether a new treatment is both safe and effective.

Often, clinical trials compare a new treatment with a standard one so that doctors can learn which is more effective. Women with breast cancer who are interested in taking part in a clinical trial should talk to their doctor.

What Is Staging?

Once breast cancer has been found, it is staged. Staging means determining how far the cancer has progressed. Through staging, the doctor can tell if the cancer has spread and, if so, to what parts of the body. More tests may be performed to help determine the stage. Knowing the stage of the disease helps the doctor plan treatment.

Staging will let the doctor know the following:

- The size of the tumor and exactly where it is in the breast
- If the cancer has spread within the breast
- If cancer is present in the lymph nodes under the arm
- If cancer is present in other parts of the body

Here are the stages of breast cancer:

- Stage 0 is very early breast cancer that has not spread within or outside the breast. Doctors often refer to this type of cancer as *in situ* or non-invasive cancer.
- Stage I and stage II also are early stages of breast cancer. Stage I means that the tumor has not spread beyond the breast. In stage II, the tumor may be larger and may have spread to the lymph nodes.
- Stage III is called locally advanced cancer. Here the tumor has spread beyond the breast to lymph nodes or to other tissues near the breast.

- Stage IV is metastatic cancer. In this stage the cancer has spread beyond the breast and the underarm lymph nodes to other parts of the body, most often the bones, lungs, liver, or brain.

The choice of treatment is based on many factors. For stage I, II or III cancers, the main goals are to treat the cancer and reduce the chance it will come back, either at the place where the tumor first occurred or elsewhere in the body. For stage IV cancer, the goal is to improve symptoms and prolong survival.

Standard Treatments

There are a number of treatments for breast cancer, but the ones women choose most often—alone or in combination—are surgery, radiation therapy, chemotherapy, and hormone therapy.

Here is what the standard cancer treatments are designed to do:

- Surgery takes out the cancer.
- Hormone therapy keeps cancer cells from getting the hormones they need to survive and grow.
- Radiation therapy uses high-energy beams to kill cancer cells and shrink tumors.
- Chemotherapy uses anti-cancer drugs to kill cancer cells.

Treatment for breast cancer may involve local or whole-body therapy. Doctors use local therapies, such as surgery or radiation, to remove or destroy breast cancer in a specific area. Whole-body, or systemic, treatments like chemotherapy, hormonal, or biological therapies are used to destroy or control cancer throughout the body. Some patients have both kinds of treatment.

If you have early-stage breast cancer, one common treatment available to you is a lumpectomy combined with radiation therapy. A lumpectomy is surgery that preserves a woman's breast.

In a lumpectomy, the surgeon removes only the tumor and a small amount of the surrounding tissue. The survival rate for a woman who has this therapy plus radiation is similar to that for a woman who chooses a radical mastectomy, which is complete removal of a breast.

If you have breast cancer that has spread locally—just to other parts of the breast—your treatment may involve a combination of chemotherapy and surgery. Doctors first shrink the tumor with chemotherapy and then remove it through surgery. Shrinking the tumor before surgery may allow a woman to avoid a mastectomy and keep her breast.

In the past, doctors would remove a lot of lymph nodes near breast tumors to see if the cancer had spread. Some doctors are also using a method called sentinel node biopsy. Using a dye or radioactive tracer, surgeons locate the first or "sentinel" lymph node closest to the tumor, and remove only that node to see if the cancer has spread.

If the breast cancer has spread to other parts of the body, such as the lung or bone, you might receive chemotherapy and/or hormonal therapy to destroy cancer cells and control the disease. Radiation therapy may also be useful to control tumors in other parts of the body.

Latest Research

Several new technologies offer hope for making future treatment easier for women with breast cancer. Using a special tool, doctors can today insert a miniature camera through the nipple and into a milk duct in the breast to examine the area for cancer. In the future, doctors may use this tool to deliver treatment.

Researchers are testing another technique to help women who have undergone weeks of conventional radiation therapy. Using a small catheter—a tube with a balloon tip—doctors can deliver tiny radioactive beads to a place on the breast where cancer tissue has been removed. This can reduce the therapy time to a matter of days.

New drug therapies also are on the horizon. Findings from several clinical trials show that the chemotherapy drug paclitaxel combined with the drugs cyclophosphamide and doxorubicin can help women with tumors that have spread to other parts of the body.

This mix of drugs may increase the length of time you will live or the length of time you will live without cancer. It may someday prove useful for some women with localized breast cancer after they have had surgery.

New research shows women with early-stage breast cancer who took the drug letrozole, an aromatase inhibitor, after they completed five years of tamoxifen therapy significantly reduced their risk of breast cancer recurrence.

Also, other new research found a test that can predict both the risk of breast cancer recurrence and who is most likely to benefit from chemotherapy such as letrozole. Herceptin® is another drug commonly used to treat women who have a certain type of breast cancer. This drug slows or stops the growth of cancer cells by blocking Her-2, a protein found on the surface of some types of breast cancer cells.

Approximately 20 percent of breast cancers produce too much Her-2. These "Her-2 positive" tumors tend to grow faster and are generally more likely to return than tumors that do not overproduce Her-2.

Cancer treatments like chemotherapy can be systemic, meaning they affect whole tissues, organs, or the entire body. Herceptin®, however, is the first drug used to target only a specific molecule involved in breast cancer.

Results from two recent clinical trials show that those patients with early-stage Her-2 positive breast cancer who received Herceptin® in combination with chemotherapy had a 52 percent decrease in risk in the cancer returning compared with patients who received chemotherapy treatment alone.

In an attempt to further specialize breast cancer treatment, The Trial Assigning Individualized Options for Treatment, or TAILORx, was recently initiated by the National Cancer Institute (NCI). This study will enroll ten thousand women to examine whether appropriate treatment can be assigned based on genes that are frequently associated with risk of recurrence of breast cancer.

The goal of TAILORx is important because the majority of women with early-stage breast cancer are advised to receive chemotherapy in addition to radiation and hormonal therapy, yet research has not demonstrated that chemotherapy benefits all of them equally.

TAILORx seeks to examine many of a woman's genes simultaneously and use this information in choosing a treatment course, thus sparing women unnecessary treatment if chemotherapy is not likely to be of substantial benefit to them.

Several methods show promise in reducing the risk of breast cancer. In October 1998, the U.S. Food and Drug Administration, or FDA, approved the drug tamoxifen to lower the chance of cancer in high-risk women.

The approval of tamoxifen followed a clinical trial sponsored by the National Cancer Institute that included more than thirteen thousand premenopausal and postmenopausal women. All of the women were considered at high risk for breast cancer.

One group of women took the drug tamoxifen and another took a placebo—an inactive pill that looked like tamoxifen. The results of the study showed a 49 percent decrease in breast cancer among women who took tamoxifen.

Tamoxifen does have side effects. The most serious in some women are an increased risk of endometrial cancer, uterine sarcoma, and an increased risk of blood clots. Women at high risk for breast cancer may want to consult their doctor to see if tamoxifen may help them.

The Study of Tamoxifen and Raloxifene (STAR) is a more recent clinical trial sponsored by the National Cancer Institute. STAR enlisted nearly twenty thousand women to compare tamoxifen to the drug raloxifene for effectiveness in reducing of breast cancer risk.

Raloxifene, marketed as Evista®, has been approved for use to lower the risk of and treat osteoporosis.

Initial results of the STAR trial show that raloxifene works as well as tamoxifen in reducing breast cancer risk for postmenopausal women at increased risk of the disease. Both drugs decrease risk by about 50 percent.

In addition, women enrolled in STAR who were assigned to take raloxifene had fewer uterine cancers, blood clots, and cataracts than those taking tamoxifen.

However, taking raloxifene raised the risk of blood clots and fatal strokes in women already at risk.

Chapter 34

Cervical Cancer

The Cervix

The cervix is part of a woman's reproductive system. It is the lower, narrow part of the uterus (womb). The uterus is a hollow, pear-shaped organ in the lower abdomen. The cervix connects the uterus to the vagina. The vagina leads to the outside of the body.

The cervical canal is a passageway. Blood flows from the uterus through the canal into the vagina during a woman's menstrual period. The cervix also produces mucus. The mucus helps sperm move from the vagina into the uterus. During pregnancy, the cervix is tightly closed to help keep the baby inside the uterus. During childbirth, the cervix dilates (opens) to allow the baby to pass through the vagina.

Understanding Cancer

Tumors can be benign or malignant.

Benign tumors are not cancer: Benign tumors are rarely life threatening. Generally, benign tumors can be removed, and they usually do not grow back. Cells from benign tumors do not invade the tissues around them or spread to other parts of the body. Polyps, cysts, and genital warts are types of benign growths on the cervix.

Malignant tumors are cancer: Malignant tumors are generally more serious than benign tumors. They may be life threatening. Malignant

---

Excerpted from "What You Need to Know about Cancer of the Cervix," National Cancer Institute, March 18, 2005.

tumors often can be removed, but sometimes they grow back. Cells from malignant tumors can invade and damage nearby tissues and organs and can spread (metastasize) to other parts of the body. Cancer cells spread by breaking away from the original (primary) tumor and entering the bloodstream or lymphatic system. The cells invade other organs and form new tumors that damage these organs. The spread of cancer is called metastasis.

Risk Factors

Studies have found a number of factors that may increase the risk of cervical cancer. These factors may act together to increase the risk even more.

Human papillomaviruses (HPVs): HPV infection is the main risk factor for cervical cancer. HPV is a group of viruses that can infect the cervix. HPV infections are very common. These viruses can be passed from person to person through sexual contact. Most adults have been infected with HPV at some time in their lives. Some types of HPV can cause changes to cells in the cervix. These changes can lead to genital warts, cancer, and other problems. Doctors may check for HPV even if there are no warts or other symptoms. If a woman has an HPV infection, her doctor can discuss ways to avoid infecting other people. The Pap test can detect cell changes in the cervix caused by HPV. Treatment of these cell changes can prevent cervical cancer. There are several treatment methods, including freezing or burning the infected tissue. Sometimes medicine also helps.

Lack of regular Pap tests: Cervical cancer is more common among women who do not have regular Pap tests. The Pap test helps doctors find precancerous cells. Treating precancerous cervical changes often prevents cancer.

Weakened immune system (the body's natural defense system): Women with human immunodeficiency virus (HIV), the virus that causes acquired immunodeficiency syndrome (AIDS), or who take drugs that suppress the immune system have a higher-than-average risk of developing cervical cancer. For these women, doctors suggest regular screening for cervical cancer.

Age: Cancer of the cervix occurs most often in women over the age of forty.

Sexual history: Women who have had many sexual partners have a higher-than-average risk of developing cervical cancer. Also, a woman who has had sexual intercourse with a man who has had many sexual partners may be at higher risk of developing cervical cancer. In both cases, the risk of developing cervical cancer is higher because these women have a higher-than-average risk of HPV infection.

Smoking cigarettes: Women with an HPV infection who smoke cigarettes have a higher risk of cervical cancer than women with HPV infection who do not smoke.

Using birth control pills for a long time: Using birth control pills for a long time (five or more years) may increase the risk of cervical cancer among women with HPV infection.

Having many children: Studies suggest that giving birth to many children may increase the risk of cervical cancer among women with HPV infection.

Diethylstilbestrol (DES): DES may increase the risk of a rare form of cervical cancer and certain other cancers of the reproductive system in daughters exposed to this drug before birth. DES was given to some pregnant women in the United States between about 1940 and 1971. (It is no longer given to pregnant women.)

Women who think they may be at risk for cancer of the cervix should discuss this concern with their doctor. They may want to ask about a schedule for checkups.

Screening

Screening to check for cervical changes before there are symptoms is very important. Screening can help the doctor find abnormal cells before cancer develops. Finding and treating abnormal cells can prevent most cervical cancer. Also, screening can help find cancer early, when treatment is more likely to be effective.

Doctors recommend that women help reduce their risk of cervical cancer by having regular Pap tests. A Pap test (sometimes called Pap smear or cervical smear) is a simple test used to look at cervical cells. For most women, the test is not painful. A Pap test is done in a doctor's office or clinic during a pelvic exam. The doctor or nurse scrapes a sample of cells from the cervix, and then smears the cells on a glass slide. In a new type of Pap test (liquid-based Pap test), the cells are rinsed into a small container of liquid. A special machine puts the cells onto slides. For both types of Pap test, a lab checks the cells on the slides under a microscope for abnormalities.

Pap tests can find cervical cancer or abnormal cells that can lead to cervical cancer. Doctors generally recommend that:

- Women should begin having Pap tests three years after they begin having sexual intercourse, or when they reach age twenty-one (whichever comes first).
- Most women should have a Pap test at least once every three years.
- Women aged sixty-five to seventy who have had at least three normal Pap tests and no abnormal Pap tests in the past ten years may decide, after speaking with their doctor, to stop cervical cancer screening.
- Women who have had a hysterectomy (surgery) to remove the uterus and cervix, also called a total hysterectomy, do not need to have cervical cancer screening. However, if the surgery was treatment for precancerous cells or cancer, the woman should continue with screening.

Women should talk with their doctor about when they should begin having Pap tests, how often to have them, and when they can stop having them. This is especially important for women at higher-than-average risk of cervical cancer.

Most often, abnormal cells found by a Pap test are not cancerous. However, some abnormal conditions may become cancer over time:

- **Low-grade squamous intraepithelial lesion (LSIL):** LSILs are mild cell changes on the surface of the cervix. Such changes often are caused by HPV infections. LSILs are common, especially in young women. LSILs are not cancer. Even without treatment, most LSILs stay the same or go away. However, some turn into high-grade lesions, which may lead to cancer.
- **High-grade squamous intraepithelial lesion (HSIL):** HSILs are not cancer, but without treatment they may lead to cancer. The precancerous cells are only on the surface of the cervix. They look very different from normal cells.

Symptoms

Precancerous changes and early cancers of the cervix generally do not cause pain or other symptoms. It is important not to wait to feel pain before seeing a doctor.

When the disease gets worse, women may notice one or more of these symptoms:

- Abnormal vaginal bleeding
- Bleeding that occurs between regular menstrual periods
- Bleeding after sexual intercourse, douching, or a pelvic exam
- Menstrual periods that last longer and are heavier than before
- Bleeding after menopause
- Increased vaginal discharge
- Pelvic pain
- Pain during sexual intercourse

Infections or other health problems may also cause these symptoms. Only a doctor can tell for sure. A woman with any of these symptoms should tell her doctor so that problems can be diagnosed and treated as early as possible.

Diagnosis

If a woman has a symptom or Pap test results that suggest precancerous cells or cancer of the cervix, her doctor will suggest other procedures to make a diagnosis.

These may include the following:

- **Colposcopy:** The doctor uses a colposcope to look at the cervix. The colposcope combines a bright light with a magnifying lens to make tissue easier to see. It is not inserted into the vagina. A colposcopy is usually done in the doctor's office or clinic.
- **Biopsy:** The doctor removes tissue to look for precancerous cells or cancer cells. Most women have their biopsy in the doctor's office with local anesthesia. A pathologist checks the tissue with a microscope.
- **Punch biopsy:** The doctor uses a sharp, hollow device to pinch off small samples of cervical tissue.

- **Loop electrosurgical excision procedure (LEEP):** The doctor uses an electric wire loop to slice off a thin, round piece of tissue.
- **Endocervical curettage:** The doctor uses a curette (a small, spoon-shaped instrument) to scrape a small sample of tissue from the cervical canal. Some doctors may use a thin, soft brush instead of a curette.
- **Conization:** The doctor removes a cone-shaped sample of tissue. A conization, or cone biopsy, lets the pathologist see if abnormal cells are in the tissue beneath the surface of the cervix. The doctor may do this test in the hospital under general anesthesia. Conization also may be used to remove a precancerous area.

Removing tissue from the cervix may cause some bleeding or other discharge. The area usually heals quickly. Women may also feel some pain similar to menstrual cramps. Medicine can relieve this discomfort.

Staging

If the biopsy shows that you have cancer, your doctor will do a thorough pelvic exam and may remove additional tissue to learn the extent (stage) of your disease. The stage tells whether the tumor has invaded nearby tissues, whether the cancer has spread and, if so, to what parts of the body.

These are the stages of cervical cancer:

- **Stage 0:** The cancer is found only in the top layer of cells in the tissue that lines the cervix. Stage 0 is also called carcinoma in situ.
- **Stage I:** The cancer has invaded the cervix beneath the top layer of cells. It is found only in the cervix.
- **Stage II:** The cancer extends beyond the cervix into nearby tissues. It extends to the upper part of the vagina. The cancer does not invade the lower third of the vagina or the pelvic wall (the lining of the part of the body between the hips).
- **Stage III:** The cancer extends to the lower part of the vagina. It also may have spread to the pelvic wall and nearby lymph nodes.

- **Stage IV:** The cancer has spread to the bladder, rectum, or other parts of the body.
- **Recurrent cancer:** The cancer was treated, but has returned after a period of time during which it could not be detected. The cancer may show up again in the cervix or in other parts of the body.

Getting a Second Opinion

Before starting treatment, you might want a second opinion about the diagnosis and treatment plan. Many insurance companies cover a second opinion if you or your doctor requests it. It may take some time and effort to gather medical records and arrange to see another doctor. Usually it is not a problem to take several weeks to get a second opinion. In most cases, the delay in starting treatment will not make treatment less effective. To make sure, you should discuss this delay with your doctor. Some women with cervical cancer need treatment right away.

Methods of Treatment

Women with cervical cancer may be treated with surgery, radiation therapy, chemotherapy, radiation therapy and chemotherapy, or a combination of all three methods.

At any stage of disease, women with cervical cancer may have treatment to control pain and other symptoms, to relieve the side effects of therapy, and to ease emotional and practical problems. This kind of treatment is called supportive care, symptom management, or palliative care.

You may want to talk to your doctor about taking part in a clinical trial, a research study of new treatment methods.

Surgery

Surgery treats the cancer in the cervix and the area close to the tumor.

Most women with early cervical cancer have surgery to remove the cervix and uterus (total hysterectomy). However, for very early (Stage 0) cervical cancer, a hysterectomy may not be needed. Other ways to remove the cancerous tissue include conization, cryosurgery, laser surgery, or LEEP.

Some women need a radical hysterectomy. A radical hysterectomy is surgery to remove the uterus, cervix, and part of the vagina.

With either total or radical hysterectomy, the surgeon may remove both fallopian tubes and ovaries. (This procedure is a salpingo-oophorectomy.)

The surgeon may also remove the lymph nodes near the tumor to see if they contain cancer. If cancer cells have reached the lymph nodes, it means the disease may have spread to other parts of the body.

Radiation Therapy

Radiation therapy (also called radiotherapy) uses high-energy rays to kill cancer cells. It affects cells only in the treated area.

Women have radiation therapy alone, with chemotherapy, or with chemotherapy and surgery. The doctor may suggest radiation therapy instead of surgery for the small number of women who cannot have surgery for medical reasons. Most women with cancer that extends beyond the cervix have radiation therapy and chemotherapy. For cancer that has spread to distant organs, radiation therapy alone may be used.

Chemotherapy

Chemotherapy uses anticancer drugs to kill cancer cells. It is called systemic therapy because the drugs enter the bloodstream and can affect cells all over the body. For treatment of cervical cancer, chemotherapy is generally combined with radiation therapy. For cancer that has spread to distant organs, chemotherapy alone may be used.

Anticancer drugs for cervical cancer are usually given through a vein. Women usually receive treatment in an outpatient part of the hospital, at the doctor's office, or at home. Rarely, a woman needs to stay in the hospital during treatment.

Side Effects of Treatment

Because cancer treatment often damages healthy cells and tissues, unwanted side effects are common. Side effects depend mainly on the type and extent of the treatment. Side effects may not be the same for each woman, and they may change from one treatment session to the next. Before treatment starts, your health care team will explain possible side effects and suggest ways to help you manage them.

Complementary and Alternative Medicine

Some people with cancer use complementary and alternative medicine (CAM) to ease stress or to reduce side effects and symptoms:

- An approach is generally called complementary medicine when it is used along with standard treatment.
- An approach is called alternative medicine when it is used instead of standard treatment.

Acupuncture, massage therapy, herbal products, vitamins or special diets, visualization, meditation, and spiritual healing are types of CAM. Many people say that such approaches help them feel better.

However, some types of CAM, including certain vitamins, may interfere with standard treatment. Combining CAM with standard treatment may even be harmful. Before trying any type of CAM, you should discuss its possible benefits and harmful effects with your doctor.

Some types of CAM are expensive. Health insurance may not cover the cost.

Follow-up Care

Follow-up care after treatment for cervical cancer is important. Even when the cancer seems to have been completely removed or destroyed, the disease sometimes returns because undetected cancer cells remained somewhere in the body after treatment. Your doctor will monitor your recovery and check for recurrence of the cancer. Checkups help ensure that any changes in your health are noted and treated as needed. Checkups may include a physical exam as well as Pap tests and chest x-rays. Between scheduled visits, you should contact the doctor right away if you have any health problems.

Sources of Support

Living with a serious disease such as cervical cancer is not easy. You may worry about caring for your family, keeping your job, or continuing daily activities. Concerns about treatments and managing side effects, hospital stays, and medical bills are also common. Doctors, nurses, and other members of the health care team can answer questions about treatment, working, or other activities. Meeting with a social worker, counselor, or member of the clergy can be helpful if you want to talk about your feelings or concerns. Often, a social worker can suggest resources for financial aid, transportation, home care, or emotional support.

Support groups also can help. In these groups, patients or their family members meet with other patients or their families to share what they have learned about coping with the disease and the effects of treatment. Groups may offer support in person, over the telephone, or on the internet. You may want to talk with a member of your health care team about finding a support group.

The Promise of Cancer Research

Clinical trials are designed to answer important questions and to find out whether new approaches are safe and effective. Research already has led to many advances, and researchers continue to search for more effective methods for dealing with cancer.

Researchers are testing new approaches to treatment, including anticancer drugs and drug combinations. They also are studying different methods, doses, and schedules of radiation therapy. Some trials are combining chemotherapy, surgery, and radiation therapy. Other trials are researching biological therapy.

Researchers also are studying surgery to remove sentinel lymph nodes. A sentinel lymph node is the first lymph node to which the cancer is likely to spread. Today, surgeons often have to remove many lymph nodes and check each of them for cancer. But if the research shows that it is possible to identify the sentinel lymph node (the lymph node most likely to have cancer), doctors may be able to avoid more surgery to remove other lymph nodes.

People who join clinical trials may be among the first to benefit if a new approach is effective. And even if participants do not benefit directly, they still make an important contribution to medicine by helping doctors learn more about the disease and how to control it. Although clinical trials may pose some risks, researchers do all they can to protect their patients.

Chapter 35

Ovarian Cancer

Understanding Ovarian Cancer

Cancer begins in cells, the building blocks that make up tissues. Tissues make up the organs of the body.

Normally, cells grow and divide to form new cells as the body needs them. When cells grow old, they die, and new cells take their place.

Sometimes, this orderly process goes wrong. New cells form when the body does not need them, and old cells do not die when they should. These extra cells can form a mass of tissue called a growth or tumor.

Tumors can be benign or malignant.

Benign tumors are not cancer: Benign tumors are rarely life-threatening. Generally, benign tumors can be removed. They usually do not grow back. Benign tumors do not invade the tissues around them. Cells from benign tumors do not spread to other parts of the body.

Malignant tumors are cancer: Malignant tumors are generally more serious than benign tumors. They may be life-threatening. Malignant tumors often can be removed. But sometimes they grow back. Malignant tumors can invade and damage nearby tissues and organs. Cells from malignant tumors can spread to other parts of the body. Cancer cells spread by breaking away from the original (primary) tumor and entering the lymphatic system or bloodstream. The cells invade other organs and form new tumors that damage these organs. The spread of cancer is called metastasis.

Excerpted from "What You Need to Know about Ovarian Cancer," National Cancer Institute, July 17, 2006.

Benign and Malignant Cysts

An ovarian cyst may be found on the surface of an ovary or inside it. A cyst contains fluid. Sometimes it contains solid tissue too. Most ovarian cysts are benign (not cancer).

Most ovarian cysts go away with time. Sometimes, a doctor will find a cyst that does not go away or that gets larger. The doctor may order tests to make sure that the cyst is not cancer.

Ovarian cancer can invade, shed, or spread to other organs:

- **Invade:** A malignant ovarian tumor can grow and invade organs next to the ovaries, such as the fallopian tubes and uterus.
- **Shed:** Cancer cells can shed (break off) from the main ovarian tumor. Shedding into the abdomen may lead to new tumors forming on the surface of nearby organs and tissues. The doctor may call these seeds or implants.
- **Spread:** Cancer cells can spread through the lymphatic system to lymph nodes in the pelvis, abdomen, and chest. Cancer cells may also spread through the bloodstream to organs such as the liver and lungs.

Risk Factors

Studies have found the following risk factors for ovarian cancer:

- **Family history of cancer:** Women who have a mother, daughter, or sister with ovarian cancer have an increased risk of the disease. Also, women with a family history of cancer of the breast, uterus, colon, or rectum may also have an increased risk of ovarian cancer. If several women in a family have ovarian or breast cancer, especially at a young age, this is considered a strong family history. If you have a strong family history of ovarian or breast cancer, you may wish to talk to a genetic counselor. The counselor may suggest genetic testing for you and the women in your family. Genetic tests can sometimes show the presence of specific gene changes that increase the risk of ovarian cancer.
- **Personal history of cancer:** Women who have had cancer of the breast, uterus, colon, or rectum have a higher risk of ovarian cancer.
- **Age over fifty-five:** Most women are over age fifty-five when diagnosed with ovarian cancer.

- **Never pregnant:** Older women who have never been pregnant have an increased risk of ovarian cancer.
- **Menopausal hormone therapy:** Some studies have suggested that women who take estrogen by itself (estrogen without progesterone) for ten or more years may have an increased risk of ovarian cancer.

Scientists have also studied whether taking certain fertility drugs, using talcum powder, or being obese are risk factors. It is not clear whether these are risk factors, but if they are, they are not strong risk factors.

Having a risk factor does not mean that a woman will get ovarian cancer. Most women who have risk factors do not get ovarian cancer. On the other hand, women who do get the disease often have no known risk factors, except for growing older. Women who think they may be at risk of ovarian cancer should talk with their doctor.

Symptoms

Early ovarian cancer may not cause obvious symptoms. But, as the cancer grows, symptoms may include the following:

- Pressure or pain in the abdomen, pelvis, back, or legs
- A swollen or bloated abdomen
- Nausea, indigestion, gas, constipation, or diarrhea
- Feeling very tired all the time

Less common symptoms include the following:

- Shortness of breath
- Feeling the need to urinate often
- Unusual vaginal bleeding (heavy periods, or bleeding after menopause)

Most often these symptoms are not due to cancer, but only a doctor can tell for sure. Any woman with these symptoms should tell her doctor.

Diagnosis

If you have a symptom that suggests ovarian cancer, your doctor must find out whether it is due to cancer or to some other cause. Your doctor may ask about your personal and family medical history.

You may have one or more of the following tests. Your doctor can explain more about each test:

- **Physical exam:** Your doctor checks general signs of health. Your doctor may press on your abdomen to check for tumors or an abnormal buildup of fluid (ascites). A sample of fluid can be taken to look for ovarian cancer cells.
- **Pelvic exam:** Your doctor feels the ovaries and nearby organs for lumps or other changes in their shape or size. A Pap test is part of a normal pelvic exam, but it is not used to collect ovarian cells. The Pap test detects cervical cancer. The Pap test is not used to diagnose ovarian cancer.
- **Blood tests:** Your doctor may order blood tests. The lab may check the level of several substances, including CA-125. CA-125 is a substance found on the surface of ovarian cancer cells and on some normal tissues. A high CA-125 level could be a sign of cancer or other conditions. The CA-125 test is not used alone to diagnose ovarian cancer. This test is approved by the Food and Drug Administration for monitoring a woman's response to ovarian cancer treatment and for detecting its return after treatment.
- **Ultrasound:** The ultrasound device uses sound waves that people cannot hear. The device aims sound waves at organs inside the pelvis. The waves bounce off the organs. A computer creates a picture from the echoes. The picture may show an ovarian tumor. For a better view of the ovaries, the device may be inserted into the vagina (transvaginal ultrasound).
- **Biopsy:** A biopsy is the removal of tissue or fluid to look for cancer cells. Based on the results of the blood tests and ultrasound, your doctor may suggest surgery (a laparotomy) to remove tissue and fluid from the pelvis and abdomen. Surgery is usually needed to diagnose ovarian cancer.

Although most women have a laparotomy for diagnosis, some women have a procedure known as laparoscopy. The doctor inserts a thin, lighted tube (a laparoscope) through a small incision in the abdomen. Laparoscopy may be used to remove a small, benign cyst or an early ovarian cancer. It may also be used to learn whether cancer has spread.

A pathologist uses a microscope to look for cancer cells in the tissue or fluid. If ovarian cancer cells are found, the pathologist describes the grade of the cells. Grades 1, 2, and 3 describe how abnormal the cancer cells look. Grade 1 cancer cells are not as likely as to grow and spread as Grade 3 cells.

Staging

To plan the best treatment, your doctor needs to know the grade of the tumor and the extent (stage) of the disease. The stage is based on whether the tumor has invaded nearby tissues, whether the cancer has spread, and if so, to what parts of the body.

Usually, surgery is needed before staging can be complete. The surgeon takes many samples of tissue from the pelvis and abdomen to look for cancer.

Your doctor may order tests to find out whether the cancer has spread. These are the stages of ovarian cancer:

- **Stage I:** Cancer cells are found in one or both ovaries. Cancer cells may be found on the surface of the ovaries or in fluid collected from the abdomen.
- **Stage II:** Cancer cells have spread from one or both ovaries to other tissues in the pelvis. Cancer cells are found on the fallopian tubes, the uterus, or other tissues in the pelvis. Cancer cells may be found in fluid collected from the abdomen.
- **Stage III:** Cancer cells have spread to tissues outside the pelvis or to the regional lymph nodes. Cancer cells may be found on the outside of the liver.
- **Stage IV:** Cancer cells have spread to tissues outside the abdomen and pelvis. Cancer cells may be found inside the liver, in the lungs, or in other organs.

Treatment Methods

Your doctor can describe your treatment choices and the expected results. Most women have surgery and chemotherapy. Rarely, radiation therapy is used.

Surgery

The surgeon makes a long cut in the wall of the abdomen. This type of surgery is called a laparotomy. If ovarian cancer is found, the surgeon removes the following:

- Both ovaries and fallopian tubes (salpingo-oophorectomy)
- The uterus (hysterectomy)
- The omentum (the thin, fatty pad of tissue that covers the intestines)
- Nearby lymph nodes
- Samples of tissue from the pelvis and abdomen

If the cancer has spread, the surgeon removes as much cancer as possible. This is called "debulking" surgery.

If you have early Stage I ovarian cancer, the extent of surgery may depend on whether you want to get pregnant and have children. Some women with very early ovarian cancer may decide with their doctor to have only one ovary, one fallopian tube, and the omentum removed.

You may be uncomfortable for the first few days after surgery. Medicine can help control your pain. Before surgery, you should discuss the plan for pain relief with your doctor or nurse. After surgery, your doctor can adjust the plan if you need more pain relief.

The time it takes to heal after surgery is different for each woman. You will spend several days in the hospital. It may be several weeks before you return to normal activities.

Chemotherapy

Chemotherapy uses anticancer drugs to kill cancer cells. Most women have chemotherapy for ovarian cancer after surgery. Some women have chemotherapy before surgery.

Usually, more than one drug is given.

Chemotherapy is given in cycles. Each treatment period is followed by a rest period. The length of the rest period and the number of cycles depend on the anticancer drugs used.

You may have your treatment in a clinic, at the doctor's office, or at home. Some women may need to stay in the hospital during treatment.

The side effects of chemotherapy depend mainly on which drugs are given and how much. The drugs can harm normal cells that divide rapidly:

- **Blood cells:** These cells fight infection, help blood to clot, and carry oxygen to all parts of your body. When drugs affect your blood cells, you are more likely to get infections, bruise or bleed easily, and feel very weak and tired. Your health care team checks you for low levels of blood cells. If blood tests show low levels, your health care team can suggest medicines that can help your body make new blood cells.

- **Cells in hair roots:** Some drugs can cause hair loss. Your hair will grow back, but it may be somewhat different in color and texture.
- **Cells that line the digestive tract:** Some drugs can cause poor appetite, nausea and vomiting, diarrhea, or mouth and lip sores. Ask your health care team about medicines that help with these problems.

Some drugs used to treat ovarian cancer can cause hearing loss, kidney damage, joint pain, and tingling or numbness in the hands or feet. Most of these side effects usually go away after treatment ends.

Radiation Therapy

Radiation therapy (also called radiotherapy) uses high-energy rays to kill cancer cells. A large machine directs radiation at the body.

Radiation therapy is rarely used in the initial treatment of ovarian cancer, but it may be used to relieve pain and other problems caused by the disease. The treatment is given at a hospital or clinic. Each treatment takes only a few minutes.

Follow-up Care

You will need regular checkups after treatment for ovarian cancer. Even when there are no longer any signs of cancer, the disease sometimes returns because undetected cancer cells remained somewhere in your body after treatment.

Checkups help ensure that any changes in your health are noted and treated if needed. Checkups may include a pelvic exam, a CA-125 test, other blood tests, and imaging exams.

If you have any health problems between checkups, you should contact your doctor.

Chapter 36

Uterine Cancer

The Uterus

The uterus is part of a woman's reproductive system. It is the hollow, pear-shaped organ where a baby grows. The uterus is in the pelvis between the bladder and the rectum.

The wall of the uterus has two layers of tissue. The inner layer, or lining, is the endometrium. The outer layer is muscle tissue called the myometrium.

In women of childbearing age, the lining of the uterus grows and thickens each month to prepare for pregnancy. If a woman does not become pregnant, the thick, bloody lining flows out of the body through the vagina. This flow is called menstruation.

Malignant Tumors

Malignant tumors are cancer. They are generally more serious and may be life threatening. Cancer cells can invade and damage nearby tissues and organs. Also, cancer cells can break away from a malignant tumor and enter the bloodstream or lymphatic system. That is how cancer cells spread from the original (primary) tumor to form new tumors in other organs. The spread of cancer is called metastasis.

Excerpted from "What You Need to Know About Cancer of the Uterus," National Cancer Institute, September 16, 2002. Reviewed by David A. Cooke, M.D., December 2008.

When uterine cancer spreads (metastasizes) outside the uterus, cancer cells are often found in nearby lymph nodes, nerves, or blood vessels. If the cancer has reached the lymph nodes, cancer cells may have spread to other lymph nodes and other organs, such as the lungs, liver, and bones.

The most common type of cancer of the uterus begins in the lining (endometrium). It is called endometrial cancer, uterine cancer, or cancer of the uterus. In this chapter, we will use the terms "uterine cancer" or "cancer of the uterus" to refer to cancer that begins in the endometrium.

Uterine Cancer: Who's at Risk?

No one knows the exact causes of uterine cancer. However, it is clear that this disease is not contagious. No one can "catch" cancer from another person.

Most women who have known risk factors do not get uterine cancer. On the other hand, many who do get this disease have none of these factors. Doctors can seldom explain why one woman gets uterine cancer and another does not.

Studies have found the following risk factors:

- **Age:** Cancer of the uterus occurs mostly in women over age fifty.
- **Endometrial hyperplasia:** The risk of uterine cancer is higher if a woman has endometrial hyperplasia.
- **Hormone replacement therapy (HRT):** HRT is used to control the symptoms of menopause, to prevent osteoporosis (thinning of the bones), and to reduce the risk of heart disease or stroke. Women who use estrogen without progesterone have an increased risk of uterine cancer. Long-term use and large doses of estrogen seem to increase this risk. Women who use a combination of estrogen and progesterone have a lower risk of uterine cancer than women who use estrogen alone. The progesterone protects the uterus.
- **Obesity and related conditions:** The body makes some of its estrogen in fatty tissue. That's why obese women are more likely than thin women to have higher levels of estrogen in their bodies. High levels of estrogen may be the reason that obese women have an increased risk of developing uterine cancer. The risk of this disease is also higher in women with diabetes or high blood pressure (conditions that occur in many obese women).

- **Tamoxifen:** Women taking the drug tamoxifen to prevent or treat breast cancer have an increased risk of uterine cancer. This risk appears to be related to the estrogen-like effect of this drug on the uterus. Doctors monitor women taking tamoxifen for possible signs or symptoms of uterine cancer. The benefits of tamoxifen to treat breast cancer outweigh the risk of developing other cancers. Still, each woman is different. Any woman considering taking tamoxifen should discuss with the doctor her personal and family medical history and her concerns.
- **Race:** White women are more likely than African American women to get uterine cancer.
- **Colorectal cancer:** Women who have had an inherited form of colorectal cancer have a higher risk of developing uterine cancer than other women.

Other risk factors are related to how long a woman's body is exposed to estrogen. Women who have no children, begin menstruation at a very young age, or enter menopause late in life are exposed to estrogen longer and have a higher risk.

Women with known risk factors and those who are concerned about uterine cancer should ask their doctor about the symptoms to watch for and how often to have checkups. The doctor's advice will be based on the woman's age, medical history, and other factors.

Symptoms

Uterine cancer usually occurs after menopause. But it may also occur around the time that menopause begins. Abnormal vaginal bleeding is the most common symptom of uterine cancer. Bleeding may start as a watery, blood-streaked flow that gradually contains more blood. Women should not assume that abnormal vaginal bleeding is part of menopause.

A woman should see her doctor if she has any of the following symptoms:

- Unusual vaginal bleeding or discharge
- Difficult or painful urination
- Pain during intercourse
- Pain in the pelvic area

These symptoms can be caused by cancer or other less serious conditions. Most often they are not cancer, but only a doctor can tell for sure.

Diagnosis

If a woman has symptoms that suggest uterine cancer, her doctor may check general signs of health and may order blood and urine tests. The doctor also may perform one or more of the following exams:

- **Pelvic exam:** A woman has a pelvic exam to check the vagina, uterus, bladder, and rectum. The doctor feels these organs for any lumps or changes in their shape or size. To see the upper part of the vagina and the cervix, the doctor inserts an instrument called a speculum into the vagina.
- **Pap test:** The doctor collects cells from the cervix and upper vagina. A medical laboratory checks for abnormal cells. Although the Pap test can detect cancer of the cervix, cells from inside the uterus usually do not show up on a Pap test. This is why the doctor collects samples of cells from inside the uterus in a procedure called a biopsy.
- **Transvaginal ultrasound:** The doctor inserts an instrument into the vagina. The instrument aims high-frequency sound waves at the uterus. The pattern of the echoes they produce creates a picture. If the endometrium looks too thick, the doctor can do a biopsy.
- **Biopsy:** The doctor removes a sample of tissue from the uterine lining. This usually can be done in the doctor's office. In some cases, however, a woman may need to have a dilation and curettage (D&C). A D&C is usually done as same-day surgery with anesthesia in a hospital. A pathologist examines the tissue to check for cancer cells, hyperplasia, and other conditions. For a short time after the biopsy, some women have cramps and vaginal bleeding.

Staging

If uterine cancer is diagnosed, the doctor needs to know the stage, or extent, of the disease to plan the best treatment. Staging is a careful attempt to find out whether the cancer has spread, and if so, to what parts of the body.

In most cases, the most reliable way to stage this disease is to remove the uterus (hysterectomy). After the uterus has been removed, the surgeon can look for obvious signs that the cancer has invaded the muscle of the uterus. The surgeon also can check the lymph nodes and other organs in the pelvic area for signs of cancer.

These are the main features of each stage of the disease:

- **Stage I:** The cancer is only in the body of the uterus. It is not in the cervix.
- **Stage II:** The cancer has spread from the body of the uterus to the cervix.
- **Stage III:** The cancer has spread outside the uterus, but not outside the pelvis (and not to the bladder or rectum). Lymph nodes in the pelvis may contain cancer cells.
- **Stage IV:** The cancer has spread into the bladder or rectum. Or it has spread beyond the pelvis to other body parts.

Methods of Treatment

Women with uterine cancer have many treatment options. Most women with uterine cancer are treated with surgery. Some have radiation therapy. A smaller number of women may be treated with hormonal therapy. Some patients receive a combination of therapies.

A woman may want to talk with her doctor about taking part in a clinical trial, a research study of new treatment methods. Clinical trials are an important option for women with all stages of uterine cancer.

Most women with uterine cancer have surgery to remove the uterus (hysterectomy) through an incision in the abdomen. The doctor also removes both fallopian tubes and both ovaries.

The doctor may also remove the lymph nodes near the tumor to see if they contain cancer. If cancer cells have reached the lymph nodes, it may mean that the disease has spread to other parts of the body. If cancer cells have not spread beyond the endometrium, the woman may not need to have any other treatment. The length of the hospital stay may vary from several days to a week.

In radiation therapy, high-energy rays are used to kill cancer cells. Like surgery, radiation therapy is a local therapy. It affects cancer cells only in the treated area.

Some women with stage I, II, or III uterine cancer need both radiation therapy and surgery. They may have radiation before surgery to shrink the tumor or after surgery to destroy any cancer cells that remain in the area. Also, the doctor may suggest radiation treatments for the small number of women who cannot have surgery.

Hormonal therapy involves substances that prevent cancer cells from getting or using the hormones they may need to grow. Hormones can attach to hormone receptors, causing changes in uterine tissue. Before therapy begins, the doctor may request a hormone receptor test. This special lab test of uterine tissue helps the doctor learn if estrogen and progesterone receptors are present. If the tissue has receptors, the woman is more likely to respond to hormonal therapy.

Hormonal therapy is called a systemic therapy because it can affect cancer cells throughout the body. Usually, hormonal therapy is a type of progesterone taken as a pill.

The doctor may use hormonal therapy for women with uterine cancer who are unable to have surgery or radiation therapy. Also, the doctor may give hormonal therapy to women with uterine cancer that has spread to the lungs or other distant sites. It is also given to women with uterine cancer that has come back.

Side Effects of Cancer Treatment

Because cancer treatment may damage healthy cells and tissues, unwanted side effects sometimes occur. These side effects depend on many factors, including the type and extent of the treatment. Side effects may not be the same for each person, and they may even change from one treatment session to the next. Before treatment starts, doctors and nurses will explain the possible side effects and how they will help you manage them.

Follow-up Care

Follow-up care after treatment for uterine cancer is important. Women should not hesitate to discuss follow-up with their doctor. Regular checkups ensure that any changes in health are noticed. Any problem that develops can be found and treated as soon as possible. Checkups may include a physical exam, a pelvic exam, x-rays, and laboratory tests.

Support for Women with Uterine Cancer

Living with a serious disease such as cancer is not easy. Some people find they need help coping with the emotional and practical aspects of their disease. Support groups can help. In these groups, patients or their family members get together to share what they have learned about coping with the disease and the effects of treatment. Patients may want to talk with a member of their health care team about finding a support group.

The Promise of Cancer Research

Patients who take part in clinical trials have the first chance to benefit from treatments that have shown promise in earlier research. They also make an important contribution to medical science by helping doctors learn more about the disease. Although clinical trials may pose some risks, researchers take many very careful steps to protect people who take part.

In a large trial with hundreds of women, doctors are studying a less extensive method of surgery to remove the uterus. Normally, the doctor makes an incision in the abdomen to remove the uterus. In this study, doctors use a laparoscope (a lighted tube) to help remove the uterus through the vagina. Also, the doctor can use the laparoscope to help remove the ovaries and lymph nodes and to look into the abdomen for signs of cancer.

Other researchers are looking at the effectiveness of radiation therapy after surgery, as well as at the combination of surgery, radiation, and chemotherapy. Other trials are studying new drugs, new drug combinations, and biological therapies. Some of these studies are designed to find ways to reduce the side effects of treatment and to improve the quality of women's lives.

Chapter 37

Vaginal and Vulvar Cancers

Vaginal Cancer

Vaginal cancer is a disease in which malignant (cancer) cells form in the vagina.

The vagina is the canal leading from the cervix (the opening of uterus) to the outside of the body. At birth, a baby passes out of the body through the vagina (also called the birth canal).

Vaginal cancer is not common. When found in early stages, it can often be cured. There are two main types of vaginal cancer:

- **Squamous cell carcinoma:** Cancer that forms in squamous cells, the thin, flat cells lining the vagina. Squamous cell vaginal cancer spreads slowly and usually stays near the vagina, but may spread to the lungs and liver. This is the most common type of vaginal cancer. It is found most often in women aged sixty or older.
- **Adenocarcinoma:** Cancer that begins in glandular (secretory) cells. Glandular cells in the lining of the vagina make and release

---

"Vaginal Cancer" is excerpted from "Vaginal Cancer Treatment (PDQ®): Patient Version." PDQ® Cancer Information Summary. National Cancer Institute; Bethesda, MD. Updated 05/23/2008. Available at: http://www.cancer.gov. Accessed June 11, 2008. "Vulvar Cancer" is excerpted from "Vulvar Cancer Treatment (PDQ®): Patient Version." PDQ® Cancer Information Summary. National Cancer Institute; Bethesda, MD. Updated 07/31/2008. Available at: http://www.cancer.gov. Accessed May 8, 2008.

fluids such as mucus. Adenocarcinoma is more likely than squamous cell cancer to spread to the lungs and lymph nodes. It is found most often in women aged thirty or younger.

Age and exposure to the drug diethylstilbestrol (DES) before birth affect a woman's risk of developing vaginal cancer.

Anything that increases your risk of getting a disease is called a risk factor. Risk factors for vaginal cancer include the following:

- Being aged sixty or older.
- Being exposed to DES while in the mother's womb. In the 1950s, the drug DES was given to some pregnant women to prevent miscarriage (premature birth of a fetus that cannot survive). Women who were exposed to DES before birth have an increased risk of developing vaginal cancer. Some of these women develop a rare form of cancer called clear cell adenocarcinoma.
- Having human papillomavirus (HPV) infection.
- Having a history of abnormal cells in the cervix or cervical cancer.

Possible signs of vaginal cancer include pain or abnormal vaginal bleeding.

Vaginal cancer often does not cause early symptoms and may be found during a routine Pap test. When symptoms occur they may be caused by vaginal cancer or by other conditions. A doctor should be consulted if any of the following problems occur:

- Bleeding or discharge not related to menstrual periods.
- Pain during sexual intercourse.
- Pain in the pelvic area.
- A lump in the vagina.

Tests that examine the vagina and other organs in the pelvis are used to detect and diagnose vaginal cancer.

The following tests and procedures may be used:

- **Physical exam and history:** An exam of the body to check general signs of health, including checking for signs of disease, such as lumps or anything else that seems unusual. A history of the patient's health habits and past illnesses and treatments will also be taken.

- **Pelvic exam:** An exam of the vagina, cervix, uterus, fallopian tubes, ovaries, and rectum. The doctor or nurse inserts one or two lubricated, gloved fingers of one hand into the vagina and places the other hand over the lower abdomen to feel the size, shape, and position of the uterus and ovaries. A speculum is also inserted into the vagina and the doctor or nurse looks at the vagina and cervix for signs of disease. A Pap test or Pap smear of the cervix is usually done. The doctor or nurse also inserts a lubricated, gloved finger into the rectum to feel for lumps or abnormal areas.
- **Pap smear:** A procedure to collect cells from the surface of the cervix and vagina. A piece of cotton, a brush, or a small wooden stick is used to gently scrape cells from the cervix and vagina. The cells are viewed under a microscope to find out if they are abnormal. This procedure is also called a Pap test.
- **Biopsy:** The removal of cells or tissues from the vagina and cervix so they can be viewed under a microscope by a pathologist to check for signs of cancer. If a Pap smear shows abnormal cells in the vagina, a biopsy may be done during a colposcopy.
- **Colposcopy:** A procedure in which a colposcope (a lighted, magnifying instrument) is used to check the vagina and cervix for abnormal areas. Tissue samples may be taken using a curette (spoon-shaped instrument) and checked under a microscope for signs of disease.

Certain factors affect prognosis (chance of recovery) and treatment options.

The prognosis (chance of recovery) depends on the following:

- The stage of the cancer (whether it is in the vagina only or has spread to other areas).
- The size of the tumor.
- The grade of tumor cells (how different they are from normal cells).
- Where the cancer is within the vagina.
- Whether there are symptoms.
- The patient's age and general health.
- Whether the cancer has just been diagnosed or has recurred (come back).

Treatment options depend on the following:

- The stage, size, and location of the cancer.
- Whether the tumor cells are squamous cell or adenocarcinoma.
- Whether the patient has a uterus or has had a hysterectomy.
- Whether the patient has had past radiation treatment to the pelvis.

Stages of Vaginal Cancer

After vaginal cancer has been diagnosed, tests are done to find out if cancer cells have spread within the vagina or to other parts of the body.

The process used to find out if cancer has spread within the vagina or to other parts of the body is called staging. The information gathered from the staging process determines the stage of the disease. It is important to know the stage in order to plan treatment.

The following stages are used for vaginal cancer:

- **Stage 0 (carcinoma in situ):** In stage 0, abnormal cells are found in tissue lining the inside of the vagina. These abnormal cells may become cancer and spread into nearby normal tissue. Stage 0 is also called carcinoma in situ.
- **Stage I:** In stage I, cancer has formed and is found in the vagina only.
- **Stage II:** In stage II, cancer has spread from the vagina to the tissue around the vagina.
- **Stage III:** In stage III, cancer has spread from the vagina to the lymph nodes in the pelvis or groin, or to the pelvis, or both.
- **Stage IV:** Stage IV is divided into stage IVA and stage IVB. In stage IVA, cancer may have spread to lymph nodes in the pelvis or groin and has spread to the lining of the bladder or rectum and/or beyond the pelvis. In stage IVB, cancer has spread to parts of the body that are not near the vagina, such as the lungs. Cancer may also have spread to the lymph nodes.

Recurrent Vaginal Cancer

Recurrent vaginal cancer is cancer that has recurred (come back) after it has been treated. The cancer may come back in the vagina or in other parts of the body.

Treatment Option Overview

Different types of treatments are available for patients with vaginal cancer. Some treatments are standard (the currently used treatment), and some are being tested in clinical trials. A treatment clinical trial is a research study meant to help improve current treatments or obtain information on new treatments for patients with cancer. When clinical trials show that a new treatment is better than the standard treatment, the new treatment may become the standard treatment. Patients may want to think about taking part in a clinical trial. Some clinical trials are open only to patients who have not started treatment.

Three types of standard treatment are used: surgery, radiation therapy, and chemotherapy.

Surgery: Surgery is the most common treatment of vaginal cancer. The following surgical procedures may be used:

- *Laser surgery:* A surgical procedure that uses a laser beam (a narrow beam of intense light) as a knife to make bloodless cuts in tissue or to remove a surface lesion such as a tumor.
- *Wide local excision:* A surgical procedure that takes out the cancer and some of the healthy tissue around it.
- *Vaginectomy:* Surgery to remove all or part of the vagina.
- *Total hysterectomy:* Surgery to remove the uterus, including the cervix. If the uterus and cervix are taken out through the vagina, the operation is called a vaginal hysterectomy. If the uterus and cervix are taken out through a large incision (cut) in the abdomen, the operation is called a total abdominal hysterectomy. If the uterus and cervix are taken out through a small incision in the abdomen using a laparoscope, the operation is called a total laparoscopic hysterectomy.
- *Lymphadenectomy:* A surgical procedure in which lymph nodes are removed and checked under a microscope for signs of cancer. This procedure is also called lymph node dissection. If the cancer is in the upper vagina, the pelvic lymph nodes may be removed. If the cancer is in the lower vagina, lymph nodes in the groin may be removed.
- *Pelvic exenteration:* Surgery to remove the lower colon, rectum, and bladder. In women, the cervix, vagina, ovaries, and nearby

lymph nodes are also removed. Artificial openings (stoma) are made for urine and stool to flow from the body into a collection bag.

Skin grafting may follow surgery, to repair or reconstruct the vagina. Skin grafting is a surgical procedure in which skin is moved from one part of the body to another. A piece of healthy skin is taken from a part of the body that is usually hidden, such as the buttock or thigh, and used to repair or rebuild the area treated with surgery.

Even if the doctor removes all the cancer that can be seen at the time of the surgery, some patients may be given radiation therapy after surgery to kill any cancer cells that are left. Treatment given after the surgery, to increase the chances of a cure, is called adjuvant therapy.

Radiation therapy: Radiation therapy is a cancer treatment that uses high-energy x-rays or other types of radiation to kill cancer cells or keep them from growing. There are two types of radiation therapy. External radiation therapy uses a machine outside the body to send radiation toward the cancer. Internal radiation therapy uses a radioactive substance sealed in needles, seeds, wires, or catheters that are placed directly into or near the cancer. The way the radiation therapy is given depends on the type and stage of the cancer being treated.

Chemotherapy: Chemotherapy is a cancer treatment that uses drugs to stop the growth of cancer cells, either by killing the cells or by stopping them from dividing. When chemotherapy is taken by mouth or injected into a vein or muscle, the drugs enter the bloodstream and can affect cancer cells throughout the body (systemic chemotherapy). When chemotherapy is placed directly into the spinal column, an organ, or a body cavity such as the abdomen, the drugs mainly affect cancer cells in those areas (regional chemotherapy). The way the chemotherapy is given depends on the type and stage of the cancer being treated.

Topical chemotherapy for squamous cell vaginal cancer may be applied to the vagina in a cream or lotion.

New types of treatment are being tested in clinical trials.

Radiosensitizers: Radiosensitizers are drugs that make tumor cells more sensitive to radiation therapy. Combining radiation therapy with radiosensitizers may kill more tumor cells.

Clinical Trials

Patients may want to think about taking part in a clinical trial.

For some patients, taking part in a clinical trial may be the best treatment choice. Clinical trials are part of the cancer research process. Clinical trials are done to find out if new cancer treatments are safe and effective or better than the standard treatment.

Many of today's standard treatments for cancer are based on earlier clinical trials. Patients who take part in a clinical trial may receive the standard treatment or be among the first to receive a new treatment.

Patients who take part in clinical trials also help improve the way cancer will be treated in the future. Even when clinical trials do not lead to effective new treatments, they often answer important questions and help move research forward.

Patients can enter clinical trials before, during, or after starting their cancer treatment.

Some clinical trials only include patients who have not yet received treatment. Other trials test treatments for patients whose cancer has not gotten better. There are also clinical trials that test new ways to stop cancer from recurring (coming back) or reduce the side effects of cancer treatment.

Follow-up Care

Follow-up tests may be needed.

Some of the tests that were done to diagnose the cancer or to find out the stage of the cancer may be repeated. Some tests will be repeated in order to see how well the treatment is working. Decisions about whether to continue, change, or stop treatment may be based on the results of these tests. This is sometimes called re-staging.

Some of the tests will continue to be done from time to time after treatment has ended. The results of these tests can show if your condition has changed or if the cancer has recurred (come back). These tests are sometimes called follow-up tests or check-ups.

Vulvar Cancer

Vulvar cancer is a rare disease in which malignant (cancer) cells form in the tissues of the vulva.

Vulvar cancer forms in a woman's external genitalia. The vulva includes the inner and outer lips of the vagina, the clitoris (sensitive tissue between the lips), and the opening of the vagina and its glands.

Vulvar cancer most often affects the outer vaginal lips. Less often, cancer affects the inner vaginal lips or the clitoris.

Vulvar cancer usually develops slowly over a period of years. Abnormal cells can grow on the surface of the vulvar skin for a long time. This precancerous condition is called vulvar intraepithelial neoplasia (VIN) or dysplasia. Because it is possible for VIN or dysplasia to develop into vulvar cancer, treatment of this condition is very important.

Human papillomavirus (HPV) infection and older age can affect the risk of developing vulvar cancer.

Risk factors include the following:

- Having HPV infection
- Older age

Possible signs of vulvar cancer include bleeding or itching.

Vulvar cancer often does not cause early symptoms. When symptoms occur, they may be caused by vulvar cancer or by other conditions. A doctor should be consulted if any of the following problems occur:

- A lump in the vulva
- Itching that does not go away in the vulvar area
- Bleeding not related to menstruation (periods)
- Tenderness in the vulvar area

Tests that examine the vulva are used to detect (find) and diagnose vulvar cancer.

The following tests and procedures may be used:

- **Physical exam and history:** An exam of the body to check general signs of health, including checking the vulva for signs of disease, such as lumps or anything else that seems unusual. A history of the patient's health habits and past illnesses and treatments will also be taken.
- **Biopsy:** The removal of cells or tissues from the vulva so they can be viewed under a microscope by a pathologist to check for signs of cancer.

Certain factors affect prognosis (chance of recovery) and treatment options:

- The stage of the cancer
- The patient's age and general health
- Whether the cancer has just been diagnosed or has recurred (come back)

Stages of Vulvar Cancer

After vulvar cancer has been diagnosed, tests are done to find out if cancer cells have spread within the vulva or to other parts of the body.

The process used to find out if cancer has spread within the vulva or to other parts of the body is called staging. The information gathered from the staging process determines the stage of the disease. It is important to know the stage in order to plan treatment.

The following stages are used for vulvar cancer:

- **Stage 0 (carcinoma in situ):** In stage 0, abnormal cells are found on the surface of the vulvar skin. These abnormal cells may become cancer and spread into nearby normal tissue. Stage 0 is also called carcinoma in situ.
- **Stage I:** In stage I, cancer has formed and is found in the vulva only or in the vulva and perineum (area between the rectum and the vagina). The tumor is two centimeters or smaller and has spread to tissue under the skin. Stage I vulvar cancer is divided into stage IA and stage IB. In stage IA the tumor has spread one millimeter or less into the tissue of the vulva. In stage IB the tumor has spread more than one millimeter into the tissue of the vulva.
- **Stage II:** In stage II, cancer is found in the vulva or the vulva and perineum (space between the rectum and the vagina), and the tumor is larger than two centimeters.
- **Stage III:** In stage III vulvar cancer, the cancer is of any size and either is found only in the vulva or the vulva and perineum and has spread to nearby lymph nodes on one side of the groin, or has spread to nearby tissues such as the lower part of the urethra and/or vagina or anus, and may have spread to nearby lymph nodes on one side of the groin.
- **Stage IV:** Stage IV is divided into stage IVA and stage IVB, based on where the cancer has spread. In stage IVA, cancer has spread to nearby lymph nodes on both sides of the groin, or has

spread beyond nearby tissues to the upper part of the urethra, bladder, or rectum, or has attached to the pelvic bone and may have spread to lymph nodes. In stage IVB, cancer has spread to distant parts of the body.

Recurrent Vulvar Cancer

Recurrent vulvar cancer is cancer that has recurred (come back) after it has been treated. The cancer may come back in the vulva or in other parts of the body.

Treatment Option Overview

Different types of treatments are available for patients with vulvar cancer. Some treatments are standard (the currently used treatment), and some are being tested in clinical trials. Before starting treatment, patients may want to think about taking part in a clinical trial. A treatment clinical trial is a research study meant to help improve current treatments or obtain information on new treatments for patients with cancer. When clinical trials show that a new treatment is better than the standard treatment, the new treatment may become the standard treatment.

Four types of standard treatment are used: laser therapy, surgery, radiation therapy, and chemotherapy.

Laser therapy: Laser therapy is a cancer treatment that uses a laser beam (a narrow beam of intense light) to kill cancer cells.

Surgery: Surgery is the most common treatment for cancer of the vulva. The goal of surgery is to remove all the cancer without any loss of the woman's sexual function. One of the following types of surgery may be done:

- *Wide local excision:* A surgical procedure to remove the cancer and some of the normal tissue around the cancer.
- *Radical local excision:* A surgical procedure to remove the cancer and a large amount of normal tissue around it. Nearby lymph nodes in the groin may also be removed.
- *Vulvectomy:* A surgical procedure to remove part or all of the vulva. This may be done as a skinning vulvectomy, where the top layer of vulvar skin where the cancer is found is removed and skin grafts from other parts of the body may be needed to cover

the area; a simple vulvectomy, where the entire vulva is removed; a modified radical vulvectomy, where the vulva containing cancer and some of the normal tissue around it is removed; or a radical vulvectomy, where the entire vulva, including the clitoris, and nearby tissue is removed, sometimes along with nearby lymph nodes.

- *Pelvic exenteration:* A surgical procedure to remove the lower colon, rectum, and bladder. The cervix, vagina, ovaries, and nearby lymph nodes are also removed. Artificial openings (stoma) are made for urine and stool to flow from the body into a collection bag.

Even if the doctor removes all the cancer that can be seen at the time of the surgery, some patients may have chemotherapy or radiation therapy after surgery to kill any cancer cells that are left. Treatment given after the surgery, to increase the chances of a cure, is called adjuvant therapy.

Radiation therapy: Radiation therapy is a cancer treatment that uses high-energy x-rays or other types of radiation to kill cancer cells. There are two types of radiation therapy. External radiation therapy uses a machine outside the body to send radiation toward the cancer. Internal radiation therapy uses a radioactive substance sealed in needles, seeds, wires, or catheters that are placed directly into or near the cancer. The way the radiation therapy is given depends on the type and stage of the cancer being treated.

Chemotherapy: Chemotherapy is a cancer treatment that uses drugs to stop the growth of cancer cells, either by killing the cells or by stopping the cells from dividing. When chemotherapy is taken by mouth or injected into a vein or muscle, the drugs enter the bloodstream and can reach cancer cells throughout the body (systemic chemotherapy). When chemotherapy is placed directly into the spinal column, an organ, a body cavity such as the abdomen, or onto the skin, the drugs mainly affect cancer cells in those areas (regional chemotherapy). The way the chemotherapy is given depends on the type and stage of the cancer being treated.

Topical chemotherapy for vulvar cancer may be applied to the skin in a cream or lotion.

Chapter 38

Other Common Cancers in Women

Chapter Contents

Section 38.1

Lung Cancer: The Leading Cause of Cancer Death Among Women

From "Facts about Lung Cancer," reprinted courtesy of the Illinois Department of Public Health (www.idph.state.il.us). This document is available online at http://www.idph.state.il.us/about/womenshealth/factsheets/lung.htm; accessed May 12, 2008.

How common is lung cancer in women?

Lung cancer is the largest single cause of cancer deaths in the United States. For years, men were at higher risk for lung cancer because of higher smoking rates. However, with more women smoking, lung cancer surpassed breast cancer in 1987 as the leading cause of cancer deaths among women. Over the last two decades, lung cancer deaths have increased 150 percent in women, compared to an increase of about 20 percent in men. In fact, with all outside factors being equal, women have a greater risk of developing lung cancer than men. Several studies have suggested that estrogen may help lung cancers to grow, increasing the risk of lung cancer developing in women.

What causes lung cancer?

Smoking is by far the leading risk factor for lung cancer. Tobacco smoke causes more than eight out of ten cases of lung cancer. The longer a person has been smoking and the more packs per day smoked, the greater the risk. If a person stops smoking before lung cancer develops, the lung tissue will slowly return to normal. Cigar and pipe smoking are almost as likely to cause lung cancer as is cigarette smoking.

People who do not smoke but who breathe the smoke of others (secondhand smoke) also have a higher risk of lung cancer. Secondhand smoke is the third leading cause of preventable death in America, yet nearly half of all nonsmoking Americans are still regularly exposed to it. Nonsmokers exposed to secondhand smoke at home or work increase their risk of developing lung cancer by 20 to 30 percent.

Asbestos is another risk factor. People who work with asbestos have a higher risk of getting lung cancer. If they also smoke, the risk is greatly increased. Arsenic and radon, as well as other cancer-causing agents in the workplace, are also risk factors. Other factors that increase a person's risk include having had radiation therapy to the lung; personal and family history; diet; and air pollution.

What is the current treatment for lung cancer?

The best way to avoid death from lung cancer is never to smoke or to stop smoking. Once lung cancer is diagnosed, there are several treatment options, including radiation, various chemotherapies, and surgery. Survival rates have improved for non–small cell lung cancer because of advances in combination radiation/chemotherapy treatment. However, small cell lung cancer (most often found in people who smoke cigarettes) is still very difficult to treat. Small cell is the most aggressive of lung cancers, and many patients have advanced disease by the time it is diagnosed. Small cell lung cancer is responsive to both chemotherapy and radiation, yet nearly all these patients eventually relapse and need additional treatment.

There is a clear need for more effective treatments for lung cancer. New advances in research have recently led to new drugs that can protect normal cells from being destroyed from chemotherapy.

Early detection remains the key to successful therapy. If you have a history of chronic coughing, coughing up blood, chest pain, shortness of breath, hoarseness or wheezing, on-going problems with bronchitis or pneumonia, swelling of the neck and face, loss of appetite or weight loss, or fatigue, you should be evaluated by your physician as soon as possible. Lung cancer is not the only smoking-related cause of death in women. The World Health Organization states that at least 25 percent of women smokers will die of smoking-related disease such as cardiovascular disease and chronic obstructive pulmonary disease (COPD).

How can I prevent lung cancer?

The best way to prevent lung cancer is to avoid smoking. If you currently smoke, ask your health care provider to assist you in finding resources to help you quit smoking. It is also important to try to avoid secondhand tobacco smoke, radon, asbestos, and pollution, which can increase a person's risk of developing lung cancer. Controlling other lung diseases, such as tuberculosis, can help prevent lung cancer, since there is evidence that lung cancer tends to develop in scarred areas of the lung. Finally, eating a good diet with lots of fruits and vegetables also may help prevent lung cancer.

Section 38.2

Skin Cancer: The Most Prevalent Type of Cancer

Skin cancer is the most prevalent of all types of cancers. It is estimated that more than one million Americans develop skin cancer every year.

Fair-skinned people who sunburn easily are at a particularly high risk for developing skin cancer. Other less important factors include repeated medical and industrial x-ray exposure, scarring from diseases or burns, occupational exposure to compounds such as coal tar and arsenic, and family history.

Actinic Keratoses (AK)

Actinic keratoses or solar keratoses are considered the earliest stage in the development of skin cancer. They are small, scaly spots most commonly found on the face, ears, neck, lower arms, and back of the hands in fair-skinned individuals who have had significant sun exposure. Actinic keratoses can be treated by cryotherapy (freezing), topical chemotherapy (applying a cream or lotion), chemical peeling, dermabrasion, laser surgery, curettage, photodynamic therapy (a chemical is applied to the skin prior to exposure to a light source), or other dermatologic surgical procedures. Some actinic keratoses may progress to advanced stages which require more extensive treatment. Proper use of sunscreens can help prevent actinic keratoses even after extensive sun damage has already occurred.

Basal Cell Carcinoma (BCC)

Basal cell carcinoma is the most common type of skin cancer and appears frequently on the head, neck, and hands as a small, fleshy bump, nodule, or red patch. Other parts of the body may be affected as well. Basal cell carcinomas are frequently found in fair-skinned people and rarely occur in dark skin. They usually do not grow quickly. It can take many months or years for one to grow to a diameter of one-half inch. Untreated, the cancer often will begin to bleed, crust over, heal, and repeat the cycle, and can extend below the skin to the bone and nerves, causing considerable local damage.

Squamous Cell Carcinoma (SCC)

Squamous cell carcinoma is the second most common skin cancer; it is primarily found in fair-skinned people and rarely in dark-skinned individuals. Typically located on the rim of the ear, the face, lips, and mouth, this cancer may appear as a bump, or as a red, scaly patch. SCC can develop into large masses and become invasive. Unlike basal cell carcinoma, this form of cancer can metastasize (spread to other parts of the body); therefore, it is important to get early treatment.

When found early and treated properly, the cure rate for both basal cell and squamous cell carcinomas is over 95 percent.

Malignant Melanoma

Malignant Melanoma is the most deadly of all skin cancers. Every year, an estimated 8,000 Americans will die from melanoma; it is projected that greater than 108,000 Americans will develop melanoma annually. The death rate is declining because melanoma is usually curable when detected in its early stages and patients are seeking help sooner.

Melanoma begins in melanocytes, the skin cells that produce the dark protective pigment called melanin which makes the skin tan. Since melanoma cells usually continue to produce melanin, the cancer appears in mixed shades of tan, brown, and black; although it can also be red or white. Melanoma can metastasize (spread), making treatment essential.

Melanoma may appear suddenly or begin in or near a mole or another dark spot in the skin. It is important to know the location and appearance of the moles on the body to detect changes early. Any changing mole must be examined by a dermatologist. Early melanoma can be removed while still in the curable stage.

Excessive sun exposure, especially sunburn, is the most important preventable cause of melanoma. Light-skinned individuals are at particular risk. Heredity also plays a part. A person has an increased chance of developing melanoma if a relative or close family member has had melanoma. Atypical moles, which may run in families, and a large number of moles, can serve as markers for people at increased risk for developing melanoma.

Dark skin is not a guarantee against melanoma. People with skin of color can develop melanoma, especially on the palms, soles, under the nails, in the mouth, or on the genitalia.

The ABCDs of Melanoma

Consult a dermatologist immediately if any of your moles or pigmented spots exhibit:

- **Asymmetry:** One half does not match the other half in size, shape, color, or thickness.
- **Border irregularity:** The edges are ragged, scalloped, or poorly defined.
- **Color:** The pigmentation is not uniform. Shades of tan, brown, and black are present. Dashes of red, white, and blue add to the mottled appearance.
- **Diameter:** While melanomas are usually greater than six millimeters in diameter (the size of a pencil eraser) when diagnosed, they can be smaller. If you notice a mole different from others, or which changes, itches, or bleeds (even if it is small), you should see a dermatologist.

Warning signs of melanoma include:

- Changes in the surface of a mole. Scaliness, oozing, bleeding, or the appearance of a new bump.
- Spread of pigment from the border of a mole into surrounding skin.
- Change in sensation including itchiness, tenderness, or pain.

Treatment of Skin Cancer

If a skin biopsy reveals cancer, the dermatologist has an array of medical and surgical procedures as treatment, depending upon the type of cancer, its location, and the needs of the individual.

Dermatologic surgical treatments include: surgical excision; electrodesiccation and curettage (ED&C), which involves alternately scraping or burning the tumor in combination with low levels of electricity; cryosurgery (freezing using liquid nitrogen); and laser surgery. Mohs micrographic surgery is a special procedure used to remove the whole tumor while sparing as much normal skin as possible.

Other dermatologic treatments include radiation therapy and photodynamic therapy (a chemical is applied to the skin prior to exposure to a light source). Topical chemotherapy products may also be used.

Early Detection Is the Surest Way to a Cure

Develop a regular routine to inspect your body for any skin changes. If a growth, mole, sore, or skin discoloration appears suddenly, or begins to change, see a dermatologist. It is wise to have an annual skin examination by a dermatologist, especially for adults with significant past sun exposure or a family history of skin cancer.

How to Protect Yourself from Ultraviolet Light

Sun exposure is the most preventable risk factor for all skin cancers, including melanoma.[1,2] You can have fun in the sun and decrease your risk of skin cancer. Here's how to Be Sun Smart℠:

- Generously apply a water-resistant sunscreen with a sun protection factor (SPF) of at least 15 that provides broad-spectrum protection from both ultraviolet A (UVA) and ultraviolet B (UVB) rays to all exposed skin. Reapply every two hours, even on cloudy days, and after swimming or sweating. Look for the American Academy of Dermatology (AAD) Seal of Recognition™ on products that meet these criteria.
- Wear protective clothing, such as a long-sleeved shirt, pants, a wide-brimmed hat, and sunglasses, where possible.
- Seek shade when appropriate, remembering that the sun's rays are strongest between 10 a.m. and 4 p.m. If your shadow is shorter than you are, seek shade.
- Protect children from sun exposure by playing in the shade, using protective clothing, and applying sunscreen.
- Use extra caution near water, snow, and sand as they reflect the damaging rays of the sun, which can increase your chance of sunburn.
- Get vitamin D safely through a healthy diet that may include vitamin supplements. Don't seek the sun.[3]
- Avoid tanning beds. Ultraviolet light from the sun and tanning beds can cause skin cancer and wrinkling. If you want to look

like you've been in the sun, consider using a sunless self-tanning product, but continue to use sunscreen with it.

- Check your birthday suit on your birthday. If you notice anything changing, growing, or bleeding on your skin, see a dermatologist. Skin cancer is very treatable when caught early.

Periodic Self-Examination

Early detection and removal offer the best chance for a cure. Periodic self-examinations aid in recognition of any new or developing lesion. Get familiar with your skin and your own pattern of moles, freckles, and "beauty marks." Make sure to look at the entire body every month or two. Watch for changes in the number, size, shape, and color of pigmented areas. Consult a dermatologist promptly if any changes are noticed. Individuals at high risk should be examined by a dermatologist on a regular basis. It is beneficial to get assistance from a partner in performing skin self exams.

1. Examine body front and back in mirror, then right and left sides, arms raised.
2. Bend elbows, look carefully at forearms, back of upper arms, and palms.
3. Next, look at backs of legs and feet, spaces between toes, and soles.
4. Examine back of neck and scalp with a hand mirror. Part hair to lift.
5. Finally, check back and buttocks with a hand mirror.

References

1. American Cancer Society. 2008 Cancer Facts and Figures. http://www.cancer.org/downloads/STT/2008CAFFfinalsecured.pdf
2. Robinson, JK. Sun Exposure, Sun Protection and Vitamin D. *JAMA* 2005; 294: 1541–43.
3. Hemminki K, Dong C. Subsequent cancers after in situ and invasive squamous cell carcinoma of the skin. *Arch Dermatol* 2000;136:647–51.

Section 38.3

Cancer of the Thyroid: Affects More Women than Men

From "Cancer of the Thyroid," © 2005 American Thyroid Association (www.thyroid.org). Reprinted with permission.

Thyroid cancer is the most common endocrine-related cancer; however, it is rare compared to other cancers. In the United States there are only about 20,000 new patients annually. Even though the diagnosis of cancer is terrifying, the outlook for patients with thyroid cancer is usually excellent. First, most thyroid cancer is easily curable with surgery. Second, thyroid cancer rarely causes pain or disability. Third, effective and well-tolerated treatment is available for the most common forms of thyroid cancer.

What are the symptoms of thyroid cancer?

The key sign of thyroid cancer is a lump (nodule) in the thyroid, and most thyroid cancers do not cause any symptoms. Instead, your doctor may discover the nodule during a routine physical examination or you may notice a lump in your neck while looking in a mirror. A few patients with thyroid cancer complain of pain in the neck, jaw, or ear. If the cancer is large enough, it may cause difficulty swallowing or cause a "tickle in the throat" or shortness of breath if it is pressing on the windpipe. Rarely, hoarseness can be caused if the cancer irritates a nerve to the voice box.

What causes thyroid cancer?

Thyroid cancer is more common in people who have a history of exposure of the thyroid gland to radiation, have a family history of thyroid cancer, and are older than forty years of age. However, for most patients, we do not know the specific reason why they develop thyroid cancer.

Exposure of the thyroid to radiation causes thyroid cancer in susceptible patients, especially if the exposure occurred as a child. Many years ago (i.e., in the 1940s and 1950s), radiation exposure included x-ray treatments for acne, inflamed tonsils, adenoids, lymph nodes, or an enlarged thymus gland. X-rays also were used to measure foot sizes in shoe stores. Currently, x-ray exposure is usually limited to treatment of serious cancers such as Hodgkin disease (cancer of the lymph nodes). Routine x-ray exposure (e.g., dental x-rays, chest x-rays, mammograms) does not cause thyroid cancer.

Thyroid cancer can be caused by absorbing radioactive iodine released during a nuclear power plant emergency, such as the 1986 nuclear accident at the Chernobyl power plant in Russia. Children who were exposed were the most affected, and cancers were seen within a few years of that disaster. You can be protected from developing thyroid cancer due to a nuclear power plant emergency by taking potassium iodide, which blocks your thyroid from absorbing radioactive iodine. The United States government is currently developing guidelines to distribute potassium iodide to people living near nuclear power plants.

How is thyroid cancer diagnosed?

A diagnosis of thyroid cancer is made on the basis of a biopsy of a thyroid nodule or after the nodule is removed during surgery. Although thyroid nodules are very common, less than one in ten harbor a thyroid cancer.

What are the types of thyroid cancer?

Papillary thyroid cancer: Papillary thyroid cancer is the most common type, making up about 70 to 80 percent of all thyroid cancers. Papillary thyroid cancer can occur at any age. There are only about twelve thousand new cases of papillary cancer in the United States each year, but because these patients have such a long life expectancy, we estimate that one in a thousand people in the United States have or have had this form of cancer. Papillary cancer tends to grow slowly and to spread first to lymph glands in the neck. Unlike some other tumors, the generally excellent outlook for papillary cancer is usually not affected by spread of the cancer to the lymph nodes.

Follicular thyroid cancer: Follicular thyroid cancer, which makes up about 10 to 15 percent of all thyroid cancers in the United States, tends to occur in somewhat older patients than does papillary cancer. As with papillary cancer, follicular cancer first can grow into lymph nodes in the neck. Follicular cancer is also more likely than papillary cancer to grow into blood vessels and from there to spread to distant areas, particularly the lungs and bones.

Medullary thyroid cancer: Medullary thyroid cancer, which accounts for 5 to 10 percent of all thyroid cancers, is more likely to run in families and be associated with other endocrine problems. In fact, medullary thyroid cancer is the only thyroid cancer that can be diagnosed by genetic testing of the blood cells. In family members of an affected person, a positive test for the RET proto-oncogene can lead to an early diagnosis of medullary thyroid cancer and, subsequently, curative surgery to remove it.

Anaplastic thyroid cancer: Anaplastic thyroid cancer is the most advanced and aggressive thyroid cancer and is the least likely to respond to treatment. Fortunately, anaplastic thyroid cancer is rare and found in less than 5 percent of patients with thyroid cancer.

What is the treatment for thyroid cancer?

Surgery: The primary therapy for all forms of thyroid cancer is surgery. The generally accepted approach is to remove the entire thyroid gland, or as much of it as can be safely removed. After surgery, patients need to be on thyroid hormone for the rest of their life. Often the thyroid cancer is cured by surgery alone, especially if the cancer is small. If the cancer is large within the thyroid or if it has spread to lymph nodes or if your doctor feels that you are at high risk for recurrent cancer, radioactive iodine can be used as a "magic bullet" to destroy thyroid cancer cells after removal of the thyroid gland by surgery.

Radioactive iodine therapy: A major reason for the usually excellent prognosis for patients with papillary and follicular thyroid cancer is that radioactive iodine can be used as a magic bullet to seek out and destroy thyroid cancer cells with little or no damage to other tissues in the body. Thyroid cells normally concentrate iodine from the bloodstream to use to produce the thyroid hormones. By contrast, thyroid cancer cells usually take up only tiny amounts of iodine. However, high levels of thyroid stimulating hormone (TSH) can arouse thyroid cancer cells to take up significant amounts of iodine.

If your doctor recommends radioactive iodine therapy, high levels of TSH will be produced in your body by making you hypothyroid for a short time—either by not starting thyroid hormone pills after the thyroid gland is removed or by stopping your thyroid hormone pills if you are already on medication. Sometimes, to minimize your symptoms of hypothyroidism, your doctor may prescribe Cytomel® (T3) to take while you are becoming hypothyroid. Also, you may be asked to go on a low-iodine diet before the treatment to increase the effectiveness of the radioactive iodine. Once the TSH level is high enough, a whole-body iodine scan is done by administering a small dose of radioactive iodine to determine if there are remaining thyroid cells that need to be destroyed. If enough cells show up on the whole-body iodine scan, a large dose of radioactive iodine (I131) is given, and then the thyroid pills are restarted. Radioactive iodine therapy has proved to be safe and well tolerated, and it has even been able to cure cases of thyroid cancer that had already spread to the lungs.

What is the follow-up for patients with thyroid cancer?

Periodic follow-up examinations are essential for all patients with thyroid cancer because the thyroid cancer can return—sometimes many years after the apparently successful initial treatment. These follow-up visits include a careful history and physical examination, with particular attention to the neck area, as well as blood tests to determine if any changes of your thyroid hormone dose are needed. In particular, blood tests are done to measure the levels of T4 and TSH as well as a thyroid cell protein, thyroglobulin, which serves as a thyroid cancer marker. The thyroid hormone dose is adjusted to lower the TSH level into the low range. If the thyroglobulin level is still detectable despite a TSH in the low range, it means that there still are potential thyroid cancer cells functioning in the body. This finding may lead to additional tests and possible further treatment with radioactive iodine and/or surgery. Unfortunately, in some thyroid cancer patients the presence of interfering antibodies in the blood may prevent accurate thyroglobulin measurement.

In addition to routine blood tests, your doctor may want to repeat periodically a whole-body iodine scan to determine if any thyroid cells remain. This can be done after your TSH level is raised, either by stopping your thyroid hormone and your becoming hypothyroid (see above) or by administering Thyrogen® (synthetic human TSH) injections.

What is the prognosis of thyroid cancer?

Overall, the prognosis of thyroid cancer is very good. In general, the prognosis is better in younger patients than in those over forty years of age. Patients with papillary carcinoma who have a primary tumor that is confined to the thyroid gland itself have an excellent outlook: only one out of every one hundred such patients have died of thyroid cancer by twenty-five years later. The prognosis is not quite as good in patients over the age of forty, or in patients with tumors larger than four centimeters (1.5 inches) in diameter. Still, even those patients who are unable to be cured of their thyroid cancer are able to live a long time and feel well despite their cancer.

Chapter 39

Questions and Answers about Hormone Replacement Therapy Use and Cancer in Women

What is menopause?

Menopause is the time in a woman's life when menstruation (having a period) ends. It is part of a biological process that begins, for most women, in their mid-thirties. During this time, the ovaries gradually produce lower levels of natural sex hormones—estrogen and progesterone. Estrogen promotes the normal development of a woman's breasts and uterus, controls the cycle of ovulation (when an ovary releases an egg into a fallopian tube), and affects many aspects of a woman's physical and emotional health. Progesterone controls menstruation and prepares the lining of the uterus to receive the fertilized egg.

"Natural menopause" occurs when a woman has her last menstrual period, or stops menstruating, and is considered complete when menstruation has stopped for one year. This usually occurs between ages forty-five and fifty-five, with variations in timing from woman to woman. Women who undergo surgery to remove both ovaries (an operation called bilateral oophorectomy) experience "surgical menopause"—an immediate end to menstruation caused by lack of hormones produced by the ovaries.

By the time a woman has reached natural menopause, estrogen output has decreased significantly. Even though low levels of this

---

Reprinted from "Menopausal Hormone Replacement Therapy Use and Cancer: Questions and Answers," National Cancer Institute, October 5, 2007.

hormone are produced by other organs after menopause, these levels are only about one-tenth of the level found in premenopausal women. Progesterone is nearly absent in menopausal women.

What are menopausal hormones and why are they used?

Doctors may recommend menopausal hormones to counter some of the problems often associated with the onset of menopause (hot flashes, night sweats, sleeplessness, and vaginal dryness) or to prevent some long-term conditions that are more common in postmenopausal women, such as osteoporosis (a condition characterized by a decrease in bone mass and density, causing bones to become fragile). Menopausal hormone use (sometimes referred to as hormone replacement therapy or postmenopausal hormone use) usually involves treatment with either estrogen alone or estrogen in combination with progesterone or progestin, a synthetic hormone with effects similar to those of progesterone. Among women who are prescribed menopausal hormones, women who have undergone a hysterectomy (surgery to remove the uterus and, sometimes, the cervix) are generally given estrogen alone. Women who have not undergone this surgery are given estrogen plus progestin, which is known to have a lower risk of causing endometrial cancer (cancer of the lining of the uterus).

How does medical research determine the benefits and risks of taking menopausal hormones?

Researchers commonly conduct two very different, yet important types of studies with people to examine the benefits and risks of hormone use: clinical trials and observational studies. In clinical trials, the participants are given either hormones or placebos (look-alike pills that do not contain any drug) to determine the effect of the hormones on various conditions and diseases. In observational studies, the investigators do not try to affect the outcome; they compare the health status of women taking hormones to that of women not taking hormones.

What has medical research found out about the risks and benefits of hormone use after menopause?

The most comprehensive evidence about the risks and benefits of taking hormones after menopause to prevent disease comes from the Women's Health Initiative (WHI) Hormone Program, which was sponsored by the National Heart, Lung, and Blood Institute (NHLBI) and the National Cancer Institute (NCI), parts of the National Institutes of Health (NIH). This research program examined the effects of menopausal hormones on women's health. The WHI Hormone Program involved two studies—the use of estrogen plus progestin for women with a uterus (the Estrogen-plus-Progestin Study), and the use of estrogen alone for women without a uterus (the Estrogen-Alone Study). In both hormone therapy studies, women were randomly assigned to receive either the hormone medication being studied or the placebo.

The WHI Estrogen-plus-Progestin Study was stopped in July 2002, when investigators reported that the overall risks of estrogen plus progestin, specifically Prempro®, outweighed the benefits.[1] The researchers found that use of this estrogen-plus-progestin pill increased the risk of breast cancer, heart disease, stroke, blood clots, and urinary incontinence. However, the risk of colorectal cancer and hip fractures was lower among women using estrogen plus progestin than among those taking the placebo.[1] In addition, the WHI Memory Study showed that estrogen plus progestin doubled the risk for developing dementia (a decline in mental ability in which the patient can no longer function independently on a day-to-day basis) in postmenopausal women age sixty-five and older. The risk increased for all types of dementia, including Alzheimer disease.[2]

The WHI Estrogen-Alone Study, which involved Premarin®, was stopped in February 2004, when the researchers concluded that estrogen alone increased the risk of stroke and blood clots. In contrast with the WHI Estrogen-plus-Progestin Study, the risk of breast cancer was decreased in women using estrogen alone compared with those taking the placebo. Use of estrogen alone did not increase or decrease the risk of colorectal cancer.[3] Similar to the results seen in the Estrogen-plus-Progestin Study, women using estrogen alone had an increased risk of urinary incontinence and a decreased risk of hip fractures.

Another large epidemiologic study, the Million Women Study, enrolled 1.3 million women in the United Kingdom. This study evaluated health outcomes in women using and not using menopausal hormones. Several analyses have been published to date, and many more are expected in the future.[4, 5, 6]

How does menopausal hormone use affect breast cancer risk and survival?

The WHI Estrogen-plus-Progestin Study concluded that estrogen plus progestin increases the risk of invasive breast cancer. After five years of follow-up, women taking these hormones had a 24 percent increase in breast cancer risk compared with women taking the placebo. The increase amounted to an additional eight cases of breast cancer for every ten thousand women taking estrogen plus progestin for one year compared with ten thousand women taking the placebo.[7]

A detailed analysis of data from the WHI Estrogen-plus-Progestin Study showed that, among women taking estrogen plus progestin, the breast cancers were slightly larger and diagnosed at more advanced stages compared with breast cancers in women taking the placebo. Among women taking estrogen plus progestin, 25.4 percent of the cancers had spread outside the breast to nearby organs or lymph nodes compared with 16.0 percent among non-users. Women taking estrogen plus progestin also had more abnormal mammograms (breast x-rays that require additional evaluation) than the women taking the placebo.[7]

The WHI Estrogen-Alone Study concluded that taking estrogen did not increase the risk of breast cancer in women with a prior hysterectomy, at least for the seven years of follow-up in the study. Further analysis of data from the study indicated a 20 percent decrease in risk of breast cancer in women taking estrogen alone, although this decrease was seen mainly in the occurrence of early-stage breast cancer and ductal breast cancer (a specific type that begins in the lining of the milk ducts in the breast.[8] The observed reduction amounted to six fewer cases of breast cancer for every ten thousand women taking estrogen for one year compared with ten thousand non-users, but this lower incidence was not statistically significant; i.e., the lower incidence could have arisen by chance rather than being related to estrogen-alone use.[8] The Estrogen-Alone Study also showed a substantial increase in the frequency of abnormal mammograms.[8]

A comprehensive review of data from fifty-one epidemiological (population) studies published in the 1980s and 1990s found a statistically significant increase in breast cancer risk among current or recent users of any hormone replacement therapy compared with the risk among non-users. Most women in the analysis (88 percent) had used estrogen alone, and data for estrogen-plus-progestin users was not analyzed separately. Analysis of the pooled data also showed that the risk of breast cancer increased with increasing duration of hormone use, and this effect was more prominent in women with low body weight or a low body mass index. However, breast cancers in hormone users were less likely to have spread to other parts of the body compared with the breast cancers in non-users. The increase in breast cancer risk largely, if not completely, disappeared about five years after cessation of hormone use.[9]

As part of the Million Women Study, researchers examined six types of breast cancer among users and nonusers of menopausal hormones. The results showed that the effects of hormone use varied among breast cancer types. Overall, breast cancer risk was significantly increased among current users, although the risk was lower among women with higher body mass index.[5]

What are the effects of hormone use on the risk of endometrial cancer?

Studies have shown that long-term exposure of the uterus to estrogen alone increases a woman's risk of endometrial cancer. The risk associated with estrogen plus progestin appears to be much less, but some data suggest that the risk is still increased compared with the risk for non-users. The long-term effects of estrogen plus progestin on endometrial cancer risk remain uncertain.[10]

The WHI Estrogen-plus-Progestin Study showed that endometrial cancer rates for women taking estrogen plus progestin daily were the same as or possibly less than those for women taking the placebo pill. Uterine bleeding, however, was a common side effect, leading to more frequent biopsies and ultrasounds for women taking estrogen plus progestin compared with those taking a placebo.[11]

The Million Women Study confirmed a lower risk of endometrial cancer in women taking estrogen plus progestin in comparison with those taking estrogen only or tibolone, a synthetic steroid that is not available in the United States.[6]

How does menopausal hormone use affect the risk of ovarian cancer?

Several observational studies have found that the use of estrogen alone is associated with a slightly increased risk of ovarian cancer for women who used this hormone for ten or more years. One observational study that followed 44,241 menopausal women for approximately twenty years concluded that women who used estrogen alone for ten or more years were twice as likely to develop ovarian cancer compared with women who did not use menopausal hormones.[12] Another large observational study also found an association between estrogen use and death due to ovarian cancer. In this study, the increased risk appeared to be limited to women who used estrogen for ten or more years.[13]

The results from the Million Women Study showed that women currently using menopausal hormones had an increased risk of developing ovarian cancer and a 20 percent likelihood of dying from the disease compared with non-users. However, the increased risk disappeared after hormone use stopped.[4]

Data from the WHI Estrogen-plus-Progestin Study indicate that there may be an increased risk of ovarian cancer with use of estrogen plus progestin.[11] After 5.6 years of follow-up, a 58 percent increased risk of ovarian cancer was reported in women using estrogen plus progestin compared with non-users, but the increased risk was not statistically significant. One observational study suggested that regimens of estrogen plus progestin do not increase the risk of ovarian cancer if progestin is used for more than fifteen days per month,[14] but this study was too small to draw firm conclusions. More research is needed to clarify the relationship between menopausal hormone use, particularly for estrogen plus progestin, and the risk of ovarian cancer.

How does menopausal hormone use affect the risk of colorectal cancer?

After five years of follow-up of women taking estrogen plus progestin, the WHI Estrogen-plus-Progestin Study reported a 37 percent reduction in colorectal cancer cases compared with women taking the placebo.[1] On average, the researchers found that if a group of ten thousand women takes estrogen plus progestin for a year, six fewer cases of colon cancer will occur than in a group of non-users. These findings are consistent with observational studies, which have suggested that the use of postmenopausal hormones may reduce the risk of colorectal cancer.[1, 15] The WHI Estrogen-Alone Study concluded that estrogen alone had no significant effect on colorectal cancer risk.[3]

Should women with a history of cancer take menopausal hormones?

One of the roles of naturally occurring estrogen is to promote the normal growth of cells in the breast and uterus. For this reason, it is generally believed that menopausal estrogen use by women who have already been diagnosed with breast cancer may promote further tumor growth. Studies of hormone use to treat menopausal symptoms in breast cancer survivors have produced conflicting results.

In one trial, 434 breast cancer survivors receiving either estrogen alone or estrogen plus progestin were followed for two years before the study was stopped because researchers concluded that even short-term use of hormone replacement therapy posed an unacceptable risk of breast cancer recurrence. Among these study participants, 26 women in the group receiving hormone replacement therapy had another occurrence of breast cancer compared with 7 women in the group receiving no hormone replacement therapy.[16] In another study, which included 378 women who were followed for four years, 11 women receiving hormone replacement therapy had another occurrence of breast cancer compared with 13 women receiving no hormone replacement therapy, so the risk of breast cancer recurrence was not increased.[17] A review of fifteen studies comprising a total of 1,416 breast cancer survivors and 1,998 women without a history of breast cancer found no increase in risk of cancer recurrence with hormone replacement therapy use.[18]

There is limited research on the risks associated with menopausal hormone use by women who have had other cancers, particularly gynecological cancers. One review of the published research found that no firm conclusion could be drawn about the safety of hormone use in women with a history of cancer. However, survivors of gastric and bladder cancer and meningioma may be at higher risk of a recurrence. Survivors of gynecological cancers may be at higher risk because these cancers tend to be more hormone-dependent, but more studies are needed.[19]

Does the way in which hormones are administered make a difference?

Most of the data on the long-term health effects of hormones come from studies in which hormones (estrogen alone or estrogen plus progestin) are administered orally in the form of pills. Hormones in the form of transdermal patches or gels are also used to treat menopause-related symptoms. Estrogen-containing vaginal creams and rings can be used specifically for vaginal dryness. Progesterone is also available as a pill or gel. The amount of estrogen that enters the bloodstream from estrogen-containing vaginal creams and rings depends on the types of hormones and the dose. Generally, vaginal administration of hormones results in lower levels of circulating hormones compared with an equivalent oral dose. Because the vaginal epithelium (thin layer of tissue that covers the vagina) responds to very small doses of estrogen, low-dose estrogen-containing creams or gels can be used.

What should women do if they are concerned about taking menopausal hormones?

Although menopausal hormones have short-term benefits such as relief from hot flashes and vaginal dryness, several health concerns are associated with their use. Women should discuss with their health care provider whether to take menopausal hormones and what alternatives may be appropriate for them. The U.S. Food and Drug Administration (FDA) currently advises women to use menopausal hormones for the shortest time and at the lowest dose possible to control symptoms.

What are the alternatives for women who choose not to take menopausal hormones?

To decrease the risk of chronic disease, women can adopt a healthy lifestyle by exercising regularly, eating a healthy diet, limiting the consumption of alcohol, and not starting to smoke or, for smokers, trying to quit. Eating foods rich in calcium and vitamin D or taking dietary supplements containing these nutrients can help prevent osteoporosis. Results from the WHI showed that taking calcium and vitamin D supplements provided some benefit in preserving bone mass and preventing hip fractures, particularly in women age sixty and older. Although generally well tolerated, these supplements were associated with an increased risk of kidney stones. Other drugs, such as alendronate (Fosamax®), raloxifene (Evista®), and risedronate (Actonel®), have been shown to prevent bone loss. In addition, parathyroid hormone (Forteo®) is approved by the FDA for osteoporosis treatment.

Short-term menopause-related problems may go away on their own and frequently require no therapy at all. Local therapy for specific symptoms, such as vaginal dryness and urinary bladder conditions, is available. Some women seek relief from menopausal symptoms with nonprescription complementary and alternative therapies containing estrogen-like compounds. Some sources of these estrogen-like compounds include soy-based products, whole grain cereal, oilseeds (primarily flaxseed), legumes, and the botanical black cohosh. The benefits and risks of most of these agents have not been proven, however.

One NIH-funded study, the Herbal Alternatives (HALT) for Menopause Study, involved 351 women, some of whom were postmenopausal while others were approaching menopause. All of these women experienced hot flashes and night sweats and were given herbal supplements, menopausal hormones, or no therapy. Women in the herbal supplement groups received black cohosh alone, a multibotanical supplement (including black cohosh), or the multibotanical supplement plus counseling to increase their intake of dietary soy. Women in the herbal supplement groups had no significant reduction in the number of hot flashes and night sweats compared with women who received no therapy. The women who received menopausal hormones had significantly fewer menopausal symptoms compared with the women who received no therapy.[20]

Women should talk with their doctor about the option best for them.

What research still needs to be done?

Unresolved questions include whether different forms of the hormones, lower doses, different hormones, or different methods of administration are safer or more effective; whether risks and/or benefits persist after women stop taking hormones; whether women might be able to take hormones safely for a short period of time; and whether certain subgroups of women, including women with a history of cancer, might be at higher or lower risk than the general population.

The WHI continues to evaluate the longer-term effects of calcium and vitamin D supplements on preserving bone mass, preventing hip fractures, and reducing colon cancer risk, and continues long-term follow-up of women in the hormone trials.

The NIH continues to sponsor research to evaluate the effects of estrogen-like compounds on menopausal symptoms and long-term health after menopause. Several NCI-sponsored studies are evaluating the effectiveness of nonhormonal treatments, such as the botanical St. John's wort and the antidepressant drug citalopram hydrobromide, in reducing hot flashes in women with a history of breast cancer.

Selected References

1. Rossouw JE, Anderson GL, Prentice RL, et al. Risks and benefits of estrogen plus progestin in healthy postmenopausal women: Principal results from the Women's Health Initiative randomized controlled trial. *Journal of the American Medical Association* 2002; 288(3):321–33.

2. Shumaker SA, Legault C, Rapp SR, et al. Estrogen plus progestin and the incidence of dementia and mild cognitive impairment in postmenopausal women: The Women's Health Initiative Memory Study: A randomized controlled trial. *Journal of the American Medical Association* 2003; 289(20):2651–62.

3. Anderson GL, Limacher M, Assaf AR, et al. Effects of conjugated equine estrogen in postmenopausal women with hysterectomy:

The Women's Health Initiative randomized controlled trial. *Journal of the American Medical Association* 2004; 291(14):1701–12.

4. Beral V, Million Women Study Collaborators. Ovarian cancer and hormone replacement therapy in the Million Women Study. *Lancet* 2007; 369:1703–10.

5. Reeves GK, Beral V, Green J, Gathani T, Bull D. Hormonal therapy for menopause and breast cancer risk by histological type: A cohort study and meta-analysis. *Lancet Oncology* 2006; 7:910–18.

6. Beral V, Bull D, Reeves G, Million Women Study Collaborators. Endometrial cancer and hormone-replacement therapy in the Million Women Study. *Lancet* 2005; 365(9470):1543–51.

7. Chlebowski RT, Hendrix SL, Langer RD, et al. Influence of estrogen plus progestin on breast cancer and mammography in healthy postmenopausal women: The Women's Health Initiative randomized trial. *Journal of the American Medical Association* 2003; 289(24):3243–53.

8. Stefanick ML, Anderson GL, Margolis KL, et al. Effects of conjugated equine estrogens on breast cancer and mammography screening in postmenopausal women with hysterectomy. *Journal of the American Medical Association* 2006; 295(14):1647–57.

9. Collaborative Group on Hormonal Factors in Breast Cancer. Breast cancer and hormone replacement therapy: Collaborative reanalysis of data from 51 epidemiological studies of 52,705 women with breast cancer and 108,411 women without breast cancer. *Lancet* 1997; 350(9084):1047–59.

10. Grady D, Gebretsadik T, Kerlikowske K, Ernster V, Petitti D. Hormone replacement therapy and endometrial cancer risk: A meta-analysis. *Obstetrics and Gynecology* 1995; 85(2):304–13.

11. Anderson GL, Judd HL, Kaunitz AM, et al. Effects of estrogen plus progestin on gynecologic cancers and associated diagnostic procedures: The Women's Health Initiative randomized trial. *Journal of the American Medical Association* 2003; 290(13): 1739–48.

12. Lacey JV Jr., Mink PJ, Lubin JH, et al. Menopausal hormone replacement therapy and risk of ovarian cancer. *Journal of the American Medical Association* 2002; 288(3):334–41.

13. Rodriguez C, Patel AV, Calle EE, Jacob EJ, Thun MJ. Estrogen replacement therapy and ovarian cancer mortality in a large prospective study of US women. *Journal of the American Medical Association* 2001; 285(11):1460–65.

14. Riman T, Dickman PW, Nilsson S, et al. Hormone replacement therapy and the risk of invasive epithelial ovarian cancer in Swedish women. *Journal of the National Cancer Institute* 2002; 94(7):497–504.

15. Grodstein F, Newcomb PA, Stampfer MJ. Postmenopausal hormone therapy and the risk of colorectal cancer: A review and meta-analysis. *American Journal of Medicine* 1999; 106:574–82.

16. Holmberg L, Anderson H. HABITS (hormonal replacement therapy after breast cancer—is it safe?), a randomised comparison: Trial stopped. *Lancet* 2004; 363(9407):453–55.

17. von Schoultz E, Rutqvist LE. Menopausal hormone therapy after breast cancer: The Stockholm randomized trial. *Journal of the National Cancer Institute* 2005; 97(7):533–35.

18. Batur P, Blixen CE, Moore HC, Thacker HL, Xu M. Menopausal hormone therapy (HT) in patients with breast cancer. *Maturitas* 2006; 53(2):123–32.

19. Biglia N, Gadducci A, Ponzone R, Roagna R, Sismondi P. Hormone replacement therapy in cancer survivors. *Maturitas* 2004; 48(4):333–46.

20. Newton KM, Reed SD, LaCroix AZ, et al. Treatment of vasomotor symptoms of menopause with black cohosh, multibotanicals, soy, hormone therapy, or placebo: A randomized trial. *Annals of Internal Medicine* 2006; 145(12):869–79.

Part Five

Other Chronic Health Conditions of Special Concern to Women

Chapter 40

Arthritis

What is arthritis?

Arthritis literally means joint inflammation, but it is often used to identify a group of more than one hundred rheumatic diseases that may cause pain, stiffness, and swelling in the joints and in areas close to the joints.

How many people have arthritis?

More than forty million people in the United States have some form of arthritis, and many have chronic pain that limits daily activity. Osteoarthritis is by far the most common form of arthritis, affecting more than twenty million people.

Rheumatoid arthritis is the most disabling form of arthritis. More than two million people have this disease. Gout occurs in approximately 840 out of every 100,000 people. It is rare in children and young adults.

What is osteoarthritis?

Osteoarthritis is the most common form of arthritis among older people. It affects hands, low back, neck, and weight-bearing joints such as knees, hips, and feet.

Osteoarthritis occurs when cartilage, the tissue that cushions the ends of the bones within the joints, breaks down and wears away. This

---

Excerpted from "Arthritis," NIH Senior Health, August 15, 2006 causes bones to rub together, causing pain, swelling, and loss of motion of the joint.

What causes osteoarthritis?

Osteoarthritis often results from years of wear and tear on joints. This wear and tear mostly affects the cartilage, the tissue that cushions the ends of bones within the joint. Osteoarthritis occurs when the cartilage begins to fray, wear away, and decay.

Putting too much stress on a joint that has been repeatedly injured may lead to the development of osteoarthritis, too. A person who is overweight is more likely to develop osteoarthritis because of too much stress on the joints. Also, improper joint alignment may lead to the development of osteoarthritis.

How can I reduce my chances of developing osteoarthritis?

Maintaining a healthy weight, avoiding injury, and engaging in moderate daily physical activity are all ways to decrease your chances of developing osteoarthritis.

What are some common symptoms of osteoarthritis?

Common symptoms of osteoarthritis include joint pain, swelling, or tenderness; stiffness after getting out of bed; and a crunching feeling or sound of bone rubbing on bone. Not everyone with osteoarthritis develops symptoms. In fact, only a third of people with x-ray evidence of osteoarthritis report pain or other symptoms.

How is osteoarthritis diagnosed?

The doctor will use a combination of tests to try to determine if osteoarthritis is causing the symptoms. These may include a medical history, a physical examination, x-rays, and laboratory tests. A patient's attitudes, daily activities, and levels of anxiety or depression have a lot to do with how much the symptoms of osteoarthritis affect day-to-day living.

Is there a cure for osteoarthritis?

There is no cure for osteoarthritis and no way to reverse the joint damage once it occurs. However, current treatments can relieve symptoms.

Exercise is one of the best treatments. Exercise can improve mood and outlook, decrease pain, and assist in maintaining a healthy weight.

Warm towels, hot packs, or a warm bath or shower can provide temporary pain relief. Medications such as nonsteroidal anti-inflammatory drugs, or NSAIDs, help reduce pain and inflammation that result from osteoarthritis.

Can glucosamine and chondroitin sulfate relieve symptoms of osteoarthritis?

For some people, glucosamine and chondroitin sulfate may help relieve the symptoms of osteoarthritis. Scientific studies have shown that these supplements may have some benefit for people with osteoarthritis. However, the effectiveness of these supplements is still under investigation.

The National Institutes of Health (NIH) is currently funding the Glucosamine and Chondroitin Arthritis Intervention Trial, or GAIT, to test whether or not glucosamine and/or chondroitin have a beneficial effect for people with knee osteoarthritis. The results of the recently completed first phase of the study indicate that these supplements have a limited effectiveness for most patients with osteoarthritis.

What is rheumatoid arthritis?

Rheumatoid arthritis is an inflammatory disease that causes pain, swelling, stiffness, and loss of function in the joints. It can cause mild to severe symptoms.

People with rheumatoid arthritis may feel sick, tired, and sometimes feverish. Sometimes rheumatoid arthritis attacks tissue in the skin, lungs, eyes, and blood vessels.

The disease generally occurs in a symmetrical pattern. If one knee or hand is involved, usually the other one is, too. It can occur at any age, but often begins between ages forty and sixty. About two to three times as many women as men have rheumatoid arthritis.

What causes rheumatoid arthritis?

Scientists believe that rheumatoid arthritis results from the interaction of many factors such as genetics, hormones, and the environment. Although rheumatoid arthritis sometimes runs in families, the actual cause of rheumatoid arthritis is still unknown.

Research suggests that a person's genetic makeup is an important part of the picture, but not the whole story. Some evidence shows that infectious agents, such as viruses and bacteria, may trigger rheumatoid arthritis in people with an inherited tendency to develop the disease. The exact agent or agents, however, are not yet known.

It is important to note that rheumatoid arthritis is not contagious. A person cannot catch it from someone else.

What are some common symptoms of rheumatoid arthritis?

Rheumatoid arthritis is characterized by inflammation of the joint lining. This inflammation causes warmth, redness, swelling, and pain around the joints.

The pain of rheumatoid arthritis varies greatly from person to person, for reasons that doctors do not yet understand completely. Factors that contribute to the pain include swelling within the joint, the amount of heat or redness present, or damage that has occurred within the joint.

How is rheumatoid arthritis diagnosed?

Rheumatoid arthritis can be difficult to diagnose in its early stages because the full range of symptoms develops over time, and only a few symptoms may be present in the early stages.

As part of the diagnosis, your doctor will look for symptoms such as swelling, warmth, pain, and limitations in joint motion throughout your body. Your doctor may ask you questions about the intensity of your pain symptoms, how often they occur, and what makes the pain better or worse.

There is no single, definitive test for rheumatoid arthritis. One common test is for rheumatoid factor, an antibody that is eventually present in the blood of most rheumatoid arthritis patients. An antibody is a special protein made by the immune system that normally helps fight foreign substances in the body. Not all people with rheumatoid arthritis test positive for rheumatoid factor, however, especially early in the disease.

Another test is the citrulline antibody test. Other common tests include one called the erythrocyte sedimentation rate that indicates the presence of inflammation in the body, a white blood cell count, and a blood test for anemia.

X-rays are often used to determine the degree of joint destruction. They are not useful in the early stages of rheumatoid arthritis before bone damage is evident, but they can be used later to monitor the progression of the disease.

How is rheumatoid arthritis treated?

Medication, exercise, and, in some cases, surgery are common treatments for this disease. Most people who have rheumatoid arthritis take medications. Some drugs only provide relief for pain; others reduce inflammation.

People with rheumatoid arthritis can also benefit from exercise, but they need to maintain a good balance between rest and exercise. They should get rest when the disease is active and get more exercise when it is not.

In some cases, a doctor will recommend surgery to restore function or relieve pain in a damaged joint. Several types of surgery are available to patients with severe joint damage. Joint replacement and tendon reconstruction are examples.

What are some non-drug therapies that can help people with rheumatoid arthritis?

Both rest and exercise can help people with rheumatoid arthritis. Rest helps reduce active joint inflammation and pain and fights tiredness. Exercise can help people sleep well, reduce pain, and maintain a positive attitude. An overall nutritious diet with the right amount of calories, protein, and calcium is important.

Some people find that using a splint for a short time around a painful joint reduces pain and swelling by supporting the joint and letting it rest. Assistive devices may help reduce stress and lessen pain in the joints. Examples include zipper pullers and aids to help with moving in and out of chairs and beds.

What kind of surgery is available for people with rheumatoid arthritis or osteoarthritis?

Several types of surgery, including joint replacement and tendon reconstruction, are available to people with rheumatoid arthritis and osteoarthritis. A doctor may perform surgery to smooth out, fuse, or reposition bones, or to replace joints.

The purpose of these procedures is to reduce pain, improve joint function, and improve a person's ability to perform activities of daily living. For people with arthritis, surgery is one way to help relieve pain and disability.

If you are considering surgery for osteoarthritis or rheumatoid arthritis, there are important factors to discuss with your doctor beforehand.

These include your age and occupation, the extent of your disability and pain, and how much the disease interferes with your everyday life.

Today, most surgery for osteoarthritis involves replacing the hip or knee joint. Surgeons may replace affected joints with artificial ones called prostheses.

What is gout?

Gout is one of the most painful rheumatic diseases. It occurs when needle-like crystals of uric acid build up in connective tissue, in the joint space between two bones, or in both.

Adult men, particularly those between the ages of forty and fifty, are more likely than women to develop gout. Women rarely develop the disease while still menstruating.

Sometime during the course of the disease, gout will affect the big toe in about 75 percent of patients. Gout frequently affects joints in the lower part of the body such as knee, ankles, or toes.

What causes gout?

Researchers have discovered several key risk factors for developing gout. In addition to inherited traits, diet, weight, and alcohol play a role in the development of gout. Up to 8 percent of people with gout have a family history of the disease.

Most people with gout have too much uric acid in their blood, a condition called hyperuricemia. Uric acid is a substance that results from the breakdown of purines, which are part of all human tissue and are found in many foods. Hyperuricemia occurs when high levels of uric acid build up in the bloodstream.

What are some common symptoms of gout?

Gout frequently first attacks the joints in the big toe. The affected joint may become swollen, red, or warm. Attacks usually occur at night.

How is gout diagnosed?

To confirm a diagnosis of gout, the doctor inserts a needle into the inflamed joint and draws a sample of synovial fluid, the substance that lubricates a joint. A laboratory technician places some of the fluid on a slide and looks for uric acid crystals under a microscope. If uric acid crystals are found in the fluid surrounding the joint, the person usually has gout.

What are the most common treatments for an acute attack of gout?

Physicians often prescribe high doses of nonsteroidal anti-inflammatory drugs, or NSAIDs, or steroids for a sudden attack of gout. NSAIDs are taken by mouth and corticosteroids are either taken by mouth or injected into the affected joint. Patients often begin to improve within a few hours of treatment, and the attack usually goes away completely within a week or so.

Chapter 41

Autoimmune and Related Diseases

Chapter Contents

Section 41.1

Autoimmune Diseases: An Overview

Excerpted from "Autoimmune Diseases: Overview," National Women's Health Information Center, January 2005.

What are autoimmune diseases?

Our bodies have an immune system that protects us from disease and infection. But if you have an autoimmune disease, your immune system attacks itself by mistake, and you can get sick. Autoimmune diseases can affect connective tissue in your body (the tissue which binds together body tissues and organs). Autoimmune disease can affect many parts of your body, like your nerves, muscles, endocrine system (system that directs your body's hormones and other chemicals), and digestive system.

Who is at risk for getting autoimmune diseases?

Most autoimmune diseases occur in women, and most often during their childbearing years. Some of these diseases also affect African American, American Indian, and Latina women more than white women. These diseases tend to run in families, so your genes, along with the way your immune system responds to certain triggers or things in the environment, affect your chances of getting one of these diseases. If you think you may have an autoimmune disease, ask your family members if they have had symptoms like yours. The good news is that if you have an autoimmune disease, there *are* things you can do to feel better!

What are the most common symptoms of autoimmune diseases?

There are more than eighty types of autoimmune diseases. Learning the symptoms of some of the more common autoimmune diseases can help you recognize the signs if you get one. But some autoimmune diseases share similar symptoms. This makes it hard for doctors to find out if you really have one of these diseases, and which one it might be.

This can make your trip to doctors long and stressful. But if you are having symptoms that bother you, you need to persist to make sure you get relief. Below are descriptions of some common autoimmune diseases.

Table 41.1. Common Autoimmune Diseases (*continued on next page*)

Disease	**Symptoms**	**Tests to Help Find Out If You Have It**
Hashimoto thyroiditis (underactive thyroid)	• tiredness • depression • sensitivity to cold • weight gain • muscle weakness and cramps • dry hair • tough skin • constipation • sometimes there are no symptoms	• blood test for thyroid stimulating hormone (TSH)
Graves disease (overactive thyroid)	• insomnia (not able to sleep) • irritability • weight loss without dieting • heat sensitivity • sweating • fine brittle hair • weakness in your muscles • light menstrual periods • bulging eyes • shaky hands • sometimes there are no symptoms	• blood test for thyroid stimulating hormone (TSH)
Lupus	• swelling and damage to the joints, skin, kidneys, heart, lungs, blood vessels, and brain • "butterfly" rash across the nose and cheeks • rashes on other parts of the body • painful and swollen joints • sensitivity to the sun	• exam of your body • lab tests (antinuclear antibody [ANA] test, blood tests, and urine tests)

Table 41.1. Common Autoimmune Diseases (*continued*)

Disease	Symptoms	Tests to Help Find Out If You Have It
Multiple sclerosis (MS)	• weakness and trouble with coordination, balance, speaking, and walking • paralysis • tremors • numbness and tingling feeling in arms, legs, hands, and feet	• exam of your body • exam of your brain, spinal cord, and nerves (neurological exam) • x-ray tests (magnetic resonance imaging [MRI] and magnetic resonance spectroscopy [MRS]) • other tests on the brain and spinal cord fluid to look for things linked to these diseases
Rheumatoid arthritis	• inflammation begins in the tissue lining your joints and then spreads to the whole joint (hand joints are the most common site, but it can affect most joints in the body) • muscle pain • deformed joints • weakness • fatigue • loss of appetite • weight loss • becoming confined to bed in severe cases	• blood tests may show that you have anemia (when your body does not have enough red blood cells) and an antibody called rheumatoid factor (RF). (Some people with RF never get this disease, and others with the disease never have RF.)

Are chronic fatigue syndrome and fibromyalgia autoimmune diseases?

Chronic fatigue syndrome (CFS) and fibromyalgia (FM) are not autoimmune diseases, but they often have symptoms—like being tired all the time and pain—that may seem like other autoimmune diseases.

CFS can cause you to be very tired, have trouble concentrating, feel weak, and have muscle pain. Symptoms of CFS come and go. The cause of CFS is not known.

FM is a disorder with symptoms of widespread muscle pain, fatigue (feeling tired and having low energy), and multiple tender points. Tender points are located in the neck, spine, shoulders, hips, and knees and are painful when pressure is applied to them. FM mainly occurs in women of childbearing age, but children, the elderly, and men are sometimes diagnosed with FM. The cause is not known.

What are flare-ups?

Symptoms of autoimmune diseases can come and go, ranging in how bad they are, or all go away for a while (called remission). Flare-ups, or the sudden and severe onset of symptoms, can also happen. It's best to work closely and often with your doctor and other members of your health care team to manage your illness. If you have a flare-up, it is best to first call your doctor. Don't try a "cure" you heard about from a friend or relative.

Are there medicines to treat autoimmune diseases?

You can take medicines to help your symptoms, which your doctor(s) will talk with you about. The type of medicine you take depends on which disease you have and what your symptoms are. Some people can take over-the-counter drugs, like aspirin and ibuprofen, for pain. Others with more severe symptoms may have to take certain kinds of prescription drugs that can help with pain, swelling, depression, anxiety, sleep problems, fatigue, or rashes. You also might be able to take medicine to help slow the progress of your disease. New treatments for autoimmune diseases are being studied all the time.

How can I manage my life now that I have an autoimmune disease?

Although there is no cure for autoimmune diseases, you can treat your symptoms and learn to manage your disease, so you can enjoy life! Women with autoimmune diseases lead full, active lives. Your life goals should not have to change. It is important, though, to see a doctor who specializes in these types of diseases.

What are some things I can do to feel better?

If you are living with an autoimmune disease, there are things you can do each day to feel better:

- **Eat a healthy diet:** Keep your immune system as healthy as can be! The list of nutrients that you need for a healthy immune system is long. But don't try to overload on vitamins because that could be worse for your health. Try to get all you need from food, rather than from vitamin pills. Eat balanced meals with foods from all of the food groups. Include yummy fruits and vegetables and whole grains. Also eat calcium-rich foods, such as fat-free or low-fat milk and yogurt. Avoid fatty foods.

- **Get regular exercise (but be careful not to overdo it):** Thirty minutes most days of the week is best, but talk with your doctor about what types of exercise you can do. A gradual and gentle exercise program often works well for people with long-lasting muscle and joint pain. Some types of yoga or tai chi exercises may be helpful.
- **Get enough rest:** Rest allows your body tissues and joints the time they need to repair. Sleeping is a great way you can help both your body and mind. If you don't get enough sleep, your stress level and your symptoms could get worse. You also can't fight off sickness as well when you sleep poorly. With enough sleep, you can tackle your problems better and lower your risk for illness. Try to get at least seven hours of sleep every night.
- **Reduce stress and try "self" pain management:** You also might be able to lessen your pain or muscle spasms and deal with other aspects of living with your disease if you try meditation or self-hypnosis. You can learn to do these through self-help books, tapes, or with the help of an instructor. You also can use imagery (use the power of your thoughts to "destroy" your pain) or distract your focus on your pain by doing a hobby or something else you enjoy.

What kinds of doctors will I need to treat my autoimmune disease?

Juggling your health care needs among different doctors and other types of health care providers can be hard. But visiting other types of health care workers, along with your main doctor, may be helpful in managing some symptoms of your autoimmune disease. If you are visiting many types of health care workers, make sure you have a supportive main doctor to help you. Often, your family doctor may help you coordinate care. Here are some other kinds of health care workers that may be useful:

- **Nephrologist:** A doctor who will look at how well your kidneys are working. Kidneys are organs that clean the blood and produce urine.

- **Rheumatologist:** A doctor who specializes in arthritis and other diseases.
- **Endocrinologist:** A doctor who specializes in diseases that affect your glands (organs in your body that make hormones). Glands help control the body's reproduction, energy levels, weight, food and waste production, and growth and development.
- **Physical therapist:** A health care worker who can help you with stiffness, weakness, restricted body movement, and with finding out the proper level of exercise for your body.
- **Occupational therapist:** A health care worker who can help you find devices or make changes in your home or workplace to make life easier for you. They also can teach you ways to do all you have to despite your pain and other health problems.
- **Speech therapist:** A health care worker who can be helpful for people with MS who have speech problems.
- **Vocational therapist:** A health care worker who offers job training for people who cannot do their current jobs because of their illness or other health problems. You can find this type of person through both public and private agencies.
- **Counselor for emotional support:** A health care worker who is specially trained to help you to find ways to cope with your illness. You can work through your feelings of anger, fear, denial, and frustration.
- **Support groups:** Some women find that talking with others who have the same health problem is helpful in finding new ways to cope with it.
- **Chiropractor:** A type of doctor who might be helpful in relieving some of your symptoms, such as muscle spasms and backaches. But you should only see this type of doctor along with your regular autoimmune disease doctor, not in place of him or her.

Section 41.2

Lupus

Reprinted from "Do I Have Lupus?" National Institute of Arthritis and Musculoskeletal and Skin Diseases, March 2003. Revised by David A. Cooke, MD, December 2008.

If you have lupus, you probably have many questions. Lupus isn't a simple disease with an easy answer. You can't take a pill and make it go away. The people you live with and work with may have trouble understanding that you're sick. Lupus doesn't have a clear set of signs that people can see. You may know that something's wrong, even though it may take a while to be diagnosed.

Lupus has many shades. It can affect people of different races, ethnicities, and ages, both men and women. It can look like different diseases. It's different for every person who has it.

The good news is that you can get help and fight lupus. Learning about it is the first step. Ask questions. Talk to your doctor, family, and friends. People who look for answers are more likely to find them.

Understanding Lupus

Lupus is an autoimmune disease. Your body's immune system is like an army with hundreds of soldiers. The immune system's job is to fight foreign substances in the body, like germs and viruses. But in autoimmune diseases, the immune system is out of control. It attacks healthy tissues, not germs.

You can't catch lupus from another person. It isn't cancer, and it isn't related to acquired immunodeficiency syndrome (AIDS).

Lupus is a disease that can affect many parts of the body. Everyone reacts differently. One person with lupus may have swollen knees and fever. Another person may be tired all the time or have kidney trouble. Someone else may have rashes. Lupus can involve the joints, the skin, the kidneys, the lungs, the heart, and/or the brain. If you have lupus, it may affect two or three parts of your body. Usually, one person doesn't have all the possible symptoms.

There are three main types of lupus:

- Systemic lupus erythematosus is the most common form. It's sometimes called SLE, or just lupus. The word "systemic" means that the disease can involve many parts of the body such as the heart, lungs, kidneys, and brain. Almost any part of the body can be affected, but most patients will only have problems with a few. SLE symptoms can be mild or serious.
- Discoid lupus erythematosus mainly affects the skin. A red rash may appear, or the skin on the face, scalp, or elsewhere may change color.
- Drug-induced lupus is triggered by a few medicines. It's like SLE, but symptoms are usually milder. Most of the time, the disease goes away when the medicine is stopped. More men develop drug-induced lupus because the drugs that cause it, hydralazine and procainamide, are used to treat heart conditions that are more common in men.

Signs and Symptoms of Lupus

Lupus may be hard to diagnose. It's often mistaken for other diseases. For this reason, lupus has been called the "great imitator." The signs of lupus differ from person to person. Some people have just a few signs; others have more.

Common signs of lupus are as follows:

- Red rash or color change on the face, often in the shape of a butterfly across the nose and cheeks
- Painful or swollen joints
- Unexplained fever
- Chest pain with deep breathing
- Swollen glands
- Extreme fatigue (feeling tired all the time)
- Unusual hair loss (mainly on the scalp)
- Pale or purple fingers or toes from cold or stress
- Sensitivity to the sun
- Low blood count
- Depression, trouble thinking, and/or memory problems

Other signs are mouth sores, unexplained seizures (convulsions), "seeing things" (hallucinations), repeated miscarriages, and unexplained kidney problems.

A Lupus Flare

When symptoms appear, it's called a "flare." These signs may come and go. You may have swelling and rashes one week and no symptoms at all the next. You may find that your symptoms flare after you've been out in the sun or after a hard day at work.

Even if you take medicine for lupus, you may find that there are times when the symptoms become worse. Learning to recognize that a flare is coming can help you take steps to cope with it. Many people feel very tired or have pain, a rash, a fever, stomach discomfort, headache, or dizziness just before a flare. Steps to prevent flares, such as limiting the time you spend in the sun and getting enough rest and quiet, can also be helpful.

Lupus can cause many different types of symptoms, and some of them may seem quite strange, especially if they have never happened before. It's important to let your doctor know immediately if you develop new or odd symptoms; they might be signs of a flare. Your doctor will be better able to tell whether or not a symptom is a reason for worry.

Preventing a Flare

- Learn to recognize that a flare is coming.
- Talk with your doctor.
- Try to set realistic goals and priorities.
- Limit the time you spend in the sun.
- Maintain a healthy diet.
- Develop coping skills to help limit stress.
- Get enough rest and quiet.
- Moderately exercise when possible.
- Develop a support system by surrounding yourself with people you trust and feel comfortable with (family, friends, etc.).

Causes of Lupus

We don't know what causes lupus. There is no cure, but in most cases lupus can be managed. Lupus sometimes seems to run in families, which suggests the disease may be hereditary. Having the genes isn't the whole story, though. The environment, sunlight, stress, and certain medicines may trigger symptoms in some people. Other people who have similar genetic backgrounds may not get signs or symptoms of the disease. Researchers are trying to find out why.

Lupus Risk Factors

Anyone can get lupus. But nine out of ten people who have it are women. African American women are three times more likely to get lupus than white women. It's also more common in Hispanic/Latino, Asian, and American Indian women.

Both African Americans and Hispanics/Latinos tend to develop lupus at a younger age and have more symptoms at diagnosis (including kidney problems).

They also tend to have more severe disease than whites. For example, African American patients have more seizures and strokes, while Hispanic/Latino patients have more heart problems. We don't understand why some people seem to have more problems with lupus than others.

Diagnosing Lupus

- **Medical history:** Telling a doctor about your symptoms and other problems you have had can help him or her understand your situation. Your history can provide clues to your disease.
- **Complete physical exam:** The doctor will look for rashes and other signs that something is wrong.
- **Laboratory testing of blood and urine samples:** Blood and urine samples often show if your immune system is overactive.
- **Skin or kidney biopsy:** In a biopsy, tissue that is removed by a minor surgical procedure is examined under a microscope. Skin or kidney tissue examined in this way can show signs of an autoimmune disease.

Lupus is most common in women between the ages of fifteen and forty-four. These are roughly the years when most women are able to have babies. Scientists think a woman's hormones may have something to do with getting lupus. Women who have had children are at higher risk of developing lupus. But it's important to remember that men and older people can get it, too.

It's less common for children under age fifteen to have lupus. One exception is babies born to women with lupus. These children may have heart, liver, or skin problems caused by lupus. With good care, most women with lupus can have a normal pregnancy and a healthy baby.

What Doctors Can Do

Go see a doctor. He or she will talk to you and take a history of your health problems. Many people have lupus for a long time before they find out they have it. It's important that you tell the doctor or nurse about your symptoms. This information, along with a physical examination and the results of laboratory tests, helps the doctor decide whether you have lupus or something else.

A rheumatologist is a doctor who specializes in treating diseases that affect the joints and muscles, like lupus. You may want to ask your regular doctor for a referral to a rheumatologist.

In some cases, a dermatologist, a doctor who specializes in treating diseases that affect the skin, may be involved in diagnosis and treatment. No single test can show that you have lupus. Your doctor may have to run several tests and study your medical history. It may take time for the doctor to diagnose lupus.

Medications for Lupus

Remember that each person has different symptoms. Treatment depends on the symptoms. The doctor may give you aspirin or a similar medicine to treat swollen joints and fever. Creams may be prescribed for a rash. For more serious problems, stronger medicines such as antimalaria drugs, corticosteroids, and chemotherapy drugs are used. Your doctor will choose a treatment based on your symptoms and needs.

Always tell your doctor if you have problems with your medicines. Let your doctor know if you take herbal or vitamin supplements. Your medicines may not mix well with these supplements. You and your doctor can work together to find the best way to treat all of your symptoms.

Most of the medications used to treat lupus suppress the immune system. This helps control the lupus, but also makes you more vulnerable to infections. You should discuss with your doctor what steps you should take to protect yourself from infection.

Coping with Lupus

You need to find out what works best for you. You may find that a rheumatologist has the best treatment plan for you. Other health professionals who can help you deal with different aspects of lupus include psychologists, occupational therapists, dermatologists, and dietitians. You might find that doing exercises with a physical therapist makes you feel better. The important thing is to follow up with your health care team on a regular basis, even when your lupus is quiet and all seems well.

Dealing with a long-lasting disease like lupus can be hard on the emotions. You might think that your friends, family, and co-workers do not understand how you feel. Sadness and anger are common reactions.

People with lupus have limited energy and must manage it wisely. Ask your health care team about ways to cope with fatigue. Most people feel better if they manage their rest and work and take their medicine. If you're depressed, medicine and counseling can help.

Also do the following:

- Pay attention to your body. Slow down or stop before you're too tired.
- Learn to pace yourself. Spread out your work and other activities.
- Don't blame yourself for your fatigue. It's part of the disease.
- Consider support groups and counseling. They can help you realize that you're not alone. Group members teach one another how to cope.
- Consider other support from your family as well as faith-based and other community groups.

It's true that staying healthy is harder when you have lupus. You need to pay close attention to your body, mind, and spirit. Having a chronic disease is stressful. People cope with stress differently. Some approaches that may help are as follows:

- Staying involved in social activities
- Practicing techniques such as meditation and yoga
- Setting priorities for spending time and energy

Exercising is another approach that can help you cope with lupus. Types of exercise that you can practice include the following:

- Range-of-motion (for example, stretching) exercises help maintain normal joint movement and relieve stiffness. This type of exercise helps maintain or increase flexibility.

- Strengthening (for example, weight-lifting) exercises help keep or increase muscle strength. Strong muscles help support and protect joints affected by lupus.
- Aerobic or endurance (for example, brisk walking or jogging) exercises improve cardiovascular fitness, help control weight, and improve overall function.

People with chronic diseases like lupus should check with their health care professional before starting an exercise program.

Learning about lupus may also help. People who are well informed and take part in planning their own care report less pain. They also may make fewer visits to the doctor, have more self-confidence, and remain more active.

Women who want to start a family should work closely with their health care team; for example, doctors, physical therapists, and nurses. Your obstetrician and your lupus doctor should work together to find the best treatment plan for you.

Hope Through Research

Scientists are working to find out what causes lupus and how it can best be treated. Here are some of the questions they are trying to answer:

- Who gets lupus and why?
- Why are women more likely to get lupus than men?
- Why are there more cases of lupus among certain racial and ethnic groups?
- What goes wrong in the immune system and why?
- What genes play a role in lupus?
- How can we fix an immune system that isn't working well?
- How can lupus symptoms best be treated?

The National Institutes of Health (NIH) supports research on health and disease. The National Institute of Arthritis and Musculoskeletal and Skin Diseases (NIAMS) supports research on the bones, joints, muscles, connective tissue, and skin. These are the parts of the body that can be affected by lupus. Research supported by NIAMS is looking at these issues:

- Certain genes make some people more likely to have serious complications, such as kidney disease. NIAMS researchers have found a gene linked to a higher risk of lupus kidney disease in African Americans. Changes in this gene keep the immune system from removing harmful germ-fighters from the body after they've done their job. Other genes may also play a role.
- Lupus is more common in women than in men. Researchers are looking into the role of hormones and other male-female differences.
- Studies are underway to determine whether certain medications or combinations of medications are better for controlling lupus, or have fewer side effects. There are also new medications being tested that might be safer or more effective than current treatments.

Section 41.3

Chronic Fatigue Syndrome

"Facts about Chronic Fatigue Syndrome," reprinted courtesy of the Illinois Department of Public Health (www.idph.state.il.us). The text of this document is available online at http://www.idph.state.il.us/about/womenshealth/factsheets/cfsyndrome.htm; accessed May 12, 2008.

What is chronic fatigue syndrome?

Chronic fatigue syndrome (CFS) is not the normal ups and downs experienced in everyday life. The early sign of this illness is a strong and noticeable fatigue that comes on suddenly and often comes and goes or never stops. It is not improved by bed rest and may be worsened by physical or mental activity. Persons with CFS most often function at a substantially lower level of activity than they were capable of before the onset of the illness. CFS is diagnosed two to four times more often in women than in men, possibly because of biological, psychological and social influences.

What are the symptoms/warning signs of chronic fatigue syndrome?

In order to be diagnosed with CFS a patient must satisfy two criteria. Severe chronic fatigue must have lasted at least six months with other known medical conditions excluded by clinical diagnoses. Also, a person must concurrently have four or more of the following symptoms: substantial impairment in short-term memory or concentration; sore throat; tender lymph nodes; muscle pain; multi-joint pain without swelling or redness; headaches of a new type, pattern, or severity; unrefreshing sleep; and post-exertional malaise lasting more than twenty-four hours. The symptoms must have persisted or recurred during six or more consecutive months and must not have predated the fatigue.

What causes chronic fatigue syndrome?

Despite a vigorous search, the cause(s) for CFS remain unknown. One possibility may be that CFS represents an endpoint of disease resulting from multiple precipitating causes. Some conditions that have been proposed to trigger the development of CFS include viral infections or other transient traumatic conditions, stress, and toxins.

Are there any risk factors?

Research indicates that CFS is most common in people in their forties and fifties and women are more likely than men to be affected.

Is there any treatment?

There is currently no cure for CFS. The therapies for this disorder are directed at symptom relief. It is important to maintain good health by eating a balanced diet and getting adequate rest, exercising regularly without causing more fatigue, and pacing oneself because too much stress can aggravate the symptoms of CFS. Working with a physician to develop a program that provides the greatest benefits also will help in reducing frustration with the illness.

Nonpharmacological therapies include acupuncture, aquatic therapy, chiropractic, cranial-sacral, light exercise, massage, self-hypnosis, stretching, tai chi, therapeutic touch, and yoga. Certain psychotherapies such as cognitive behavioral therapy also have shown promise for facilitating patient coping and for alleviating some of the distress associated with CFS.

In pharmacological therapy there are a variety of medications that can relieve specific symptoms. It is important to begin with low doses and to escalate the dosage gradually as necessary.

Some CFS patients may also find it therapeutic to meet with other people who have this illness, and this can be accomplished by joining a local CFS support group. Support groups are not appropriate for everyone, and may actually add to their stress rather than relieving it.

What is the prognosis?

The clinical course of CFS varies considerably among persons who have the disorder. The actual percentage of patients who recover is unknown, and even the definition of what should be considered recovery is subject to debate. Some patients recover to the point where they can resume work and other activities, but continue to experience various or periodic CFS symptoms. Some patients recover completely with time, and some grow progressively worse. CFS follows a cyclical course, alternating between periods of illness and relative well being.

Section 41.4

Fibromyalgia

Reprinted from "Fibromyalgia," National Women's Health Information Center, May 2006.

What is fibromyalgia (FM)?

Fibromyalgia is a disorder that causes aches and pain all over the body. People with FM also are tender throughout the body, which is most pronounced at certain regions termed "tender points." Tender points are specific places on the neck, shoulders, back, hips, arms, and legs. These points hurt when pressure is put on them.

What are the symptoms of fibromyalgia?

People with FM could have the following symptoms:

- Muscle pain
- Fatigue
- Trouble sleeping
- Joint pain, stiffness (sometimes worse in the morning)
- Headaches
- Restless legs
- Tingling or numbness in hands and feet
- Problems with thinking and memory (sometimes called "fibro fog")
- Leg cramps
- Feeling nervous
- Depression
- Feeling dizzy or lightheaded
- Painful cramping during your period
- Jaw pain
- Upset stomach, cramping, bloating, feeling constipated, or diarrhea
- Trouble swallowing
- Frequent or painful urination

How common is fibromyalgia? Who is mainly affected?

FM affects as many as one in fifty Americans. Most people with FM are women (about 80 to 90 percent). However, men and children also can have the disorder. Most people are diagnosed during middle age. FM can occur by itself, but people with certain other diseases, such as rheumatoid arthritis and other types of arthritis, may be more likely to have FM. Individuals who have a close relative with FM are more likely to develop FM.

What causes fibromyalgia?

The causes of FM are not known. Researchers think a number of factors might be involved. FM has been linked to the following:

- Having a family history of fibromyalgia (i.e. genetics)
- Being exposed to stressful or traumatic events, such as car accidents, injuries to the body caused by performing the same action

over and over again, infections or illnesses, or being deployed to war

How is fibromyalgia diagnosed?

People with FM often see many doctors before being diagnosed. One reason for this may be that pain and fatigue, the main symptoms of FM, also are symptoms of many other conditions. Therefore, doctors often must rule out other possible causes of these symptoms before making a diagnosis of FM. FM cannot be detected by a lab test either.

A doctor who knows about FM, however, can make a diagnosis based upon two criteria:

- A history of widespread pain lasting more than three months. Pain must be present in both the right and left sides of the body as well as above and below the waist.
- Presence of tender points. The body has eighteen sites that are possible tender points. For FM diagnosis a person must have eleven or more tender points. To be deemed a tender point, pain must be felt when pressure is applied to the site. People who have FM may feel pain at other sites, too, but those eighteen sites on the body are used for diagnosis.

The previous criteria were developed for use to standardize research studies and are not necessary to diagnose individual patients, but if you feel your doctor doesn't know a lot about FM or has doubts about whether it is a "real" illness, see another doctor for a second opinion. Contact a local university medical school or research center for help finding a doctor who has helped others with FM.

How is fibromyalgia treated?

FM can be hard to treat. It's important to find a doctor who has treated others with FM. Many family doctors, general internists, or rheumatologists can treat FM. Rheumatologists are doctors who treat arthritis and other conditions that affect the joints and soft tissues.

Treatment often requires a team approach. The team may include your doctor, a physical therapist, and possibly other health care providers. A pain or rheumatology clinic can be a good place to get treatment.

The U.S. Food and Drug Administration has not yet approved any medicines to treat FM. Doctors treat FM with medicines approved for other purposes. Pain medicines and antidepressants are often used in treatment.

What is the difference between fibromyalgia and chronic fatigue syndrome?

Chronic fatigue syndrome (CFS) and FM are alike in many ways. In fact, it is not uncommon for a person to have both FM and CFS. Some experts believe that FM and CFS are in fact the same disorder, but expressed in slightly different ways. Both CFS and FM have pain and fatigue as symptoms.

The main symptom of CFS is extreme tiredness. CFS often begins after having flu-like symptoms. But people with CFS do not have the tender points that people with FM have. To be diagnosed with CFS, a person must have the following:

- Extreme fatigue for at least six months that cannot be explained by medical tests and
- Have four or more of the following symptoms:
  - Forgetting things or having a hard time focusing
  - Feeling tired even after sleeping
  - Muscle pain or aches
  - Pain or aches in joints without swelling or redness
  - Feeling discomfort or "out-of- sorts" for more than twenty-four hours after being active
  - Headaches of a new type, pattern, or strength
  - Tender lymph nodes in the neck or under the arm
  - Sore throat

Is there anything I can do to help me feel better?

Besides taking medicine prescribed by your doctor, there are many things you can do to lessen the impact of FM on your life:

- **Get enough sleep:** Getting enough sleep and the right kind of sleep can help ease the pain and fatigue of FM
- **Get moving:** Though pain and fatigue may make exercise and daily activities hard, being active as possible is important. People who have a lot of pain or fatigue should begin with walking or

other gentle exercises and slowly build up to more demanding workouts.

- **Make changes at work:** Most people with FM continue to work, but they may have to make big changes to do so. For example, some people cut down the number of hours, switch to a less demanding job, or adapt a current job.
- **Eat right:** Try to add more fruits, vegetables, and whole grains to your diet.

What if I can't work because of fibromyalgia?

If you cannot work because of your FM, contact the Social Security Administration for help with disability benefits.

What research is being done on fibromyalgia?

The National Institute of Arthritis and Musculoskeletal and Skin Diseases sponsors research to help understand FM and find better ways to diagnose, treat, and prevent it. Researchers are studying the following things:

- Why people with FM have are highly sensitive to pain
- The role of stress hormones in the body
- Medicines and behavioral treatments
- Whether there is a gene or genes that make a person more likely to have FM

Chapter 42

Cardiovascular Disorders

Chapter Contents

Section 42.1

Heart Disease

Excerpted from "Heart Disease," National Women's Health Information Center, February 2007.

What is heart disease?

Heart disease is a number of abnormal conditions affecting the heart and the blood vessels in the heart. Types of heart disease include the following:

- **Coronary artery disease (CAD):** This is the most common type and is the leading cause of heart attacks. When you have CAD, your arteries become hard and narrow. Blood has a hard time getting to the heart, so the heart does not get all the blood it needs. CAD can lead to the following:
  - **Angina:** Angina is chest pain or discomfort that happens when the heart does not get enough blood. It may feel like a pressing or squeezing pain, often in the chest, but sometimes the pain is in the shoulders, arms, neck, jaw, or back. It can also feel like indigestion (upset stomach). Angina is not a heart attack, but having angina means you are more likely to have a heart attack.
  - **Heart attack:** A heart attack occurs when an artery is severely or completely blocked, and the heart does not get the blood it needs for more than twenty minutes.
- **Heart failure:** This occurs when the heart is not able to pump blood through the body as well as it should. This means that other organs, which normally get blood from the heart, do not get enough blood. It does *not* mean that the heart stops. Signs of heart failure include shortness of breath (feeling like you can't get enough air); swelling in feet, ankles, and legs; and extreme tiredness.
- **Heart arrhythmias:** These are changes in the beat of the heart. Most people have felt dizzy, faint, out of breath or had

chest pains at one time. These changes in heartbeat are, for most people, harmless. As you get older, you are more likely to have arrhythmias. Don't panic if you have a few flutters or if your heart races once in a while. If you have flutters *and* other symptoms such as dizziness or shortness of breath (feeling like you can't get enough air), call 911 right away.

Do women need to worry about heart disease?

Yes. One in three American women dies of heart disease. In 2003, almost twice as many women died of cardiovascular disease (both heart disease and stroke) than from all cancers combined. The older a woman gets, the more likely she is to get heart disease. But women of all ages should be concerned about heart disease. All women should take steps to prevent heart disease.

Both men and women have heart attacks, but more women who have heart attacks die from them. Treatments can limit heart damage but they must be given as soon as possible after a heart attack starts. Ideally, treatment should start within one hour of the first symptoms.

What can I do to prevent heart disease?

You can reduce your chances of getting heart disease by taking these steps:

- **Know your blood pressure:** Your heart moves blood through your body. If it is hard for your heart to do this, your heart works harder, and your blood pressure will rise. People with high blood pressure often have no symptoms, so have your blood pressure checked every one to two years. If you have high blood pressure, your doctor may suggest you make some lifestyle changes, such as eating less salt (DASH eating plan) and exercising more. Your doctor may also prescribe medicine to help lower your blood pressure.
- **Don't smoke:** If you smoke, try to quit. If you're having trouble quitting, there are products and programs that can help, such as nicotine patches and gums, support groups, and programs to help you stop smoking. Ask your doctor or nurse for help.
- **Get tested for diabetes:** People with diabetes have high blood glucose (often called blood sugar). People with high blood sugar often have no symptoms, so have your blood sugar checked regularly. Having diabetes raises your chances of getting heart

disease. If you have diabetes, your doctor will decide if you need diabetes pills or insulin shots. Your doctor can also help you make a healthy eating and exercise plan.

- **Get your cholesterol and triglyceride levels tested:** High blood cholesterol can clog your arteries and keep your heart from getting the blood it needs. This can cause a heart attack. Triglycerides are a form of fat in your blood stream. High levels of triglycerides are linked to heart disease in some people. People with high blood cholesterol or high blood triglycerides often have no symptoms, so have your blood cholesterol and triglyceride levels checked regularly. If your cholesterol or triglyceride levels are high, talk to your doctor about what you can do to lower them. You may be able to lower your cholesterol and triglyceride levels by eating better and exercising more. Your doctor may prescribe medication to help lower your cholesterol.
- **Maintain a healthy weight:** Being overweight raises your risk for heart disease. Calculate your body mass index (BMI) to see if you are at a healthy weight. Eat a healthy diet and exercise at a moderate intensity for at least thirty minutes most days of the week. Start by adding more fruits, vegetables, and whole grains to your diet. Take a brisk walk on your lunch break or take the stairs instead of the elevator.
- **If you drink alcohol, limit it to no more than one drink (one 12-ounce beer, one 5-ounce glass of wine, or one 1.5-ounce shot of hard liquor) a day.**
- **Find healthy ways to cope with stress:** Lower your stress level by talking to your friends, exercising, or writing in a journal.

What does high cholesterol have to do with heart disease?

Cholesterol is a waxy substance found in all parts of the body. When there is too much cholesterol in your blood, cholesterol can build up on the walls of your arteries and cause blood clots. Cholesterol can clog your arteries and keep your heart from getting the blood it needs. This can cause a heart attack.

There are two types of cholesterol:

- Low-density lipoprotein (LDL) is often called the "bad" type of cholesterol because it can clog the arteries that carry blood to your heart. For LDL, lower numbers are better.

- High-density lipoprotein (HDL) is known as "good" cholesterol because it takes the bad cholesterol out of your blood and keeps it from building up in your arteries. For HDL, higher numbers are better.

All women age twenty and older should have their blood cholesterol and triglyceride levels checked at least once every five years.

What do my cholesterol and triglyceride numbers mean?

With total cholesterol level, lower is better. A total cholesterol level of less than 200 mg/dL is desirable; of 200 to 239 mg/dL is borderline high; and of 240 or above is high.

With LDL (bad) cholesterol, lower is better. An LDL level of less than 100 mg/dL is optimal; of 100–129 mg/dL is near or above optimal; of 130–159 mg/dL is borderline high; of 160–189 mg/dL is high; and of 190 mg/dL and above is very high.

With HDL (good) cholesterol, higher is better. More than 60 mg/dL is best.

With triglyceride levels, lower is better. Less than 150 mg/dL is best.

How can I lower my cholesterol?

You can lower your cholesterol by taking these steps:

- **Maintain a healthy weight:** If you are overweight, losing weight can help lower your total cholesterol and LDL ("bad cholesterol") levels. Calculate your body mass index (BMI) to see if you are at a healthy weight. If not, try making small changes like eating an apple instead of potato chips, taking the stairs instead of the elevator, or parking farther away from the entrance to your office, the grocery store, or the mall. (But be sure to park in a safe, well-lit spot.)

- **Eat better:** Eat foods low in saturated fats, trans fats, and cholesterol. Eat more fish, poultry (chicken, turkey—breast meat or drumstick is best), and lean meats (round, sirloin, loin). Broil, bake, roast, or poach foods. Remove the fat and skin before eating. Eat skim (fat-free) or low-fat (1%) milk and cheeses, and low-fat or nonfat yogurt. Eat more fruits and vegetables (try for 5 a day) and eat cereals, breads, rice, and pasta made from whole grains (such as "whole-wheat" or "whole-grain" bread and pasta, rye bread, brown rice, and oatmeal). Eat fewer organ meats (liver, kidney, brains), egg yolks, fats (butter, lard) and oils, and packaged and processed foods.

- **Get moving:** Exercise can help lower LDL ("bad cholesterol") and raise HDL ("good cholesterol"). Exercise at a moderate intensity for at least thirty minutes most days of the week. Take a brisk walk on your lunch break or take the stairs instead of the elevator.
- **Take your medicine:** If your doctor has prescribed medicine to lower your cholesterol, take it exactly as you have been told to.

How do I know if I have heart disease?

Heart disease often has no symptoms. But, there are some signs to watch for. Chest or arm pain or discomfort can be a symptom of heart disease and a warning sign of a heart attack. Shortness of breath (feeling like you can't get enough air), dizziness, nausea (feeling sick to your stomach), abnormal heartbeats, or feeling very tired also are signs. Talk with your doctor if you're having any of these symptoms. Your doctor will take a medical history, do a physical exam, and may order tests.

What are the signs of a heart attack?

Not everyone has all of the warning signs of heart attack. And, sometimes these signs can go away and come back.

Symptoms of a heart attack include the following:

- Pain or discomfort in the center of the chest
- Pain or discomfort in other areas of the upper body, including the arms, back, neck, jaw, or stomach
- Other symptoms, such as shortness of breath (feeling like you can't get enough air), breaking out in a cold sweat, nausea (feeling sick to your stomach), or feeling faint or woozy

Some women have more vague symptoms such as the following:

- Unusual tiredness
- Trouble sleeping
- Problems breathing
- Indigestion (upset stomach)
- Anxiety (feeling uneasy or worried)

If you think you, or someone else, may be having a heart attack, wait no more than a few minutes—five at most—before calling 911.

Should I take a daily aspirin to prevent heart attack?

Aspirin may be helpful for women at high risk, such as women who have already had a heart attack. Aspirin can have serious side effects and may be harmful when mixed with certain medicines. If you're thinking about taking aspirin, talk to your doctor first. If your doctor thinks aspirin is a good choice for you, be sure to take it exactly as your doctor tells you to.

Does taking birth control pills increase my risk for heart disease?

Taking birth control pills is generally safe for young, healthy women. But birth control pills can pose heart disease risks for some women, especially women older than thirty-five; women with high blood pressure, diabetes, or high cholesterol; and women who smoke. Talk with your doctor if you have questions about the pill.

Does using the birth control patch increase my risk for heart disease?

The patch is generally safe for young, healthy women. The patch can pose heart disease risks for some women, especially women older than thirty-five; women with high blood pressure, diabetes, or high cholesterol; and women who smoke.

Recent studies show that women who use the patch may be exposed to more estrogen (the female hormone in birth control pills and the patch that keeps users from becoming pregnant) than women who use the birth control pill. Research is underway to see if the risk for blood clots (which can lead to heart attack or stroke) is higher in patch users. Talk with your doctor if you have questions about the patch.

Does hormone replacement therapy (HRT) increase a woman's risk for heart disease?

Hormone replacement therapy (HRT) can help with some symptoms of menopause, including hot flashes, vaginal dryness, mood swings, and bone loss, but there are risks, too. For some women, taking hormones can increase their chances of having a heart attack or stroke. If you decide to use hormones, use them at the lowest dose that helps for the shortest time needed. Talk with your doctor if you have questions about HRT.

Section 42.2

High Blood Pressure (Hypertension)

"High Blood Pressure," reprinted courtesy of the Illinois Department of Public Health (www.idph.state.il.us). The text of this document is available online at http://www.idph.state.il.us/public/hb/hbhype.htm; accessed May 12, 2008.

What is high blood pressure?

Blood pressure is the force of blood as it moves through the blood vessels. If blood cannot flow easily through the vessels, the force increases. If the force is too great, you have high blood pressure.

High blood pressure is a serious disease. It increases the workload on the heart and blood vessels and can lead to heart disease, stroke, kidney problems, and even blindness.

The medical term for high blood pressure is hypertension. High blood pressure is dangerous because it makes the heart work too hard and contributes to atherosclerosis (hardening of the arteries). It increases the risk of heart disease and stroke, the first and third leading causes of death among Americans.

How can I tell if I have high blood pressure?

High blood pressure usually has no symptoms. In fact, many people have high blood pressure for years without knowing it. That's why it's called the "silent killer." In 90 to 95 percent of cases, the cause of high blood pressure is unknown.

A single elevated blood pressure reading doesn't mean you have high blood pressure, but it's a sign that further observation is required. The only way to find out if you have high blood pressure is to have your blood pressure checked.

Who is affected?

High blood pressure affects about fifty million (or one in four) American adults. It is especially common among African Americans, who tend to develop it earlier and more often than whites. Also, many Americans tend to develop high blood pressure as they get older; however hypertension is not a part of healthy aging. About 60 percent of all Americans age sixty and older have high blood pressure.

Others at high risk of developing hypertension are persons who are overweight, those with a family history of high blood pressure, and those with a high-normal blood pressure.

Does smoking tobacco cause high blood pressure?

No. However, it can temporarily raise blood pressure, and it does increase the risk of heart and blood vessel diseases. Smoking injures blood vessel walls and speeds up the process of hardening of the arteries. If you smoke, quit. Your risk of having a heart attack is reduced after the first year.

What do blood pressure numbers indicate?

The higher (systolic) number represents the pressure while the heart is beating.

The lower (diastolic) number represents the pressure when the heart is resting between beats.

The systolic pressure is always stated first and the diastolic pressure second. For example; if a person's blood pressure is 122/76 (122 over 76), the systolic pressure is 122 and the diastolic pressure is 76.

Table 42.1. Categories for Blood Pressure Levels in Adults Ages 18 Years and Older

	Blood Pressure Level (mm Hg)	
Category	**Systolic**	**Diastolic**
Normal	<120 and	<80
Prehypertension	120–139 or	80–89
Hypertension, Stage 1	140–159 or	90–99
Hypertension, Stage 2	≥160 or	≥100

Source: From the Seventh Report of the Joint National Committee on Prevention, Detection, Evaluation, and Treatment of High Blood Pressure (JNC7)

How often should I have my blood pressure checked?

If you do not have high blood pressure then you should have your pressure checked at least every two years. If you have high blood pressure consult with your health care provider.

What are factors that contribute to high blood pressure?

Because medical science doesn't understand why most cases of high blood pressure occur, it's hard to say how to prevent it. However, we do know of several factors that may contribute to high blood pressure and put you at risk for heart attack and stroke.

Controllable risk factors are as follows:

- **Obesity:** People with a body mass index (BMI) of 30.0 or higher are more likely to develop high blood pressure. BMI is used to define nutritional status and is derived from the following formula: BMI = 703 x Body Weight ÷ (Height x Height) (in pounds) (in inches). The standards are the same for men and women. A BMI of 25 to 29.9 is considered overweight.
- **Eating too much salt:** This increases blood pressure in some people.
- **Alcohol:** Heavy and regular use of alcohol can increase blood pressure dramatically.
- **Lack of exercise:** An inactive lifestyle makes it easier to become overweight and increases the chance of high blood pressure.
- **Stress:** This is often mentioned as a risk factor. However, stress levels are hard to measure, and responses to stress vary from person to person.

Uncontrollable risk factors are as follows:

- **Race:** African Americans develop high blood pressure more often than whites, and it tends to occur earlier and be more severe.
- **Heredity:** A tendency to have high blood pressure runs in families. If your parents or other close blood relatives have it, you're more likely to develop it.
- **Age:** In general, the older you get, the greater your chance of developing high blood pressure. It occurs most often in people

over age thirty-five. Men seem to develop it most often between age thirty-five and fifty. Women are more likely to develop it after menopause.

Section 42.3

Stroke

Excerpted from "Stroke," National Women's Health Information Center, May 2006.

What is a stroke?

A stroke occurs when part of the brain doesn't get the blood it needs. There are two types of stroke:

- **Ischemic stroke (most common type):** This type of stroke happens when blood is blocked from getting to the brain. This often happens because the artery is clogged with fatty deposits (atherosclerosis) or a blood clot.
- **Hemorrhagic stroke:** This type of stroke happens when a blood vessel in the brain bursts, and blood bleeds into the brain. This type of stroke can be caused by an aneurysm—a thin or weak spot in an artery that balloons out and can burst.

Both types of stroke can cause brain cells to die. This may cause a person to lose control of their speech, movement, and memory. If you think you are having a stroke, call 911.

What is a "mini-stroke"?

A "mini-stroke," also called a transient ischemic attack or (TIA), happens when, for a short time, less blood than normal gets to the brain. You may have some signs of stroke or you may not notice any signs. A "mini-stroke" lasts from a few minutes up to a day and can be a sign of a full stroke to come. If you think you are having a "mini-stroke," call 911.

What are the signs of a stroke?

A stroke happens fast. Most people have two or more signs. The most common signs are:

- Sudden numbness or weakness of face, arm, or leg (mainly on one side of the body)
- Sudden trouble seeing in one or both eyes
- Sudden trouble walking, dizziness, or loss of balance
- Sudden confusion or trouble talking or understanding speech
- Sudden bad headache with no known cause

Women may have unique symptoms:

- Sudden face and arm or leg pain
- Sudden hiccups
- Sudden nausea (feeling sick to your stomach)
- Sudden tiredness
- Sudden chest pain
- Sudden shortness of breath (feeling like you can't get enough air)
- Sudden pounding or racing heartbeat

If you have any of these symptoms, call 911.

How is stroke diagnosed?

The doctor will usually start by asking the patient what happened and when the symptoms began. Then the doctor will ask the patient some questions to see if she or he is thinking clearly. The doctor also will test the patient's reflexes to see if she or he may have had any physical damage. This helps the doctor find out which tests are needed.

What are the effects of stroke?

It depends on the type of stroke, the area of the brain where the stroke occurs, and the extent of brain injury. A mild stroke can cause little or no brain damage. A major stroke can cause severe brain damage and even death.

A stroke in the right half of the brain can cause the following:

- **Problems judging distances:** The stroke survivor may misjudge distances and fall or be unable to guide her hands to pick something up.
- **Impaired judgment and behavior:** The stroke survivor may try to do things that she should not do, such as driving a car.
- **Short-term memory loss:** The stroke survivor may be able to remember events from thirty years ago, but not what she ate for breakfast that morning.

A stroke in the left half of the brain can cause the following:

- **Speech and language problems:** The stroke survivor may have trouble speaking or understanding others.
- **Slow and cautious behavior:** The stroke survivor may need a lot of help to complete tasks.
- **Memory problems:** The stroke survivor may not remember what she did ten minutes ago or she may have a hard time learning new things.

A stroke in the cerebellum, or the part of the brain that controls balance and coordination, can cause the following:

- Abnormal reflexes of the head and upper body
- Balance problems
- Dizziness, nausea (feeling sick to your stomach), and vomiting

Strokes in the brain stem are very harmful because the brain stem controls all our body's functions that we don't have to think about, such as eye movements, breathing, hearing, speech, and swallowing. Since impulses that start in the brain must travel through the brain stem on their way to the arms and legs, patients with a brain stem stroke may also develop paralysis, or not be able to move or feel on one or both sides of the body.

In many cases, a stroke weakens the muscles, making it hard to walk, eat, or dress without help. Some symptoms may improve with time and rehabilitation or therapy.

Who is at risk for stroke?

A person of any age can have a stroke. But, stroke risk does increase with age. For every ten years after the age of fifty-five, the risk of stroke doubles, and two-thirds of all strokes occur in people over sixty-five years old. Stroke also seems to run in some families. Stroke risk doubles for a woman if someone in her immediate family (mom, dad, sister, or brother) has had a stroke.

Compared to white women, African American women have more strokes and have a higher risk of disability and death from stroke. This is partly because more African American women have high blood pressure, a major stroke risk factor. Women who smoke or who have high blood pressure, atrial fibrillation (a kind of irregular heartbeat), heart disease, or diabetes are more likely to have a stroke. Hormonal changes with pregnancy, childbirth, and menopause are also linked to an increased risk of stroke.

How do I prevent a stroke?

Experts think that up to 80 percent of strokes can be prevented. You can reduce your chances of having a stroke by taking these steps:

- **Know your blood pressure:** Your heart moves blood through your body. If it is hard for your heart to do this, your heart works harder, and your blood pressure will rise. People with high blood pressure often have no symptoms, so have your blood pressure checked every one to two years. If you have high blood pressure, your doctor may suggest you make some lifestyle changes, such as eating less salt (DASH Eating Plan) and exercising more. Your doctor may also prescribe medicine to help lower your blood pressure.
- **Don't smoke:** If you smoke, try to quit. If you are having trouble quitting, there are products and programs, including nicotine patches and gums, support groups, and programs to help you stop smoking, that can help. Ask your doctor or nurse for help.
- **Get tested for diabetes:** People with diabetes have high blood glucose (often called blood sugar). People with high blood sugar often have no symptoms, so have your blood sugar checked regularly. Having diabetes raises your chances of having a stroke. If you have diabetes, your doctor will decide if you need diabetes pills or insulin shots. Your doctor can also help you make a healthy eating and exercise plan.
- **Get your cholesterol and triglyceride levels tested:** Cholesterol is a waxy substance found in all parts of your body. When there is too much cholesterol in your blood, cholesterol can build

up on the walls of your arteries. Cholesterol can clog your arteries and keep your brain from getting the blood it needs. This can cause a stroke. Triglycerides are a form of fat in your blood stream. High levels of triglycerides are linked to stroke in some people. People with high blood cholesterol or high blood triglycerides often have no symptoms, so have your blood cholesterol and triglyceride levels checked regularly. If your cholesterol or triglyceride levels are high, talk to your doctor about what you can do to lower them. You may be able to lower your cholesterol and triglyceride levels by eating better and exercising more. Your doctor may prescribe medication to help lower your cholesterol.

- **Maintain a healthy weight:** Being overweight raises your risk for stroke. Calculate your body mass index (BMI) to see if you are at a healthy weight. Eat a healthy diet and exercise at a moderate intensity for at least thirty minutes most days of the week. Start by adding more fruits, vegetables, and whole grains to your diet. Take a brisk walk on your lunch break or take the stairs instead of the elevator.
- **If you drink alcohol, limit it to no more than one drink (one 12 ounce beer, one 5 ounce glass of wine, or one 1.5 ounce shot of hard liquor) a day.**
- **Find healthy ways to cope with stress:** Lower your stress level by talking to your friends, exercising, or writing in a journal.

Should I take a daily aspirin to prevent stroke?

Aspirin may be helpful for women at high risk, such as women who have already had a stroke. Aspirin can have serious side effects and may be harmful when mixed with certain medications. If you're thinking about taking aspirin, talk to your doctor first. If your doctor thinks aspirin is a good choice for you, be sure to take it exactly as your doctor tells you to.

Does taking birth control pills increase my risk for stroke?

Taking birth control pills is generally safe for young, healthy women. But birth control pills can raise the risk of stroke for some women, especially women over thirty-five; women with high blood pressure, diabetes, or high cholesterol; and women who smoke. Talk with your doctor if you have questions about the pill.

Does using the birth control patch increase my risk for stroke?

The patch is generally safe for young, healthy women. The patch can raise the risk of stroke for some women, especially women over thirty-five; women with high blood pressure, diabetes, or high cholesterol; and women who smoke.

Recent studies show that women who use the patch may be exposed to more estrogen (the female hormone in birth control pills and the patch that keeps users from becoming pregnant) than women who use the birth control pill. Research is underway to see if the risk for blood clots (which can lead to heart attack or stroke) is higher in patch users. Talk with your doctor if you have questions about the patch.

How is stroke treated?

Strokes caused by blood clots can be treated with clot-busting drugs such as TPA, or tissue plasminogen activator. TPA must be given within three hours of the start of a stroke to work, and tests must be done first. This is why it is so important for a person having a stroke to get to a hospital fast.

Other medicines are used to treat and to prevent stroke. Anticoagulants, such as warfarin, and antiplatelet agents, such as aspirin, block the blood's ability to clot and can help prevent a stroke in patients with high risk, such as a person who has atrial fibrillation (a kind of irregular heartbeat).

Surgery is sometimes used to treat or prevent stroke. Carotid endarterectomy is a surgery to remove fatty deposits clogging the carotid artery in the neck, which could lead to a stroke. For hemorrhagic stroke, a doctor may perform surgery to place a metal clip at the base of an aneurysm (a thin or weak spot in an artery that balloons out and can burst) or remove abnormal blood vessels.

What about rehabilitation?

Rehabilitation is a very important part of recovery for many stroke survivors. The effects of stroke may mean that you must change, relearn, or redefine how you live. Stroke rehabilitation is designed to help you return to independent living.

Section 42.4

Varicose Veins and Spider Veins

Excerpted from "Varicose Veins and Spider Veins," National Women's Health Information Center, December 2005.

What are varicose veins and spider veins?

Varicose veins are enlarged veins that can be flesh colored, dark purple, or blue. They often look like cords and appear twisted and bulging. They are swollen and raised above the surface of the skin. Varicose veins are commonly found on the backs of the calves or on the inside of the leg. During pregnancy, varicose veins called hemorrhoids can form in the vagina or around the anus.

Spider veins are similar to varicose veins, but they are smaller. They are often red or blue and are closer to the surface of the skin than varicose veins. They can look like tree branches or spider webs with their short jagged lines. Spider veins can be found on the legs and face. They can cover either a very small or very large area of skin.

What causes varicose veins and spider veins?

The heart pumps blood filled with oxygen and nutrients to the whole body. Arteries carry blood from the heart toward the body parts. Veins carry oxygen-poor blood from the body back to the heart.

The squeezing of leg muscles pumps blood back to the heart from the lower body. Veins have valves that act as one-way flaps. These valves prevent the blood from flowing backward as it moves up the legs. If the one-way valves become weak, blood can leak back into the vein and collect there. This problem is called venous insufficiency. Pooled blood enlarges the vein and it becomes varicose. Spider veins can also be caused by the backup of blood. Hormone changes, inherited factors, and exposure to the sun can also cause spider veins.

What are the signs of varicose veins?

Some common symptoms of varicose veins include the following:

- Aching pain

- Easily tired legs
- Leg heaviness
- Swelling in the legs
- Darkening of the skin (in severe cases)
- Numbness in the legs
- Itching or irritated rash in the legs

How can I prevent varicose veins and spider veins?

Not all varicose and spider veins can be prevented. But some things can reduce your chances of getting new varicose and spider veins. These same things can help ease discomfort from the ones you already have:

- Wear sunscreen to protect your skin from the sun and to limit spider veins on the face.
- Exercise regularly to improve your leg strength, circulation, and vein strength. Focus on exercises that work your legs, such as walking or running.
- Control your weight to avoid placing too much pressure on your legs.
- Do not cross your legs when sitting.
- Elevate your legs when resting as much as possible.
- Do not stand or sit for long periods of time. If you must stand for a long time, shift your weight from one leg to the other every few minutes. If you must sit for long periods of time, stand up and move around or take a short walk every thirty minutes.
- Wear elastic support stockings and avoid tight clothing that constricts your waist, groin, or legs.
- Eat a low-salt diet rich in high-fiber foods. Eating fiber reduces the chances of constipation, which can contribute to varicose veins. High-fiber foods include fresh fruits and vegetables and whole grains, like bran. Eating too much salt can cause you to retain water or swell.

Should I see a doctor about varicose veins?

Remember these important questions when deciding whether to see your doctor: Has the varicose vein become swollen, red, or very tender or warm to the touch? If yes, see your doctor. If no, are there sores or a rash on the leg or near the ankle with the varicose vein, or do you think there may be circulation problems in your feet? If yes, see your doctor. If no, continue to follow the self-care tips above.

How are varicose and spider veins treated?

Some available treatments include sclerotherapy, laser surgery, endovenous techniques, and surgery.

Sclerotherapy: This is the most common treatment for both spider veins and varicose veins. The doctor injects a solution into the vein that causes the vein walls to swell, stick together, and seal shut. This stops the flow of blood and the vein turns into scar tissue. In a few weeks, the vein should fade. The same vein may need to be treated more than once.

This treatment is very effective if done the right way. Most patients can expect a 50 to 90 percent improvement. Microsclerotherapy uses special solutions and injection techniques that increase the success rate for removal of spider veins. Sclerotherapy does not require anesthesia, and can be done in the doctor's office.

Laser surgery: New technology in laser treatments can effectively treat spider veins in the legs. Laser surgery sends very strong bursts of light onto the vein. This can makes the vein slowly fade and disappear. Lasers are very direct and accurate. So the proper laser controlled by a skilled doctor will usually only damage the area being treated. Most skin types and colors can be safely treated with lasers.

Laser treatments last for fifteen to twenty minutes. Depending on the severity of the veins, two to five treatments are generally needed to remove spider veins in the legs. Patients can return to normal activity right after treatment, just as with sclerotherapy. For spider veins larger than three millimeters, laser therapy is not very practical.

Endovenous techniques (radiofrequency and laser): These methods for treating the deeper varicose veins of the legs (the saphenous veins) have been a huge breakthrough. They have replaced surgery for the vast majority of patients with severe varicose veins. This technique is not very invasive and can be done in a doctor's office.

The doctor puts a very small tube called a catheter into the vein. Once inside, the catheter sends out radiofrequency or laser energy that shrinks and seals the vein wall. Healthy veins around the closed vein restore the normal flow of blood. As this happens, symptoms from the varicose vein improve. Veins on the surface of the skin that are connected to the treated varicose vein will also usually shrink after treatment. When needed, these connected varicose veins can be treated with sclerotherapy or other techniques.

Surgery: Surgery is used mostly to treat very large varicose veins. Types of surgery for varicose veins include surgical ligation and stripping, ambulatory phlebectomy, and endoscopic vein surgery.

With surgical ligation and stripping, problematic veins are tied shut and completely removed from the leg. Removing the veins does not affect the circulation of blood in the leg. Veins deeper in the leg take care of the larger volumes of blood. Most varicose veins removed by surgery are surface veins and collect blood only from the skin. This surgery requires either local or general anesthesia and must be done in an operating room on an outpatient basis. Significant pain in the leg and recovery time of one to four weeks depending on the extent of the surgery is typical.

With ambulatory phlebectomy, a special light source marks the location of the vein. Tiny cuts are made in the skin, and surgical hooks pull the vein out of the leg. This surgery requires local or regional anesthesia. The vein usually is removed in one treatment. Very large varicose veins can be removed with this treatment while leaving only very small scars. Patients can return to normal activity the day after treatment.

With endoscopic vein surgery, a small video camera is used to see inside the veins. Then varicose veins are removed through small cuts. People who have this surgery must have some kind of anesthesia including epidural, spinal, or general anesthesia. Patients can return to normal activity within a few weeks.

Chapter 43

Carpal Tunnel Syndrome

What is carpal tunnel syndrome (CTS)?

Carpal tunnel syndrome (CTS) is the name for a group of problems that includes swelling, pain, tingling, and loss of strength in your wrist and hand. Your wrist is made of small bones that form a narrow groove or carpal tunnel. Tendons and a nerve called the median nerve must pass through this tunnel from your forearm into your hand. The median nerve controls the feelings and sensations in the palm side of your thumb and fingers. Sometimes swelling and irritation of the tendons can put pressure on the wrist nerve, causing the symptoms of CTS. A person's dominant hand is the one that is usually affected. However, nearly half of CTS sufferers have symptoms in both hands.

CTS has become more common in the United States and is quite costly in terms of time lost from work and expensive medical treatment. The U.S. Department of Labor reported that in 2003 the average number of missed days of work due to CTS was twenty-three days, costing over $2 billion a year. It is thought that about 3.7 percent of the general public in this country suffer from CTS.

What are the symptoms of CTS?

Typically, CTS begins slowly with feelings of burning, tingling, and numbness in the wrist and hand. The areas most affected are the

---

Reprinted from "Carpal Tunnel Syndrome," National Women's Health Information Center, June 2005.

thumb, index and middle fingers. At first, symptoms may happen more often at night. Many CTS sufferers do not make the connection between a daytime activity that might be causing the CTS and the delayed symptoms. Also, many people sleep with their wrist bent, which may cause more pain and symptoms at night. As CTS gets worse, the tingling may be felt during the daytime too, along with pain moving from the wrist to your arm or down to your fingers. Pain is usually felt more on the palm side of the hand.

Another symptom of CTS is weakness of the hands that gets worse over time. Some people with CTS find it difficult to grasp an object, make a fist, or hold onto something small. The fingers may even feel like they are swollen even though they are not. Over time, this feeling will usually happen more often.

If left untreated, those with CTS can have a loss of feeling in some fingers and permanent weakness of the thumb. Thumb muscles can actually waste away over time. Eventually, CTS sufferers may have trouble telling the difference between hot and cold temperatures by touch.

What causes CTS and who is more likely to develop it?

Women are three times more likely to have CTS than men. Although there is limited research on why this is the case, scientists have several ideas. It may be that the wrist bones are naturally smaller in most women, creating a tighter space through which the nerves and tendons must pass. Other researchers are looking at genetic links that make it more likely for women to have musculoskeletal injuries such as CTS. Women also deal with strong hormonal changes during pregnancy and menopause that make them more likely to suffer from CTS. Generally, women are at higher risk of CTS between the ages of forty-five and fifty-four. Then, the risk increases for both men and women as they age.

There are other factors that can cause CTS, including certain health problems and, in some cases, the cause is unknown.

These are some of the things that might raise your chances of developing CTS:

- **Genetic predisposition:** The carpal tunnel is smaller in some people than others.
- **Repetitive movements:** People who do the same movements with their wrists and hands over and over may be more likely to develop CTS. People with certain types of jobs are more likely to

have CTS, including manufacturing and assembly line workers, grocery store checkers, violinists, and carpenters. Some hobbies and sports that use repetitive hand movements can also cause CTS, such as golfing, knitting, and gardening. Whether or not long-term typing or computer use causes CTS is still being debated. Limited research points to a weak link, but more research is needed.

- **Injury or trauma:** A sprain or a fracture of the wrist can cause swelling and pressure on the nerve, increasing the risk of CTS. Forceful and stressful movements of the hand and wrist can also cause trauma, such as strong vibrations caused by heavy machinery or power tools.
- **Pregnancy:** Hormonal changes during pregnancy and buildup of fluid can put pregnant women at greater risk of getting CTS, especially during the last few months. Most doctors treat CTS in pregnant women with wrist splits or rest, rather than surgery, as CTS almost always goes away following childbirth.
- **Menopause:** Hormonal changes during menopause can put women at greater risk of getting CTS. Also, in some postmenopausal women, the wrist structures become enlarged and can press on the wrist nerve.
- **Breast cancer:** Some women who have a mastectomy get lymphedema, the buildup of fluids that go beyond the lymph system's ability to drain it. In mastectomy patients, this causes pain and swelling of the arm. Although rare, some of these women will get CTS due to pressure on the nerve from this swelling.
- **Medical conditions:** People who have diabetes, hypothyroidism, lupus, obesity, and rheumatoid arthritis are more likely to get CTS. In some of these patients, the normal structures in the wrist can become enlarged and lead to CTS.

Also, smokers with CTS usually have worse symptoms and recover more slowly than nonsmokers.

How is CTS treated?

It is important to be treated by a doctor for CTS in order to avoid permanent damage to the wrist nerve and muscles of the hand and thumb. Underlying causes such as diabetes or a thyroid problem should be addressed first. Left untreated, CTS can cause nerve damage that leads to loss of feeling and less hand strength. Over time, the muscles of the thumb can become weak and damaged. You can even lose the ability to feel hot and cold by touch. Permanent injury occurs in about 1 percent of those with CTS.

CTS is much easier to treat early on. Most CTS patients get better after first-step treatments and the following tips for protecting the wrist. Treatments for CTS include the following:

- **Wrist splint:** A splint can be worn to support and brace your wrist in a neutral position so that the nerves and tendons can recover. A splint can be worn twenty-four hours a day or only at night. Sometimes, wearing a splint at night helps to reduce the pain. Splinting can work the best when done within three months of having any symptoms of CTS.
- **Rest:** For people with mild CTS, stopping or doing less of a repetitive movement may be all that is needed. Your doctor will likely talk to you about steps that you should take to prevent CTS from coming back.
- **Medication:** The short-term use of nonsteroidal anti-inflammatory drugs (NSAIDs) may be helpful to control CTS pain. NSAIDs include aspirin, ibuprofen, and other nonprescription pain relievers. In severe cases, an injection of cortisone may help to reduce swelling. Your doctor may also give you corticosteroids in a pill form. But, these treatments only relieve symptoms temporarily. If CTS is caused by another health problem, your doctor will probably treat that problem first. If you have diabetes, it is important to know that long-term corticosteroid use can make it hard to control insulin levels.
- **Physical therapy:** A physical therapist can help you do special exercises to make your wrist and hand stronger. There are also many different kinds of treatments that can make CTS better and help relieve symptoms. Massage, yoga, ultrasound, chiropractic manipulation, and acupuncture are just a few such options that have been found to be helpful. You should talk with your doctor before trying these alternative treatments.
- **Surgery:** CTS surgery is one of the most common surgeries done in the United States. Generally, surgery is only an option for severe cases of CTS and after other treatments have failed for a period of at least six months. Open release surgery is a

common approach to CTS surgery and involves making a small incision in the wrist or palm and cutting the ligament to enlarge the carpal tunnel. This surgery is done under a local anesthetic to numb the wrist and hand area and is an outpatient procedure.

What is the best way to prevent CTS?

Current research is focused on figuring out what causes CTS and how to prevent it. The National Institute of Neurological Disorders and Stroke (NINDS) and the National Institute of Arthritis and Musculoskeletal and Skin Diseases (NIAMS) support research on work-related factors that may cause CTS. Scientists are also researching better ways to detect and treat CTS, including alternative treatments such as acupuncture.

The following steps can help to prevent CTS:

- **Prevent workplace musculoskeletal injury:** Make sure that your workspace and equipment are at the right height and distance for your hands and wrist to work with less strain. If you are working on a computer, the keyboard should be at a height that allows your wrist to rest comfortably without having to bend at an angle. Desk or table workspace should be about 27 to 29 inches above the floor for most people. It also helps to keep your elbows close to your sides as you type to reduce the strain on your forearm. Keeping good posture and wrist position can lower your risk of getting CTS.
- **Take breaks:** Allowing your hand and wrist to rest and recover every so often will lower your risk of swelling. Experts believe that taking a ten- to fifteen-minute break every hour is a good way to prevent CTS.
- **Vary tasks:** Avoid repetitive movements without changing up your routine. Try to do tasks that use different muscle movements during each hour. Break up tasks that require repetitive wrist and hand motion with those that do not.
- **Relax your grip:** Sometimes, people get into a habit of tensing muscles without needing to. Practice doing hand and wrist motion tasks more gently and less tightly. Stress and tension play a role in muscle strain and irritation.
- **Do exercises:** After doing repetitive movements for a while, you can sometimes cancel out the effects of those movements by

flexing and bending your wrists and hands in the opposite direction. For example, after typing with your wrist and hand extended, it is helpful to make a tight fist and hold it for a second, then stretch out the fingers and hold for a few seconds. Try repeating this several times.

- **Stay warm:** Muscles that are warm are less likely to get hurt and the risk of getting CTS is greater in a cold environment. It is important to keep your hands warm while you work, even if you must wear fingerless gloves.

Chapter 44

Diabetes

What is diabetes?

Diabetes means that your blood sugar is too high. Your blood always has some sugar in it because the body uses sugar for energy; it's the fuel that keeps you going. But too much sugar in the blood is not good for your health.

Your body changes most of the food you eat into sugar. Your blood takes the sugar to the cells throughout your body. The sugar needs insulin to get into the body's cells. Insulin is a hormone made in the pancreas, an organ near the stomach. The pancreas releases insulin into the blood. Insulin helps the sugar from food get into body cells. If your body does not make enough insulin or the insulin does not work right, the sugar can't get into the cells, so it stays in the blood. This makes your blood sugar level high, causing you to have diabetes.

If not controlled, diabetes can lead to blindness, heart disease, stroke, kidney failure, amputations (having a toe or foot removed, for example), and nerve damage. In women, diabetes can cause problems during pregnancy and make it more likely that your baby will be born with birth defects.

What is pre-diabetes?

Pre-diabetes means your blood sugar is higher than normal but lower than the diabetes range. It also means you are at risk of getting

---

Excerpted from "Diabetes," National Women's Health Information Center, June 2006.

type 2 diabetes and heart disease. The good news is: You can reduce the risk of getting diabetes and even return to normal blood sugar levels with modest weight loss and moderate physical activity. If you are told you have pre-diabetes, have your blood glucose (sugar) checked again in one to two years.

What are the different types of diabetes?

The three main types of diabetes are type 1, type 2, and gestational diabetes.

Type 1 diabetes: This is commonly diagnosed in children and young adults, but it's a lifelong condition. If you have this type of diabetes, your body does not make insulin, so you must take insulin every day. Treatment for type 1 diabetes includes taking insulin shots or using an insulin pump, eating healthy, exercising regularly, taking aspirin daily (for some), and controlling blood pressure and cholesterol.

Type 2 diabetes: This is the most common type of diabetes — about nine out of ten people with diabetes have type 2 diabetes. You can get type 2 diabetes at any age, even during childhood. In type 2 diabetes, your body makes insulin, but the insulin can't do its job, so sugar is not getting into the cells. Treatment includes taking medicine, eating healthy, exercising regularly, taking aspirin daily (for some), and controlling blood pressure and cholesterol.

Gestational diabetes: This occurs during pregnancy. This type of diabetes occurs in about one in twenty pregnancies. During pregnancy your body makes hormones that keep insulin from doing its job. To make up for this, your body makes extra insulin. But in some women this extra insulin is not enough, so they get gestational diabetes. Gestational diabetes usually goes away when the pregnancy is over. Women who have had gestational diabetes are more likely to develop type 2 diabetes later in life.

Who gets diabetes?

About 20 million Americans have diabetes, about half of whom are women. As many as one third do not know they have diabetes.

What causes diabetes?

Type 1 and type 2 diabetes: The exact causes of both types of diabetes are still not known. Type 1 diabetes tends to show up after a person is exposed to a trigger, such as a virus, which can start an attack on the cells in the pancreas that make insulin. There is no one cause for type 2 diabetes, but it seems to run in families, and most people who get type 2 diabetes are overweight.

Gestational diabetes: Changing hormones and weight gain are part of a healthy pregnancy, but these changes make it hard for your body to keep up with its need for insulin. When that happens, your body doesn't get the energy it needs from the foods you eat.

Am I at risk for diabetes?

Things that can put you at risk for diabetes include the following:

- **Age:** Being older than forty-five.
- **Overweight or obesity.**
- **Family history:** Having a mother, father, brother, or sister with diabetes.
- **Race/ethnicity:** Your family background is African American, American Indian/Alaska Native, Hispanic American/Latino, Asian American/Pacific Islander or Native Hawaiian.
- **Having a baby with a birth weight more than nine pounds.**
- **Having diabetes during pregnancy (gestational diabetes).**
- **High blood pressure:** 140/90 mm HG or higher. Both numbers are important. If one or both numbers are usually high, you have high blood pressure.
- **High cholesterol:** Total cholesterol over 240 mg/dL.
- **Inactivity:** Exercising less than three times a week.
- **Abnormal results in a prior diabetes test.**
- **Having other health conditions that are linked to problems using insulin, like polycystic ovarian syndrome (PCOS).**
- **Having a history of heart disease or stroke.**

Should I be tested for diabetes?

If you're at least forty-five years old, you should get tested for diabetes, and then you should be tested again every three years. If you're forty-five or older and overweight you may want to get tested more often. If you're younger than forty-five, overweight, and have one or more of the risk factors listed above you should get tested now. Ask your doctor for a fasting blood glucose test or an oral glucose tolerance test. Your doctor will tell you if you have normal blood glucose (blood sugar), pre-diabetes, or diabetes.

What are the signs of diabetes?

- Being very thirsty
- Urinating a lot
- Feeling very hungry
- Feeling very tired
- Losing weight without trying
- Having sores that are slow to heal
- Having dry, itchy skin
- Losing feeling in or having tingling in the hands or feet
- Having blurry vision
- Having more infections than usual

If you have one or more of these signs, see your doctor.

How can I take care of myself if I have diabetes?

Many people with diabetes live healthy and full lives. By following your doctor's instructions and eating right, you can too. Here are the things you'll need to do to keep your diabetes in check:

- **Follow your meal plan:** Eat often; eat lots of whole-grain foods, fruits, and vegetables.
- **Get moving:** try to be active for at least thirty minutes on most days.
- **Test your blood sugar:** Keep track of your blood sugar levels and talk to your doctor about ways to keep your levels on target. Many women report that their blood sugar levels go up or down around their period. If you're going through menopause, you might also notice your blood sugar levels going up and down.
- **Take your diabetes medicine exactly as your doctor tells you.**

Talk to your doctor about other things you can do to take good care of yourself. Taking care of your diabetes can help prevent serious problems in your eyes, kidneys, nerves, gums and teeth, and blood vessels.

How can I take care of myself if I have gestational diabetes?

Taking care of yourself when you have gestational diabetes is very much like taking care of yourself when you have other types of diabetes. But it can be a little scary when you're pregnant and you also have a new condition to take care of. Don't worry. Many women who've had gestational diabetes have gone on to have healthy babies. Here are the things you'll need to do:

- **Follow your meal plan:** You will meet with a dietitian or diabetes educator who will help you design a meal plan full of healthy foods for you and your baby.
- **Get moving:** Try to be active for at least thirty minutes on most days.
- **Test your blood sugar:** Your doctor may ask you to use a small device called a blood glucose meter to check your blood sugar levels. You will be shown how to use the meter to check your blood sugar. Your diabetes team will tell you what your target blood sugar range is, how often you need to check your blood sugar, and what to do if it is not where it should be.
- **Take your diabetes medicine exactly as your doctor tells you:** You may need to take insulin to keep your blood sugar at the right level. If so, your health care team will show you how to give yourself insulin. Insulin will not harm your baby—it cannot move from your bloodstream to your baby's.

Is there a cure for diabetes?

There is no cure for diabetes at this time. The National Institutes of Health (NIH) is doing research in hopes of finding cures for both type 1 and type 2 diabetes. Many different approaches to curing diabetes are being studied, and researchers are making progress.

Is there anything I can do to prevent diabetes?

Yes. The best way to prevent diabetes is to make some lifestyle changes:

- **Maintain a healthy weight:** Being overweight raises your risk for diabetes. If you're overweight, start making small changes to your eating habits by adding more whole grain foods, fruits, and vegetables. Start exercising more, even if taking a short walk is all you can do for now.
- **Eat healthy:** Eat lost of whole grains, fruits, and vegetables; choose foods low in fat and cholesterol; limit your salt intake to less than 2,300 mg each day; and limit alcohol consumption to no more than one drink (one 12-ounce beer, one 5-ounce glass of wine, or one 1.5-ounce shot of hard liquor) a day.
- **Get moving:** Try to exercise for at least thirty minutes most days of the week.

Chapter 45

Female Athlete Triad

Sports and exercise are healthy activities for girls and women of all ages. But a female athlete who focuses on being thin or lightweight may eat too little and/or exercise too much. Doing this can cause long-term damage to health, or even death. It can also hurt athletic performance and/or make it necessary to limit or stop exercise.

Three interrelated illnesses may develop when a girl or young woman goes to extremes in dieting or exercise. Together, these conditions are known as the "female athletic triad."

The three conditions are:

- **Disordered eating:** Abnormal eating habits (i.e., crash diets, binge eating) or excessive exercise keeps the body from getting enough nutrition.
- **Menstrual dysfunction:** Poor nutrition, low calorie intake, high energy demands, physical and emotional stress, or low percentage of body fat can lead to hormonal changes that stop menstrual periods (amenorrhea).
- **Osteoporosis:** Lack of periods disrupts the body's bone-building processes and weakens the skeleton, making bones more likely to break.

Females at Risk

Females in any sport can develop one or more parts of the triad. At greatest risk are those in sports that reward being thin for appearance (i.e., figure skating, gymnastics) or improved performance (i.e., distance running, rowing).

Fashion trends and advertising often encourage women to try to reach unhealthy weight levels. Some female athletes suffer low self-esteem or depression, and may focus on weight loss because they think they are heavier than they actually are. Others feel pressure to lose weight from athletic coaches or parents.

Female athletes should consider these questions:

- Are you dissatisfied with your body?
- Do you strive to be thin?
- Do you continuously focus on your weight?

If the answers are yes, you may be at risk for developing abnormal patterns of eating food (disordered eating), which can lead to menstrual dysfunction and early osteoporosis.

Disordered eating: Although they usually do not realize or admit that they are ill, people with disordered eating have serious and complex disturbances in eating behaviors. They are preoccupied with body shape and weight and have poor nutritional habits.

Females are ten times more likely to have disordered eating compared with males, and the problem is especially common in females who are athletic. The illness takes many forms. Some people starve themselves (anorexia nervosa) or engage in cycles of overeating and purging (bulimia).

Others severely restrict the amount of food they eat, fast for prolonged periods of time, or misuse diet pills, diuretics, or laxatives. People with disordered eating may also exercise excessively to keep their weight down.

Disordered eating can cause many problems, including dehydration, muscle fatigue, and weakness, an erratic heartbeat, kidney damage, and other serious conditions. Not taking in enough calcium can lead to bone loss. It is especially bad to lose bone when you are a child or teenager because that is when your body should be building bone. Hormone imbalances can lead to more bone loss through menstrual dysfunction.

Menstrual dysfunction: Missing three or more periods in a row is cause for concern. With normal menstruation, the body produces estrogen, a hormone that helps to keep bones strong. Without a menstrual cycle (amenorrhea), the level of estrogen may be lowered, causing a loss of bone density and strength (premature osteoporosis).

If this happens during youth, it may become a serious problem later in life when the natural process of bone mineral loss begins after menopause. Amenorrhea may also cause stress fractures. Normal menstruation is necessary for pregnancy.

Osteoporosis: Bone tissue wears away, making your skeleton fragile. Low bone mass puts you at increased risk for fractures.

Diagnosis

Recognizing the female athletic triad is the first step toward treating it. See your doctor right away if you think you might have disordered eating, miss several menstrual periods, or get a stress fracture in sports.

Give the doctor your complete medical history, including:

- what you do for physical activity and what you eat for nutrition;
- how old you were when you began to menstruate and whether you usually have regular periods;
- if you are sexually active, use birth control pills, or have ever been pregnant;
- if you have ever had stress fractures or other injuries;
- any changes (up or down) in your weight;
- any medications you are taking or symptoms of other medical problems;
- family history of diseases (i.e., thyroid disease, osteoporosis);
- factors that cause stress in your life.

The doctor will give you complete physical and pelvic examinations and may use laboratory tests to check for pregnancy, thyroid disease, and other medical conditions. In some cases you may also get a bone density test.

Treatment

Treatment for the female athletic triad often requires help from a team of medical professionals including your doctor, a nutritionist, and a psychological counselor.

Chapter 46

Irritable Bowel Syndrome

What is irritable bowel syndrome (IBS)?

Irritable bowel syndrome (IBS) is a collection of symptoms that occur when the nerves and muscles in a person's bowel (the colon, or large intestine) do not work like they should. With IBS, a person's bowel is extra sensitive, causing discomfort and changes in bowel activity. IBS is a chronic condition, meaning it lasts a long time.

IBS is not a disease and it does not cause cancer. IBS is a "functional" disorder, which means that the bowel doesn't work as it should. The cause of IBS is not known, and there is no cure for IBS. But there are things you can do to feel better.

For some people, IBS is simply a bother. For others, it keeps them from going out, going to work, or even traveling short distances. Most people with IBS, however, can ease their symptoms by eating better, reducing stress, or taking medicine.

Who gets IBS?

Up to one in five Americans has IBS. IBS often begins before the age of thirty-five, but it can start at any age. IBS seems to run in families—people with IBS often report having a family member with IBS. Most people diagnosed with IBS (up to 75 percent) are women. But it is not known for sure that IBS affects more women than men. It may

---

Excerpted from "Irritable Bowel Syndrome," National Women's Health Information Center, June 2006.

be that women are more likely to talk to their doctors about their symptoms.

What are the symptoms of IBS?

The main symptoms of IBS include the following:

- Crampy pain in the stomach area
- Painful constipation—infrequent stools that may be hard and dry
- Painful diarrhea—frequent loose stools

Most people have either diarrhea or constipation, but some people have both.

Other symptoms include the following:

- Mucus in the stool
- Swollen or bloated stomach area
- Feeling like you haven't finished a bowel movement
- Gas
- Heartburn
- Discomfort in the upper stomach area or feeling uncomfortably full or nauseous after eating a normal size meal

Some women with IBS have more or different symptoms during their menstrual periods. Constipation may be relieved or diarrhea may occur in the day or two before or when their period starts.

How is IBS diagnosed?

If you think you may have IBS, see your doctor. Your doctor will take a medical history and ask about your symptoms. Then your doctor will perform some medical tests.

There are no tests that can show for sure that you have IBS. But your doctor may do some medical tests to make sure you don't have any other diseases that could cause your symptoms. Other possible causes include polyps, inflammation, or intolerance of foods containing a protein called gluten.

What is the treatment for IBS?

There is no cure for IBS, but there are things you can do to feel better. Treatment may include diet changes, medicine, and stress relief.

Diet changes: Some foods make IBS worse. These include milk products, like cheese or ice cream (people who have trouble digesting lactose, or milk sugar could be extra sensitive); chocolate; alcohol; caffeine (found in coffee, tea, and some sodas); carbonated drinks like soda; Sorbitol, a sweetener found in dietetic foods and in some chewing gums; and gas-producing foods, including beans and certain vegetables like broccoli or cabbage. To find out which foods are causing your symptoms, write down what you eat during the day, what symptoms you have, when symptoms occur, and what foods always make you feel bad. Try not to eat foods that cause IBS symptoms. Or try eating less of those foods.

Some foods make IBS better. Fiber lessens IBS symptoms—mainly constipation because it makes stool soft, bulky, and easier to pass. Fiber is found in bran, bread, cereal, beans, fruits, and vegetables. Some examples of foods with fiber include apples, peaches, broccoli, raw cabbage, carrots, raw peas, kidney beans, lima beans, whole-grain bread, and whole-grain cereal. Add foods with fiber to your diet a little at a time to let your body get used to them. Too much fiber all at once might cause gas, which can trigger symptoms in a person with IBS. If you have constipation, start by adding 12 grams of fiber per day. You may have to raise or lower the amount of fiber to a maximum of 30 grams per day, based on how fiber affects your bowel function and gas production.

Besides telling you to eat more foods with fiber, your doctor might also tell you to get more fiber by taking a fiber pill or drinking water mixed with a special high-fiber powder.

How much you eat matters, too. Large meals can cause cramping and diarrhea in people with IBS. If this happens to you, try eating four or five small meals a day. Or, have your usual three meals, but eat less at each meal.

Medicine: If necessary, your doctor may give you medicine to help with symptoms, including laxatives, to treat constipation; antispasmodics, to slow contractions in the bowel, which may help with diarrhea and pain; and antidepressants, to help with severe pain.

Take your medicine exactly as your doctor tells you to. Some medicines, including laxatives, can be habit-forming, and all drugs have side effects. Remember to tell your doctor about any over-the-counter medicines you are taking.

Stress relief: Stress does not cause IBS, but it can worsen your symptoms. Learning to reduce stress can help. With less stress, you may find that you have less cramping and pain. Meditation, yoga, massage, exercise, hypnotherapy, and counseling are some things that might help. You may need to try different activities to see what works best for you.

Other things that may help include the following:

- Drink six to eight glasses of water each day.
- Exercise can help with constipation and improve your overall health. Exercise helps relieve stress and depression and helps your bowel function as it should.

Chapter 47

Lung Disease

What do healthy lungs do?

Lungs are the organs that allow us to breathe. Lungs provide a huge area (as large as a football field) for oxygen from the air to pass into the bloodstream and carbon dioxide to move out. The cells of our bodies need oxygen in order to work and grow. Our cells also need to get rid of carbon dioxide.

During a normal day, we breathe nearly twenty-five thousand times, and take in (inhale) large amounts of air. The air we take in contains mostly oxygen and nitrogen. But air also has things in it that can hurt our lungs. Bacteria, viruses, tobacco smoke, car exhaust, and other pollutants can be in the air. People with lung disease have difficulty breathing. These breathing problems may prevent the body from getting enough oxygen.

Is lung disease a common health problem?

Yes. More than thirty-five million Americans have an ongoing (or chronic) lung disease like asthma or chronic obstructive pulmonary disease (COPD). If all types of lung disease are lumped together it is the number three killer in the United States. It causes one in seven deaths in this country each year.

The term lung disease refers to many disorders affecting the lungs:

Reprinted from "Lung Disease," National Women's Health Information Center, March 2006.

- Ongoing obstructive lung diseases such as asthma, chronic bronchitis, and emphysema
- Infections like influenza, pneumonia, and tuberculosis (TB)
- Lung cancer
- Pulmonary fibrosis and sarcoidosis

Should women be worried about lung disease?

Yes. The number of women diagnosed with lung disease in the United States is on the rise. The percentage of women dying from lung disease in this country is also increasing.

Here are some other reasons why lung disease is an important health concern for women:

- Lung cancer is the leading cancer killer of women in the United States. It kills more women than breast, ovarian, and cervical cancer combined.
- Deaths from lung cancer among women have risen 150 percent in the last twenty years, while deaths among men are decreasing.
- Studies show that women are 1.5 times more likely to develop lung cancer than men.
- About sixty-four thousand women in the United States die every year from chronic obstructive pulmonary disease (COPD).
- Sixty-five percent of people who die from asthma are women.
- More than twice as many women are diagnosed with chronic bronchitis than men every year.

What types of lung disease are most common in women?

Three of the most common lung diseases in women are asthma, chronic obstructive pulmonary disease (COPD), and lung cancer. Other important but less widespread lung problems that affect women include the following:

- **Pulmonary emboli and pulmonary hypertension:** These conditions affect the blood flow and gas exchange in the lungs.
- **Sarcoidosis and pulmonary fibrosis:** People with these diseases have stiffening and scarring in the lungs.
- **Influenza (the flu):** This viral infection can affect the membrane that surrounds the lungs.

Asthma: Asthma is an ongoing or chronic disease of the airways in the lungs called bronchial tubes. Bronchial tubes carry air in and out of the lungs. In people with asthma, the walls of the airways become swollen (inflamed) and oversensitive. Asthmatic airways overreact to things like viruses, smoke, dust, mold, animal hair, roaches, and pollen. When they react they get narrower. This limits the flow of air into and out of the lungs. Asthma causes wheezing, coughing, tightness in the chest, and trouble breathing.

About 20 million Americans have asthma. Women are more likely to have asthma than men. In the United States more than 11 million women had asthma in 2003 compared to 8.2 million men.

The percentage of women, especially young women, diagnosed with asthma continues to the rise in the United States. Researchers are not sure why. But there are several theories. Many experts think that more contact with indoor and outdoor allergens and pollution plays a role in increasing the rate of asthma. Exposure to house dust mite and cockroach allergens as well as tobacco smoke is linked to an increased risk of asthma.

Chronic obstructive pulmonary disease (COPD): COPD is a term that describes related diseases—chronic obstructive bronchitis and emphysema. These conditions often occur together. Both diseases limit airflow out of the lungs and make breathing difficult. COPD gets worse with time.

In almost 90 percent of cases, smoking is the cause of COPD. The single most important thing a person can do to reduce their risk of lung disease is to stop smoking.

COPD is the fourth leading cause of death in the United States. In 2003, more than 7.2 million women had COPD in this country. More women have died from COPD than men every year since 2000.

In COPD, there is inflammation of the tubes (bronchial tubes) that carry air in and out of the lungs. This ongoing irritation thickens and scars the lining of the bronchial tubes. The irritation also causes the growth of cells that make mucus.

If the airways become thickened enough to restrict air flow to and from the lungs, the condition is called chronic obstructive bronchitis. The excess mucus leads to a constant cough typical of this illness.

But early signs of COPD are often hard to detect. People often decrease their activity level without even realizing it. And some people just assume age or weight gain is the cause of their lack of energy.

In emphysema, the walls between the air sacs (alveoli) are destroyed and the lung tissue is weakened. Normally oxygen from the air goes into the blood through these air sacs. But as the air sacs become damaged, the lung has less surface area. This interferes with the movement of oxygen from the air into the blood. So less oxygen passes into the blood of people with emphysema. Emphysema causes shortness of breath, cough, and wheezing (squeaky sound when breathing).

Still, the early signs of emphysema are often very hard to detect. Since 2004, the rate of emphysema in American women has increased by 5 percent. In contrast, the rate in men has decreased by 10 percent. In 2003, approximately 1.4 million women had emphysema.

Lung cancer: Lung cancer is a disease in which abnormal (malignant) lung cells divide without control. These cancerous cells can invade nearby tissues or spread to other parts of the body. There are two major kinds of lung cancer: non–small cell lung cancer and small cell lung cancer. Non–small cell lung cancer is the most common kind.

Lung cancer is the leading cancer killer of American women. Lung cancer will kill more than sixty-eight thousand women this year. And more and more women are being diagnosed with this disease in the United States. Smoking causes 87 percent of all cases of lung cancer.

How would I know if there was something wrong with my lungs?

Early signs of lung disease can be easy to overlook. Often people with early lung disease just say they don't have much energy.

Some common signs of lung disease include the following:

- Trouble breathing
- Shortness of breath
- Feeling like you're not getting enough air
- A decreased ability to exercise
- A cough that won't go away
- Coughing up blood or mucus
- Pain or discomfort when breathing in or out

If you have any of these symptoms, call your doctor immediately. He or she will be able to pinpoint what is wrong with you.

How can I decrease my chances of lung disease?

Things you can do to reduce your risk of all lung diseases include the following:

- **Stop smoking:** If you are a smoker, the single most important thing you can do to stay healthy is stop smoking. Talk to your doctor about the best way to quit. Smoke from all tobacco products (cigarettes, cigars, and pipes) boosts the chances of lung disease.
- **Avoid secondhand smoke:** The best thing you can do to avoid lung disease is to stay away from smoke. If you live or work with people who smoke, ask them to smoke outside. Nonsmokers have the right to a smoke-free workplace. Keep in mind that cigar and pipe smoke is just as harmful as cigarette smoke.
- **Test for radon:** Find out if there are high levels of radon gas in your home or workplace. People who work in mines are often exposed to radon. And in some parts of the United States, radon is found in houses. Kits you can buy at most hardware stores can measure the amount of radon gas in your home.
- **Steer clear of asbestos:** Some jobs expose workers to asbestos. If you work in construction, shipbuilding, asbestos mining or manufacturing, car repair (brake repair), and insulation you should always wear protective clothing, including a face mask. Federal law protects people who work with asbestos. Employers who work with asbestos must train their workers about asbestos safety, provide protective gear, and monitor the levels of radon to which workers are exposed.
- **Protect yourself from dust and chemical fumes:** Working with some chemicals like vinyl chloride and nickel chromates increases the risk of lung cancer. If you spend a lot of time working around dust and chemical fumes, protect yourself. Wear protective clothing including a gas mask and ventilate work areas.
- **Eat a healthy diet:** Limited research shows that people who eat diets rich in fruits and vegetables have a lower risk of cancer. The American Cancer Society recommends eating five to six servings of fruits and vegetables every day.
- **Ask your doctor about spirometry testing:** This test checks how well you can breathe. Some groups recommend routine spirometry testing in at-risk groups. If you're a smoker over the

age of forty-five, are exposed to lung-damaging substances at work, or have other risk factors you should consider spirometry.

See your doctor right away if you have a cough that won't go away, trouble breathing, pain or discomfort in your chest, or any of the other symptoms described in this chapter.

What causes lung disease?

There are many known causes of lung disease. Still, the causes of many lung diseases are still not known. Some known causes of lung disease include the following:

- **Smoking:** Smoke from cigarettes, cigars, and pipes is the number one cause of lung disease. So the best thing you can do to reduce your risk of lung disease is to stop smoking. If you live or work with a smoker, it is also very important to steer clear of secondhand smoke. Ask the person to smoke outdoors.
- **Radon gas:** Radon gas is the second leading cause of lung cancer. Radon is naturally present in soil and rocks. You can check your home for radon with a kit bought at many hardware stores.
- **Asbestos:** Asbestos is a natural fiber that comes from minerals. The fibers break apart easily into tiny pieces that can float in the air and stick to things. If a person inhales asbestos particles, they can stick to their lungs. Asbestos harms lungs cells, which may lead to lung cancer.
- **Air pollution:** Recent studies suggest that some air pollutants like car exhaust may contribute to asthma, lung cancer, and other lung disease. But doctors still do not fully understand the link between pollution and lung disease.

How can I find out if I have asthma?

Asthma can be hard to diagnose. This is because the signs of asthma are similar those of other lung diseases. The signs of COPD, pneumonia, bronchitis, pulmonary embolism, anxiety, and heart disease can all be confused for asthma. It is important to note that women are misdiagnosed with asthma when they really have COPD more often than men.

To figure out if asthma is causing your discomfort, the doctor will first ask about your symptoms and health history. She will then do a physical exam.

To confirm the diagnosis, the doctor may run any of the following tests:

- **Spirometry:** The doctor uses a machine called a spirometer to see how well you breathe. This test measures how much air you can blow out of your lungs. It also records how fast you can exhale it. If these measurements are lower than normal, you may have asthma. But sometimes people with asthma have normal spirometry results.
- **Bronchodilator reversibility testing:** If your spirometry test is abnormal, your doctor will ask you to inhale a medicine called a bronchodilator. Then the doctor will repeat spirometry to measure how this medicine affects your breathing. Bronchodilators relax muscles around the airways, making it easier to breathe.
- **Challenge test:** If the diagnosis is still unclear after spirometry and bronchodilator reversibility testing, doctors often suggest a challenge test. During this test you will inhale a medicine that narrows the airways in your lungs. After you inhale the medicine, the doctor will do a spirometry test. If you have asthma, the medicine will reduce the amount and speed of the air exhaled.

The doctor may also suggest other tests to make sure another disease is not causing your problems. These include the following:

- **Chest x-ray:** This allows the doctor to see the condition of your lungs. Chest x-rays can help the doctor to see if other lung diseases or infections are causing your symptoms.
- **Electrocardiogram:** An electrocardiogram is a test that records the electrical activity of the heart. An electrocardiogram allows the doctor to see if heart disease is causing your breathing problems.

How is asthma treated?

Asthma is a chronic disease that cannot be cured. But medicines and lifestyle changes can help control the symptoms. One way to help relieve asthma is to avoid things in the environment that make symptoms worse. A number of types of medicines are also used to treat asthma. Most work by opening the lung airways and reducing inflammation.

The medicines used to treat asthma fall into two groups: quick-relief and long-term control.

Quick-relief: Quick-relief medicines are used only when needed. They should be taken when symptoms are getting worse to prevent a full-blown asthma attack. They can also be used to stop attacks once they have started. These medicines relieve symptoms in minutes. Short-acting inhaled bronchodilators (albuterol and pirbuterol) are two commonly used quick-relief medicines. They quickly relax tightened muscles around the airways.

Long-term control: Long-term control medicines or controller medicines are taken every day, usually over a long period of time. Over time, these medicines relieve symptoms and prevent asthma attacks in those with mild or moderate persistent asthma.

These medications help control inflammation in the lungs. To be effective, they must be used every day. These medicines are not intended to relieve symptoms immediately. Some may even take a few weeks to have their full effect.

The following are some long-term control medicines:

- *Cromolyn and nedocromil:* These inhaled medicines keep airways from swelling when a person comes in contact with a trigger.
- *Corticosteroids:* These medicines can be inhaled or taken in a pill form. They can prevent and decrease swelling in the airways. Corticosteroids can also decrease the amount of mucus.
- *Anti-leukotrienes:* These medicines come in a pill. They open the airways, control swelling and inflammation, and reduce mucus.
- *Long-acting beta 2 bronchodilators:* Over time, these inhaled medicines help relieve symptoms. They are often combined with anti-inflammatory medicines.

Staying away from triggers, taking your medicine consistently, and regular visits to the doctor will help you take control of asthma.

I just found out I'm pregnant. Should I still take my asthma medicines?

It is very important to call your doctor as soon as you find out you're pregnant. As your doctor will explain, it is extremely important to manage your asthma symptoms when you are pregnant. Taking asthma medicines and avoiding triggers helps make sure the baby gets enough oxygen. Untreated asthma can harm a growing fetus.

Many asthma medicines seem to be safe for use during pregnancy. Inhaled medicines are usually preferred for pregnant women. These medicines are less likely to be passed on to the baby than oral medicines. However, sometimes pregnant women need oral medicines to control symptoms. Talk with your doctor about the safety of asthma medicines during pregnancy. You should also talk to your doctor about getting a flu shot after the first trimester. The flu can be very serious for pregnant women with asthma.

How do I find out if I have chronic obstructive pulmonary disease (COPD)?

If you smoke, have a cough that won't go away, and shortness of breath see your doctor. To figure out if you have COPD, doctors usually do the following:

- Ask about your family and personal health history.
- Do a physical exam.
- Run some pulmonary function tests.
- Perform spirometry testing. During this test, the doctor uses a machine called a spirometer to see how well you breathe. This test measures how much air you can blow out of your lungs (lung volume). It also records how fast you can exhale it.
- Perform bronchodilator reversibility testing. During this test you will inhale a medicine called a bronchodilator. Then the doctor uses a spirometer to measure how this medicine affects your breathing. Bronchodilators relax muscles around the airways making it easier to breathe.

Your doctor may also suggest other tests like chest x-rays to make sure something else is not causing your problems. X-rays may allow the doctor to see if another lung disease or heart disease is causing your symptoms.

How is chronic obstructive pulmonary disease (COPD) treated?

The damage to the lungs in COPD cannot be repaired. But treatment can relieve symptoms. The only thing that can slow the progress of the disease is to stop smoking. So if you're a smoker, the single most important thing you can do is stop smoking. This slows down COPD and minimizes future damage to the lungs.

Medicines can also help you feel better. Common medicines used to treat COPD include the following:

- **Bronchodilators:** These medicines open up air passages in the lungs.
- **Inhaled steroids:** These medicines relieve symptoms by reducing inflammation in the lungs.
- **Antibiotics:** These medicines are used to clear up infections in the lungs.

Sometimes doctors also recommend the following for women with COPD:

- **Get a flu shot every year:** Influenza (flu) can cause serious problems for people with COPD.
- **Get the pneumococcal vaccine:** This vaccine reduces the risk of some kinds of pneumonia.
- **Pulmonary rehabilitation:** Pulmonary rehabilitation is a program that helps people cope physically and mentally with COPD. It can include exercise, training to manage the disease, diet advice, and counseling.
- **Oxygen therapy:** Oxygen therapy helps women with severe COPD. Oxygen is inhaled through a mask or a tube connected to a tank filled with 100 percent oxygen. This extra oxygen helps them breathe easier, sleep better, and live longer.
- **Surgery:** Sometimes surgery can help people with severe COPD feel better. Lung transplant surgery is becoming more common for people with severe emphysema. Another procedure called lung volume reduction surgery is also used to treat a small subset of people with severe COPD of the emphysema type. In this surgery, a part of the lung is removed.

How do I find out if I have lung cancer?

Usually there are no warning signs of early lung cancer. But if there is a sign, it is usually a cough. By the time most women have symptoms, the lung cancer often has advanced to more serious stages.

Symptoms of lung cancer may include the following:

- A cough that doesn't go away or gets worse
- Coughing up blood
- Frequent chest pain
- Hoarseness or wheezing

- Frequent problems with bronchitis or pneumonia
- Loss of appetite or weight loss
- Exhaustion

If you have any of these problems, call your doctor as soon as possible. The doctor will ask about your personal and family health history, smoking history, and exposure to harmful substances. He or she will also do a physical exam and may suggest some tests.

Common tests for lung cancer include the following:

- **Chest x-rays:** Chest x-rays allow doctors to "see" abnormal growths in the lungs.
- **Computerized tomography scans (CT scans):** A growing number of doctors use CT scans to diagnose lung cancer. CT scans are more powerful than standard x-rays. CT images can reveal subtle signs of cancer that don't show up on x-rays. This boosts the chances of finding cancer in its early, more treatable, stages.
- **Biopsy:** In this test, the doctor removes a small piece of lung tissue and studies it under a microscope. There are many ways to take a biopsy. In bronchoscopy, doctors put a special tube called a bronchoscope into the nose or mouth and down through the throat. They can see the lungs and remove a sample of tissue with this tube. In sputum cytology, doctors study a sample of mucus that is coughed up. The mucus may contain cancer cells.

I smoke. Should I get tested for lung cancer?

Talk to your doctor. Some doctors suggest testing smokers over fifty years of age for lung cancer. But experts still are not sure if routine testing (screening) saves or prolongs lives.

Testing for cancer before a person has any symptoms is called screening. Screening tends to find cancers early when it is easier to cure and treat. Screening high-risk groups (like smokers) for lung cancer is a controversial issue.

Many studies show that using x-rays to screen smokers for lung cancer does not save lives. For this reason, the National Cancer Institute and the U.S. Preventive Services Task Force (USPSTF) do not recommend screening for lung cancer. It is important to note that the USPSTF does not recommend against screening either. More studies are needed to show the exact risks and benefits of screening for lung cancer. Some groups do recommend screening in at-risk groups including smokers over forty-five years and people exposed to lung-damaging substances at work.

Computerized tomography scans (CT scans) show promise as a screening tool. The National Cancer Institute is doing an important study called the National Lung Screening Trial (NLST) to answer important questions about routine testing for lung cancer. This study will show if screening with CT scans and/or chest x-rays can save lives.

How is lung cancer treated?

Lung cancer can be treated in a number of different ways including a combination of surgery, radiation, and chemotherapy. Most of the time treatment does not cure the cancer but stops it from spreading and relieves symptoms. Your specific treatment will depend on the following:

- Kind of lung cancer
- Where the cancer is and if it has spread to other parts of the body
- Your age and overall health.

Radiation therapy uses a machine to aim high-energy x-rays at the tumor. This energy kills cancer cells. Radiation therapy can relieve pain and make a person feel better.

Chemotherapy uses medicine to kill cancer cells. Chemotherapy medicines can be injected into a vein or taken as a pill.

Surgery is used to remove tumors.

Chapter 48

Mental Health Concerns

Chapter Contents

Section 48.1

Depression

Excerpted from "Depression," National Women's Health Information Center, April 2006.

Life is full of ups and downs. But when the down times last for weeks or months at a time or keep you from living "normal," you may be suffering from depression. Depression is a medical illness that involves the body, mood, and thoughts. It affects the way you eat and sleep, the way you feel about yourself, and the way you think about things.

It is different from feeling "blue" or down for a few hours or a couple of days. It is not a condition that can be willed or wished away.

What causes depression?

There is no single cause of depression. There are many reasons why a woman may become depressed:

- **Hormonal factors:** Menstrual cycle changes, pregnancy, miscarriage, postpartum period, perimenopause, and menopause
- **Stress:** At work and home, single parenthood, caring for children and for aging parents
- **Family history:** Inherited (it's in your genes); it can also occur in people with no family history
- **Medical illness:** Stroke, heart attack, cancer
- **Chemical imbalance:** Changes in the brain chemistry

What are the signs of depression?

Not all people with depression have the same symptoms. Some people might only have a few, and others a lot. If you have one or more of these symptoms for more than two weeks or months at a time, see your doctor:

- Feeling sad, anxious, or "empty"

- Feeling hopeless
- Loss of interest in hobbies and activities that you once enjoyed
- Decreased energy
- Difficulty staying focused, remembering, making decisions
- Sleeplessness, early morning awakening, or oversleeping and not wanting to get up
- No desire to eat and weight loss or eating to "feel better" and weight gain
- Thoughts of hurting yourself
- Thoughts of death or suicide
- Easily annoyed, bothered, or angered
- Constant physical symptoms that do not get better with treatment, such as headaches, upset stomach, and pain that doesn't go away

What if I have thoughts of hurting myself?

Depression can make you think about hurting yourself or suicide. You may hurt yourself to:

- take away emotional pain and distress;
- avoid, distract from, or hold back strong feelings;
- try to feel better;
- stop a painful memory or thought;
- punish yourself;
- release or express anger that you're afraid to express to others.

Yet, hurting yourself does just that—it hurts you. At first, it may make you feel better; but it ends up making things worse. If you are thinking about hurting or even killing yourself, *please ask for help!* Call 911, 800-273-TALK (8255) or 800-SUICIDE, or check in your phone book for the number of a suicide crisis center. The centers offer experts who can help callers talk through their problems and develop a plan of action. These hotlines can also tell you where to go for more help in person. You also can talk with a family member you trust, a clergy person or a doctor. There is nothing wrong with asking for help—everyone needs help sometimes.

How is depression treated?

Most people with depression get better when they get treatment.

Once identified, depression almost always can be treated either by therapy, medicine called antidepressants, or both. Some people with milder forms of depression do well with therapy alone. Others with moderate to severe depression might benefit from antidepressants. It may take a few weeks or months before you begin to feel a change in your mood. Some people do best with combined treatment—therapy and antidepressants.

Should I stop taking my antidepressant while I am pregnant?

The decision whether or not to stay on medications is a complicated one that should be discussed with your doctor. Medication taken during pregnancy does reach the fetus. In rare cases, some antidepressants have been associated with breathing and heart problems in newborns, as well as jitteriness after delivery. However, moms who stop medications can be at increased risk for a relapse of their depression. Talk to your doctor about the risks and benefits of taking antidepressants during pregnancy. Your doctor can help you decide what is best for you and your baby.

Should I stop taking my antidepressant while breastfeeding?

If you stopped taking your medication during pregnancy, after delivery you may need to begin taking it again. Be aware that because your medication can be passed into your breast milk, breastfeeding may pose some risk for a nursing infant.

However, a number of research studies indicate that certain antidepressants, such as some of the selective serotonin reuptake inhibitors (SSRIs, a class of antidepressants for treating depression and anxiety disorders that includes medications like Zoloft®), have been used relatively safely during breastfeeding. You should discuss with your doctor whether breastfeeding is an option or whether you should plan to feed your baby formula. Although breastfeeding has some advantages for your baby, most importantly, as a mother, you need to stay healthy so you can take care of your baby.

How can I get help for my depression?

Below are some people and places that can help you get treatment:

- Family doctor
- Counselors or social workers
- Family service, social service agencies, or clergy person
- Employee assistance programs (EAP)
- Psychologists and psychiatrists

If you are unsure where to go for help, check the Yellow Pages under "mental health," "health," "social services," "suicide prevention," "crisis intervention services," "hotlines," "hospitals," or "physicians" for phone numbers and addresses.

Section 48.2

Postpartum Depression

"Postpartum Depression," May 2007, reprinted with permission from www.kidshealth.org. Copyright © 2007 The Nemours Foundation. This information was provided by KidsHealth, one of the largest resources online for medically reviewed health information written for parents, kids, and teens. For more articles like this one, visit www.KidsHealth.org, or www.TeensHealth.org.

Whether you're becoming a mom for the first time or the fourth, the days and weeks immediately following your baby's birth can be as overwhelming as they are joyful and exciting.

Many women experience major mood shifts after childbirth, ranging from brief, mild baby blues to longer-lasting, deeper clinical depression, which is known as postpartum depression.

Feelings of sadness and depression are more common after childbirth than many people may realize. It's important for new mothers—and those who love them—to understand the symptoms of postpartum depression and to reach out to family, friends, and medical professionals for help.

With the proper support and treatment, mothers who are experiencing any degree of postpartum depression can go on to be healthy, happy parents.

Baby Blues

Up to 80 percent of women experience something called the baby blues, feelings of sadness and emotional surges that begin in the first days after childbirth. With the baby blues, a woman might feel happy one minute and tearful or overwhelmed the next. She might feel sad, blue, irritable, discouraged, unhappy, tired, or moody. Baby blues usually last only a few days—but can linger as long as a week or two.

Why It Happens

These emotional surges are believed to be a natural effect of the hormone shifts that occur with pregnancy and childbirth. Levels of estrogen and progesterone that have increased during pregnancy drop suddenly after delivery, and this can affect mood. These female hormones return to their pre-pregnancy levels within a week or so. As hormone levels normalize again, baby blues usually resolve on their own without medical treatment.

What to Do

Getting proper rest, nutrition, and support are quite important—since being exhausted or sleep deprived or feeling stressed can reinforce and fuel feelings of sadness and depression.

To cope with baby blues, new moms should try to accept help in the first days and weeks after labor and delivery. Let family and friends help with errands, food shopping, household chores, or child care. Let someone prepare a meal or watch the baby while you relax with a shower, bath, or a nap.

Get plenty of rest and eat nutritious foods. Talking to people close to you, or to other new mothers, can help you feel supported and remind you that you're not alone. You don't have to stifle the tears if you feel the need to cry a bit—but try not to dwell on sad thoughts. Let the baby blues run their course and pass.

When to Call the Doctor

If baby blues linger longer than a week or two, talk to your doctor to discuss whether postpartum depression may be the cause of your emotional lows.

Postpartum Depression

For some women, the feelings of sadness or exhaustion run deeper and last longer than baby blues. About 10 percent of new mothers experience postpartum depression, which is a true clinical depression triggered by childbirth.

Postpartum depression usually begins two to three weeks after giving birth, but can start any time during the first few days, weeks, or months post-delivery.

A woman with postpartum depression may feel sad, tearful, despairing, discouraged, hopeless, worthless, or alone. She also may:

- have trouble concentrating or completing routine tasks;
- lose her appetite or not feel interested in food;
- feel indifferent to her baby or not feel attached or bonded;
- feel overwhelmed by her situation and feel that there is no hope of things getting better;
- feel like she is just going through the motions of her day without being able to feel happy, interested, pleased, or joyful about anything.

Feelings and thoughts like these are painful for a woman to experience—especially during a time that is idealized as being full of happiness. Many women are reluctant to tell someone when they feel this way. But postpartum depression is a medical condition that requires attention and treatment.

Why It Happens

Postpartum depression can affect any woman—but some may be more at risk for developing it. Women who have battled depression at another time in their lives or have one or more relatives who have had depression might have a genetic tendency to develop postpartum depression.

Most postpartum depression is thought to be related to fluctuating hormone levels that affect mood and energy. Levels of estrogen and progesterone that have increased during pregnancy drop suddenly after delivery. In some cases a woman's thyroid hormone may decrease, too.

These rapid hormone shifts affect the brain's mood chemistry in a way that can lead to sadness, low mood, and depression that lingers. Stress hormones may have an added effect on mood. Some women may experience this more than others.

When to Call the Doctor

If feelings of sadness or depression are strong, if they linger throughout most of the day for days in a row, or if they last longer that a week or two, talk to your doctor. A new mother who feels like giving up, who feels that life is not worth living, or who has suicidal thoughts or feelings needs to tell her doctor right away.

Postpartum depression can last for several months or even longer if it goes untreated. With proper treatment, a woman can feel like herself again. Treatment may include talk therapy, medication, or both. In addition, proper diet, exercise, rest, and social support can be very helpful. Some women find yoga to be beneficial. Some research suggests that expressing thoughts and emotions through certain writing techniques can help relieve symptoms of depression.

It may take several weeks for a woman to begin to feel better once she is being treated for depression, though some women begin to feel better sooner. Ask your doctor about how soon to expect improvements and ways to take care of yourself in the meantime.

Postpartum Psychosis

A more serious and rare condition is postpartum psychosis. It affects about one in one thousand women who give birth and occurs within the first month after labor and delivery. It may include hallucinations, such as hearing voices or seeing things, or feelings of paranoia.

With postpartum psychosis, a woman can have irrational ideas about her baby—such as that the baby is possessed or that she has to hurt herself or her child. This condition can be extremely serious and disabling, and new mothers who are experiencing these symptoms need medical attention right away.

Why It Happens

Women who have other psychiatric illnesses, such as bipolar disorder or schizo-affective disorder, may be at greater risk of developing postpartum psychosis.

When to Call the Doctor

Postpartum psychosis requires immediate medical attention and, often, a brief hospitalization. If you or someone you know is experiencing symptoms, don't delay getting medical attention.

Understanding the Changes after Childbirth

New mothers experience many layers of change in the days and weeks immediately following labor and delivery. In addition to the sudden drop in estrogen and progesterone—which can affect mood—there are other huge physical, emotional, and domestic changes that can affect how a new mom feels.

Physical Changes

Pregnancy brings many physical changes, and labor and delivery are physically intense and challenging. It takes time for the body to recover, and a new mother might feel exhausted, emotionally drained, or uncomfortable after delivery.

Personal and Emotional Changes

A woman's role and responsibilities may change quite a bit when she becomes a new mother. It can take time to adjust—even if she felt prepared for the change. Some women may feel isolated, worried, or scared.

Some new mothers face added stresses related to difficult circumstances or lack of support. Enduring a tough relationship, a precarious financial situation, or some other major life event at the same time—like a move or a job loss—can add stress.

Pregnancy-related stress—such as difficulty conceiving or complications during pregnancy or labor—can add to a new mom's feeling of being depleted. Sometimes (but not always) these stresses can pave the way for depression.

Changes in Routines and Responsibilities

A newborn brings special demands on a mother's time, attention, and energy. For first-time mothers, there can be lots to learn about meeting the baby's most basic needs, like sleeping, feeding, bathing, and soothing. There are lots of new routines to establish.

The baby's sleeping, waking, and feeding schedules can make it hard for a new mom to get the sleep and rest required to help handle all these new stresses and responsibilities. And without a good night's sleep, even small things can seem overwhelming.

Getting Help and Helping Yourself

Tell your doctor if you're having trouble with postpartum moods, thoughts, or feelings. Let someone else you trust know, too. This might be your partner, a friend, or a family member. This is a time to reach out and accept help and support from people close to you.

In addition to getting treatment for postpartum depression, small things you do can make it easier to get through a difficult time. You might find it helpful to:

- **Take time for yourself:** Schedule a babysitter for a regular time. This way you'll be sure to get time for yourself and know that it's coming.
- **Focus on little things to look forward to during the day:** This might be a hot shower, relaxing bath, walk around the block, or visit with a friend.
- **Read something uplifting:** Since depression may make it difficult to concentrate, choose something light and positive that can be read a bit at a time.
- **Indulge in other simple pleasures:** Page through a magazine, listen to music you enjoy, sip a cup of tea.
- **Be with others:** Create opportunities to spend time with other adults, like family and friends, who can provide some comfort and good company.
- **Ask for help:** Don't shy away from asking for emotional support or help with caring for the baby or tackling household chores.
- **Accept help:** Accepting help doesn't make you helpless—by reaching out you help yourself and your baby.
- **Rest:** Give your child a quiet place to sleep, and try to rest when the baby does.
- **Get moving:** A daily walk can help lift mood. (Check with your doctor before starting any new exercise program.)
- **Be patient:** Know that it may take time to feel better and take one day at a time.
- **Be optimistic:** Try to think of small things you're grateful for.
- **Join a support group:** Ask your doctor or women's center about resources in your community.

Helping Someone with Postpartum Depression

If you're concerned that your partner or someone else you know is experiencing postpartum depression, it's important to encourage her to talk to her doctor and to a mental health professional. Sometimes a woman is reluctant to seek help or may not recognize her own symptoms right away.

Consider giving the new mom some information on postpartum depression, and offer to read through it together. You might offer to make an appointment for her and go with her if she wants.

Once she's receiving the care she needs, support, love, and friendship are good medicine, too. Here are a few things that you can continue do for her:

- Check in with her regularly to see how she's doing.
- Listen when she wants to talk.
- Go for a walk with her (every day if possible!).
- Make her a nutritious meal (regularly!).
- Give her some breaks from housework and child care responsibilities.
- Let her take a nap or a relaxing bath while you care for her baby.
- Be patient, be kind.
- Believe in her—and remind her of her true qualities and strengths.

Brighter Days Ahead

Like all forms of depression, postpartum depression creates a cloud of negative feelings and thoughts over a woman's view of herself, those around her, her situation, and the future. Under the cloud of depression, a woman might see herself as helpless or worthless. She might view her situation as overwhelming or hopeless. Things might seem disappointing, uninteresting, or without meaning. Keep in mind that the bleak negative perspective is part of depression.

With the right treatment and support, the cloud can be lifted. This can free a woman to feel like herself again, to regain her perspective and sense of her own strength, her energy, her joy, and her hope. With those things in place, it's easier to work with changes, to see solutions to life's challenges, and to enjoy life's pleasures again.

Section 48.3

Eating Disorders

Excerpted from "Eating Disorders," National Institute of Mental Health, April 3, 2008.

What Are Eating Disorders?

An eating disorder is marked by extremes. It is present when a person experiences severe disturbances in eating behavior, such as extreme reduction of food intake or extreme overeating, or feelings of extreme distress or concern about body weight or shape.

A person with an eating disorder may have started out just eating smaller or larger amounts of food than usual, but at some point, the urge to eat less or more spirals out of control. Eating disorders are very complex, and despite scientific research to understand them, the biological, behavioral, and social underpinnings of these illnesses remain elusive.

The two main types of eating disorders are anorexia nervosa and bulimia nervosa. A third category is "eating disorders not otherwise specified (EDNOS)," which includes several variations of eating disorders. Most of these disorders are similar to anorexia or bulimia but with slightly different characteristics. Binge-eating disorder, which has received increasing research and media attention in recent years, is one type of EDNOS.

Eating disorders frequently appear during adolescence or young adulthood, but some reports indicate that they can develop during childhood or later in adulthood. Eating disorders are real, treatable medical illnesses with complex underlying psychological and biological causes. They frequently co-exist with other psychiatric disorders such as depression, substance abuse, or anxiety disorders. People with eating disorders also can suffer from numerous other physical health complications, such as heart conditions or kidney failure, which can lead to death.

Anorexia Nervosa

Anorexia nervosa is characterized by emaciation, a relentless pursuit of thinness and unwillingness to maintain a normal or healthy weight, a distortion of body image and intense fear of gaining weight, a lack of menstruation among girls and women, and extremely disturbed eating behavior. Some people with anorexia lose weight by dieting and exercising excessively; others lose weight by self-induced vomiting, or misusing laxatives, diuretics, or enemas.

Many people with anorexia see themselves as overweight, even when they are starved or are clearly malnourished. Eating, food, and weight control become obsessions. A person with anorexia typically weighs herself or himself repeatedly, portions food carefully, and eats only very small quantities of only certain foods. Some who have anorexia recover with treatment after only one episode. Others get well but have relapses. Still others have a more chronic form of anorexia, in which their health deteriorates over many years as they battle the illness.

Many people with anorexia also have coexisting psychiatric and physical illnesses, including depression, anxiety, obsessive behavior, substance abuse, cardiovascular and neurological complications, and impaired physical development.

Other symptoms may develop over time, including the following:

- thinning of the bones (osteopenia or osteoporosis)
- Brittle hair and nails
- Dry and yellowish skin
- Growth of fine hair over body (e.g., lanugo)
- Mild anemia, and muscle weakness and loss
- Severe constipation
- Low blood pressure, slowed breathing and pulse
- Drop in internal body temperature, causing a person to feel cold all the time
- Lethargy

Treating anorexia involves three components:

- Restoring the person to a healthy weight
- Treating the psychological issues related to the eating disorder
- Reducing or eliminating behaviors or thoughts that lead to disordered eating, and preventing relapse

Some research suggests that the use of medications, such as antidepressants, antipsychotics, or mood stabilizers, may be modestly effective in treating patients with anorexia by helping to resolve mood and anxiety symptoms that often co-exist with anorexia. Recent studies, however, have suggested that antidepressants may not be effective in preventing some patients with anorexia from relapsing. In addition, no medication has shown to be effective during the critical first phase of restoring a patient to healthy weight. Overall, it is unclear if and how medications can help patients conquer anorexia, but research is ongoing.

Different forms of psychotherapy, including individual, group, and family-based, can help address the psychological reasons for the illness. Some studies suggest that family-based therapies in which parents assume responsibility for feeding their afflicted adolescent are the most effective in helping a person with anorexia gain weight and improve eating habits and moods.

Shown to be effective in case studies and clinical trials, this particular approach is discussed in some guidelines and studies for treating eating disorders in younger, nonchronic patients.

Others have noted that a combined approach of medical attention and supportive psychotherapy designed specifically for anorexia patients is more effective than just psychotherapy. But the effectiveness of a treatment depends on the person involved and his or her situation. Unfortunately, no specific psychotherapy appears to be consistently effective for treating adults with anorexia. However, research into novel treatment and prevention approaches is showing some promise. One study suggests that an online intervention program may prevent some at-risk women from developing an eating disorder.

Bulimia Nervosa

Bulimia nervosa is characterized by recurrent and frequent episodes of eating unusually large amounts of food (e.g., binge eating), and feeling a lack of control over the eating. This binge eating is followed by a type of behavior that compensates for the binge, such as purging (e.g., vomiting, excessive use of laxatives or diuretics), fasting, and/or excessive exercise.

Unlike anorexia, people with bulimia can fall within the normal range for their age and weight. But like people with anorexia, they often fear gaining weight, want desperately to lose weight, and are intensely unhappy with their body size and shape. Usually, bulimic behavior is done secretly, because it is often accompanied by feelings of disgust or shame. The binging and purging cycle usually repeats several times a week. Similar to anorexia, people with bulimia often have coexisting psychological illnesses, such as depression, anxiety, and/or substance abuse problems. Many physical conditions result from the purging aspect of the illness, including electrolyte imbalances, gastrointestinal problems, and oral and tooth-related problems.

Other symptoms include the following:

- Chronically inflamed and sore throat
- Swollen glands in the neck and below the jaw
- Worn tooth enamel and increasingly sensitive and decaying teeth as a result of exposure to stomach acids
- Gastroesophageal reflux disorder
- Intestinal distress and irritation from laxative abuse
- Kidney problems from diuretic abuse
- Severe dehydration from purging of fluids

As with anorexia, treatment for bulimia often involves a combination of options and depends on the needs of the individual.

To reduce or eliminate binge and purge behavior, a patient may undergo nutritional counseling and psychotherapy, especially cognitive behavioral therapy (CBT), or be prescribed medication. Some antidepressants, such as fluoxetine (Prozac®), which is the only medication approved by the U.S. Food and Drug Administration for treating bulimia, may help patients who also have depression and/or anxiety. It also appears to help reduce binge eating and purging behavior, reduces the chance of relapse, and improves eating attitudes.

CBT that has been tailored to treat bulimia also has shown to be effective in changing binging and purging behavior, and eating attitudes. Therapy may be individually oriented or group-based.

Binge Eating Disorder

Binge eating disorder is characterized by recurrent binge eating episodes during which a person feels a loss of control over his or her eating. Unlike bulimia, binge eating episodes are not followed by purging, excessive exercise, or fasting. As a result, people with binge eating disorder often are overweight or obese. They also experience guilt, shame, and/or distress about the binge eating, which can lead to more binge eating.

Obese people with binge eating disorder often have coexisting psychological illnesses including anxiety, depression, and personality disorders. In addition, links between obesity and cardiovascular disease and hypertension are well documented.

Treatment options for binge eating disorder are similar to those used to treat bulimia. Fluoxetine and other antidepressants may reduce binge eating episodes and help alleviate depression in some patients.

Patients with binge eating disorder also may be prescribed appetite suppressants. Psychotherapy, especially CBT, is also used to treat the underlying psychological issues associated with binge eating, in an individual or group environment.

FDA Warnings on Antidepressants

Despite the relative safety and popularity of selective serotonin reuptake inhibitors (SSRIs) and other antidepressants, some studies have suggested that they may have unintentional effects on some people, especially adolescents and young adults. In 2004, the Food and Drug Administration (FDA) conducted a thorough review of published and unpublished controlled clinical trials of antidepressants that involved nearly 4,400 children and adolescents. The review revealed that 4 percent of those taking antidepressants thought about or attempted suicide (although no suicides occurred), compared to 2 percent of those receiving placebos.

This information prompted the FDA, in 2005, to adopt a "black box" warning label on all antidepressant medications to alert the public about the potential increased risk of suicidal thinking or attempts in children and adolescents taking antidepressants. In 2007, the FDA proposed that makers of all antidepressant medications extend the warning to include young adults up through age twenty-four. A "black box" warning is the most serious type of warning on prescription drug labeling.

The warning emphasizes that patients of all ages taking antidepressants should be closely monitored, especially during the initial weeks of treatment. Possible side effects to look for are worsening depression, suicidal thinking or behavior, or any unusual changes in behavior such as sleeplessness, agitation, or withdrawal from normal social situations. The warning adds that families and caregivers should also be told of the need for close monitoring and report any changes to the physician.

Results of a comprehensive review of pediatric trials conducted between 1988 and 2006 suggested that the benefits of antidepressant medications likely outweigh their risks to children and adolescents with major depression and anxiety disorders. The study was funded in part by the National Institute of Mental Health.

How Are We Working to Better Understand and Treat Eating Disorders?

Researchers are unsure of the underlying causes and nature of eating disorders. Unlike a neurological disorder, which generally can be pinpointed to a specific lesion on the brain, an eating disorder likely involves abnormal activity distributed across brain systems. With increased recognition that mental disorders are brain disorders, more researchers are using tools from both modern neuroscience and modern psychology to better understand eating disorders.

One approach involves the study of the human genes. With the publication of the human genome sequence in 2003, mental health researchers are studying the various combinations of genes to determine if any DNA variations are associated with the risk of developing a mental disorder. Neuroimaging, such as the use of magnetic resonance imaging (MRI), may also lead to a better understanding of eating disorders.

Neuroimaging already is used to identify abnormal brain activity in patients with schizophrenia, obsessive-compulsive disorder, and depression. It may also help researchers better understand how people with eating disorders process information, regardless of whether they have recovered or are still in the throes of their illness.

Conducting behavioral or psychological research on eating disorders is even more complex and challenging. As a result, few studies of treatments for eating disorders have been conducted in the past. New studies currently underway, however, are aiming to remedy the lack of information available about treatment.

Researchers also are working to define the basic processes of the disorders, which should help identify better treatments. For example, is anorexia the result of skewed body image, self-esteem problems, obsessive thoughts, compulsive behavior, or a combination of these? Can it be predicted or identified as a risk factor before drastic weight loss occurs, and therefore avoided?

These and other questions may be answered in the future as scientists and doctors think of eating disorders as medical illnesses with certain biological causes. Researchers are studying behavioral questions, along with genetic and brain systems information, to understand risk factors, identify biological markers, and develop medications that can target specific pathways that control eating behavior. Finally, neuroimaging and genetic studies may also provide clues for how each person may respond to specific treatments.

References

Agency for Healthcare Research and Quality (AHRQ). Management of Eating Disorders, Evidence Report/Technology Assessment, Number 135, 2006; AHRQ publication number 06-E010, www.ahrq.gov.

American Psychiatric Association. *Diagnostic and Statistical Manual for Mental Disorders, fourth edition (DSM-IV).* Washington, DC: American Psychiatric Press, 1994.

American Psychiatric Association (APA). Let's Talk Facts About Eating Disorders. 2005.

American Psychiatric Association Work Group on Eating Disorders. Practice guideline for the treatment of patients with eating disorders (revision). *American Journal of Psychiatry*, 2000; 157(1 Suppl): 1–39.

Andersen AE. Eating disorders in males. In: Brownell KD, Fairburn CG, eds. *Eating disorders and obesity: a comprehensive handbook*. New York: Guilford Press, 1995; 177–87.

Anderson AE. Eating disorders in males: Critical questions. In R Lemberg (ed), *Controlling Eating Disorders with Facts, Advice and Resources*. Phoenix, AZ: Oryx Press, 1992; 20–28.

Arnold LM, McElroy SL, Hudson JI, Wegele JA, Bennet AJ, Kreck PE Jr. A placebo-controlled randomized trial of fluoxetine in the treatment of binge-eating disorder. *Journal of Clinical Psychiatry*, 2002; 63:1028–33.

Becker AE, Grinspoon SK, Klibanski A, Herzog DB. Eating Disorders. *New England Journal of Medicine*, 1999; 340(14): 1092–98.

Birmingham CL, Su J, Hlynsky JA, Goldner EM, Gao M. The mortality rate of anorexia nervosa. *International Journal of Eating Disorders*. 2005 Sep; 38(2):143–46.

Bridge JA, Iyengar S, Salary CB, Barbe RP, Birmaher B, Pincus HA, Ren L, Brent DA. Clinical response and risk for reported suicidal ideation and suicide attempts in pediatric antidepressant treatment, a meta-analysis of randomized controlled trials. *Journal of the American Medical Association*, 2007; 297(15): 1683–96.

Bryant-Waugh R, Lask B. Childhood-onset eating disorders. In CG Fairburn, KD Brownell (eds.), *Eating disorders and obesity: A comprehensive handbook*, 2nd ed. New York: Guilford Press, 2002; 210–14.

Bulik CM, Sullivan PF, Kendler KS. Medical and psychiatric comorbidity in obese women with and without binge eating disorder. *International Journal of Eating Disorders*, 2002; 32: 72–78.

Eisler I, Dare C, Hodes M, Russel G, Dodge, and Le Grange D. Family therapy for adolescent anorexia nervosa: The results of a controlled comparison of two family interventions. *Journal of Child Psychology and Psychiatry*, 2000; 1: 727–36.

Fitzgerald KD, Welsh RC, Gehring WJ, Abelson JL, Himle JA, Liberzon I, Taylor SF. Error-related hyperactivity of the anterior cingulated cortex in obsessive-compulsive disorder. *Biological Psychiatry*, February 1, 2005; 57 (3): 287–94.

Halmi CA, Agras WS, Crow S, Mitchell J, Wilson GT, Bryson S, Kraemer HC. Predictors of treatment acceptance and completion in anorexia nervosa: implications for future study designs. *Archives of General Psychiatry*; 2005; 62: 776–81.

Insel TR and Quirion R. Psychiatry as a clinical neuroscience discipline. *Journal of the American Medical Association*, November 2, 2005; 294 (17): 2221–24.

Lasater L, Mehler P. Medical complications of bulimia nervosa. *Eating Behavior*, 2001; 2:279–92.

Lock J, Agras WS, Bryson S, Kraemer, HC. A comparison of short-and long-term family therapy for adolescent anorexia nervosa, *Journal of the American Academy of Child and Adolescent Psychiatry*, 2005; 44: 632–39.

Lock J, Couturier J, Agras WS. Comparison of long-term outcomes in adolescents with anorexia nervosa treated with family therapy. *Journal of the American Academy of Child and Adolescent Psychiatry*, 2006; 45: 666–72.

Lock J, Le Grange D, Agras WS, Dare C. *Treatment Manual for Anorexia Nervosa: A Family-based Approach.* New York: Guilford Press, 2001.

McIntosh VW, Jordan J, Carter FA, Luty SE, et al. Three psychotherapies for anorexia nervosa: a randomized controlled trial. *The American Journal of Psychiatry*, Apr. 2005; 162: 741–47.

Meyer-Lindenberg AS, Olsen RK, Kohn PD, Brown T, Egan MF, Weinberger DR, et al. Regionally specific disturbance of dorsolateral prefrontal-hippocampal functional connectivity in schizophrenia. *Archives of General Psychiatry*, April 2005; 62(4).

National Institute for Clinical Excellence (NICE). Core interventions in the treatment and management of anorexia nervosa, bulimia nervosa, and binge eating disorder, 2004: London: British Psychological Society.

Pezawas L, Meyer-Lindenberg A, Drabant EM, Verchinski BA, Munoz KE, Kolachana BS, et al. 5-HTTLPR polymorphism impacts human cingulated-amygdala interactions: a genetic susceptibility mechanism for depression. *Nature Neuroscience*, June 2005; 8 (6): 828–34.

Pope HG, Gruber AJ, Choi P, Olivardi R, Phillips KA. Muscle dysmorphia: an underrecognized form of body dysmorphic disorder. *Psychosomatics*, 1997; 38: 548–57.

Romano SJ, Halmi KJ, Sarkar NP, Koke SC, Lee JS. A placebo-controlled study of fluoxetine in continued treatment of bulimia nervosa after successful acute fluoxetine treatment. *American Journal of Psychiatry*, Jan. 2002; 151(9): 96–102.

Russell GF, Szmuckler GI, Dare C, Eisler I. An evaluation of family therapy in anorexia nervosa and bulimia nervosa. *Archives of General Psychiatry*, 1987; 44: 1047–56.

Spitzer RL, Yanovski S, Wadden T, Wing R, Marcus MD, Stunkard A, Devlin M, Mitchell J, Hasin D, Horne RL. Binge eating disorder: its further validation in a multisite study. *International Journal of Eating Disorders*, 1993; 13(2): 137–53.

Steiner H, Lock J. Anorexia nervosa and bulimia nervosa in children and adolescents: a review of the past ten years. *Journal of the American Academy of Child and Adolescent Psychiatry*, 1998; 37: 352–59.

Streigel-Moore RH, Franko DL. Epidemiology of Binge Eating Disorder. *International Journal of Eating Disorders*, 2003; 21: 11–27.

Taylor CB, Bryson S, Luce KH, Cunning D, Doyle AC, Abascal LB, Rockwell R, Dev P, Winzelberg AJ, Wilfley DE. Prevention of Eating Disorders in At-risk College-age Women. *Archives of General Psychiatry*; 2006 Aug; 63(8):881–88.

Walsh et al. Fluoxetine after weight restoration in anorexia nervosa: a randomized controlled trial. *Journal of the American Medical Association*. 2006 Jun 14; 295(22): 2605–12.

Wilson GT and Shafran R. Eating disorders guidelines from NICE. *Lancet*, 2005; 365: 79–81.

Wonderlich SA, Lilenfield LR, Riso LP, Engel S, Mitchell JE. Personality and anorexia nervosa. *International Journal of Eating Disorders*, 2005; 37: S68–S71.

Section 48.4

Panic Disorders

Panic disorder is a serious condition that around one out of every seventy-five people might experience. It usually appears during the teens or early adulthood, and while the exact causes are unclear, there does seem to be a connection with major life transitions that are potentially stressful: graduating from college, getting married, having a first child, and so on. There is also some evidence for a genetic predisposition; if a family member has suffered from panic disorder, you have an increased risk of suffering from it yourself, especially during a time in your life that is particularly stressful.

Panic Attacks: The Hallmark of Panic Disorder

A panic attack is a sudden surge of overwhelming fear that comes without warning and without any obvious reason. It is far more intense than the feeling of being "stressed out" that most people experience. Symptoms of a panic attack include:

- racing heartbeat;
- difficulty breathing, feeling as though you "can't get enough air";
- terror that is almost paralyzing;
- dizziness, lightheadedness, or nausea;
- trembling, sweating, shaking;
- choking, chest pains;
- hot flashes, or sudden chills;
- tingling in fingers or toes ("pins and needles");
- fear that you're going to go crazy or are about to die.

You probably recognize this as the classic "flight or fight" response that human beings experience when we are in a situation of danger. But during a panic attack, these symptoms seem to rise from out of nowhere. They occur in seemingly harmless situations—they can even happen while you are asleep.

In addition to the above symptoms, a panic attack is marked by the following conditions:

- It occurs suddenly, without any warning and without any way to stop it.
- The level of fear is way out of proportion to the actual situation; often, in fact, it's completely unrelated.
- It passes in a few minutes; the body cannot sustain the "fight or flight" response for longer than that. However, repeated attacks can continue to recur for hours.

A panic attack is not dangerous, but it can be terrifying, largely because it feels "crazy" and "out of control." Panic disorder is frightening because of the panic attacks associated with it, and also because it often leads to other complications such as phobias, depression, substance abuse, medical complications, even suicide. Its effects can range from mild word or social impairment to a total inability to face the outside world.

In fact, the phobias that people with panic disorder develop do not come from fears of actual objects or events, but rather from fear of having another attack. In these cases, people will avoid certain objects or situations because they fear that these things will trigger another attack.

How to Identify Panic Disorder

Please remember that only a licensed therapist can diagnose a panic disorder. There are certain signs you may already be aware of, though.

One study found that people sometimes see ten or more doctors before being properly diagnosed, and that only one out of four people with the disorder receive the treatment they need. That's why it's important to know what the symptoms are, and to make sure you get the right help.

Many people experience occasional panic attacks, and if you have had one or two such attacks, there probably isn't any reason to worry. The key symptom of panic disorder is the persistent fear of having future panic attacks. If you suffer from repeated (four or more) panic attacks, and especially if you have had a panic attack and are in continued fear of having another, these are signs that you should consider finding a mental health professional who specializes in panic or anxiety disorders.

What Causes Panic Disorder: Mind, Body, or Both?

Body: There may be a genetic predisposition to anxiety disorders; some sufferers report that a family member has or had a panic disorder or some other emotional disorder such as depression. Studies with twins have confirmed the possibility of "genetic inheritance" of the disorder.

Panic disorder could also be due to a biological malfunction, although a specific biological marker has yet to be identified.

All ethnic groups are vulnerable to panic disorder. For unknown reasons, women are twice as likely to get the disorder as men.

Mind: Stressful life events can trigger panic disorders. One association that has been noted is that of a recent loss or separation. Some researchers liken the "life stressor" to a thermostat; that is, when stresses lower your resistance, the underlying physical predisposition kicks in and triggers an attack.

Both: Physical and psychological causes of panic disorder work together. Although initially attacks may come out of the blue, eventually the sufferer may actually help bring them on by responding to physical symptoms of an attack.

For example, if a person with panic disorder experiences a racing heartbeat caused by drinking coffee, exercising, or taking a certain medication, they might interpret this as a symptom of an attack and, because of their anxiety, actually bring on the attack. On the other hand, coffee, exercise, and certain medications sometimes do, in fact, cause panic attacks. One of the most frustrating things for the panic sufferer is never knowing how to isolate the different triggers of an attack. That's why the right therapy for panic disorder focuses on all aspects—physical, psychological, and physiological—of the disorder.

Can People with Panic Disorder Lead Normal Lives?

The answer to this is a resounding *yes*—if they receive treatment.

Panic disorder is highly treatable, with a variety of available therapies. These treatments are extremely effective, and most people who have successfully completed treatment can continue to experience situational avoidance or anxiety, and further treatment might be necessary in those cases. Once treated, panic disorder doesn't lead to any permanent complications.

Side Effects of Panic Disorder

Without treatment, panic disorder can have very serious consequences.

The immediate danger with panic disorder is that it can often lead to a phobia. That's because once you've suffered a panic attack, you may start to avoid situations like the one you were in when the attack occurred.

Many people with panic disorder show "situational avoidance" associated with their panic attacks. For example, you might have an attack while driving, and start to avoid driving until you develop an actual phobia towards it. In worst case scenarios, people with panic disorder develop agoraphobia—fear of going outdoors—because they believe that by staying inside, they can avoid all situations that might provoke an attack, or where they might not be able to get help. The fear of an attack is so debilitating, they prefer to spend their lives locked inside their homes.

Even if you don't develop these extreme phobias, your quality of life can be severely damaged by untreated panic disorder. A recent study showed that people who suffer from panic disorder:

- are more prone to alcohol and other drug abuse;
- have greater risk of attempting suicide;
- spend more time in hospital emergency rooms;
- spend less time on hobbies, sports, and other satisfying activities;

- tend to be financially dependent on others;
- report feeling emotionally and physically less healthy than nonsufferers;
- are afraid of driving more than a few miles away from home.

Panic disorders can also have economic effects. For example, a recent study cited the case of a woman who gave up a $40,000 a year job that required travel for one close to home that only paid $14,000 a year. Other sufferers have reported losing their jobs and having to rely on public assistance or family members.

None of this needs to happen. Panic disorder can be treated successfully, and sufferers can go on to lead full and satisfying lives.

How Can Panic Disorder Be Treated?

Most specialists agree that a combination of cognitive and behavioral therapies are the best treatment for panic disorder. Medication might also be appropriate in some cases.

The first part of therapy is largely informational; many people are greatly helped by simply understanding exactly what panic disorder is, and how many others suffer from it. Many people who suffer from panic disorder are worried that their panic attacks mean they're "going crazy" or that the panic might induce a heart attack. "Cognitive restructuring" (changing one's way of thinking) helps people replace those thoughts with more realistic, positive ways of viewing the attacks.

Cognitive therapy can help the patient identify possible triggers for the attacks. The trigger in an individual case could be something like a thought, a situation, or something as subtle as a slight change in heartbeat. Once the patient understands that the panic attack is separate and independent of the trigger, that trigger begins to lose some of its power to induce an attack.

The behavioral components of the therapy can consist of what one group of clinicians has termed "interoceptive exposure." This is similar to the systematic desensitization used to cure phobias, but what it focuses on is exposure to the actual physical sensations that someone experiences during a panic attack.

People with panic disorder are more afraid of the actual attack than they are of specific objects or events; for instance, their "fear of flying" is not that the planes will crash but that they will have a panic attack in a place, like a plane, where they can't get to help. Others won't drink coffee or go to an overheated room because they're afraid that these might trigger the physical symptoms of a panic attack.

Interoceptive exposure can help them go through the symptoms of an attack (elevated heart rate, hot flashes, sweating, and so on) in a controlled setting, and teach them that these symptoms need not develop into a full-blown attack. Behavioral therapy is also used to deal with the situational avoidance associated with panic attacks. One very effective treatment for phobias is in vivo exposure, which in its simplest terms means breaking a fearful situation down into small manageable steps and doing them one at a time until the most difficult level is mastered.

Relaxation techniques can further help someone "flow through" an attack. These techniques include breathing retraining and positive visualization. Some experts have found that people with panic disorder tend to have slightly higher than average breathing rates, learning to slow this can help someone deal with a panic attack and can also prevent future attacks.

In some cases, medications may also be needed. Anti-anxiety medications may be prescribed, as well as antidepressants, and sometimes even heart medications (such as beta blockers) that are used to control irregular heartbeats.

Finally, a support group with others who suffer from panic disorder can be very helpful to some people. It can't take the place of therapy, but it can be a useful adjunct.

If you suffer from panic disorder, these therapies can help you. But you can't do them on your own; all of these treatments must be outlined and prescribed by a psychologist or psychiatrist.

How Long Does Treatment Take?

Much of the success of treatment depends on your willingness to carefully follow the outlined treatment plan. This is often multifaceted, and it won't work overnight, but if you stick with it, you should start to have noticeable improvement within about ten to twenty weekly sessions. If you continue to follow the program, within one year you will notice a tremendous improvement.

If you are suffering from panic disorder, you should be able to find help in your area. You need to find a licensed psychologist or other mental health professional who specializes in panic or anxiety disorders. There may even be a clinic nearby that specializes in these disorders.

When you speak with a therapist, specify that you think you have panic disorder, and ask about his or her experience treating this disorder.

Keep in mind, though, that panic disorder, like any other emotional disorder, isn't something you can either diagnose or cure by yourself. An experienced clinical psychologist or psychiatrist is the most qualified person to make this diagnosis, just as he or she is the most qualified to treat this disorder.

This section is designed to answer your basic questions about panic disorder; a qualified mental health professional will be able to give you more complete information.

Panic disorder does not need to disrupt your life in any way!

Section 48.5

Seasonal Affective Disorder

"Seasonal Affective Disorder," February 2004. © 2004 NAMI: The Nation's Voice on Mental Illness (www.nami.org). Reprinted with permission. Reviewed by David A. Cooke, M.D., December 2008.

If you notice periods of depression that seem to accompany seasonal changes during the year, you may suffer from seasonal affective disorder (SAD). This condition is characterized by recurrent episodes of depression—usually in late fall and winter—alternating with periods of normal or high mood the rest of the year.

Most people with SAD are women whose illness typically begins in their twenties, although men also report SAD of similar severity and have increasingly sought treatment. SAD can also occur in children and adolescents, in which case the syndrome is first suspected by parents and teachers. Many people with SAD report at least one close relative with a psychiatric condition, most frequently a severe depressive disorder (55 percent) or alcohol abuse (34 percent).

What are the patterns of SAD?

Symptoms of winter SAD usually begin in October or November and subside in March or April. Some patients begin to slump as early as August, while others remain well until January. Regardless of the time of onset, most patients don't feel fully back to normal until early

May. Depressions are usually mild to moderate, but they can be severe. Very few patients with SAD have required hospitalization, and even fewer have been treated with electroconvulsive therapy.

The usual characteristics of recurrent winter depression include oversleeping, daytime fatigue, carbohydrate craving and weight gain, although a patient does not necessarily show these symptoms. Additionally, there are the usual features of depression, especially decreased sexual interest, lethargy, hopelessness, suicidal thoughts, lack of interest in normal activities, and social withdrawal.

Light therapy, described below, is now considered the first-line treatment intervention, and if properly dosed can produce relief within days. Antidepressants may also help, and if necessary can be used in conjunction with light.

In about one-tenth of cases, annual relapse occurs in the summer rather than winter, possibly in response to high heat and humidity. During that period, the depression is more likely to be characterized by insomnia, decreased appetite, weight loss, and agitation or anxiety. Patients with such "reverse SAD" often find relief with summer trips to cooler climates in the north. Generally, normal air conditioning is not sufficient to relieve this depression, and an antidepressant may be needed.

In still fewer cases, a patient may experience both winter and summer depressions, while feeling fine each fall and spring, around the equinoxes.

The most common characteristic of people with winter SAD is their reaction to changes in environmental light. Patients living at different latitudes note that their winter depressions are longer and more profound the farther north they live. Patients with SAD also report that their depression worsens or reappears whenever the weather is overcast at any time of the year, or if their indoor lighting is decreased.

SAD is often misdiagnosed as hypothyroidism, hypoglycemia, infectious mononucleosis, and other viral infections.

How is winter SAD treated with light?

Bright white fluorescent light has been shown to reverse the winter depressive symptoms of SAD. Early studies used expensive "full-spectrum" bulbs, but these are not especially advantageous. Bulbs with color temperatures between 3000 and 6500 degrees Kelvin all have been shown to be effective. The lower color temperatures produce "softer" white light with less visual glare, while the higher color temperatures produce a "colder" skylight hue. The lamps are encased in a box with a diffusing lens, which also filters out ultraviolet radiation. The box sits on a tabletop, preferably on a stand that raises it to eye level and above. Such an arrangement further reduces glare sensations at high intensity, and preferentially illuminates the lower half of the retina, which is rich in photoreceptors that are thought to mediate the antidepressant response. Studies show between 50 and 80 percent of users showing essentially complete remission of symptoms, although the treatment needs to continue throughout the difficult season in order to maintain this benefit.

There are three major dosing dimensions of light therapy, and optimum effect requires that the dose be individualized, just as for medications.

Light intensity: The treatment uses an artificial equivalent of early morning full daylight (2,500 to 10,000 lux), higher than projected by normal home light fixtures (50 to 300 lux). A light box should be capable of delivering 10,000 lux at eye level, which allows downward adjustments if necessary.

Light duration: Daily sessions of twenty to sixty minutes may be needed. Since light intensity and duration interact, longer sessions will be needed at lower intensities. At 10,000 lux—the current standard—thirty-minute sessions are most typical.

Time of day of exposure: The antidepressant effect, many investigators think, is mediated by light's action on the internal circadian rhythm clock. Most patients with winter depression benefit by resetting this clock earlier, which is achieved specifically with morning light exposure. Since different people have different clock phases (early types, neutral types, late types), the optimum time of light exposure can differ greatly. The Center for Environmental Therapeutics, a professional nonprofit agency, offers an on-line questionnaire on its website which can be used to calculate a recommended treatment time individually, which is then adjusted depending on response. Long sleepers may need to wake up earlier for best effect, while short sleepers can maintain their habitual sleep-wake schedule.

Side effects of light therapy are uncommon. Some patients complain of irritability, eyestrain, headaches, or nausea. Those who have histories of hypomania in spring or summer are at risk for switching states under light therapy, in which case light dose needs to be reduced. There is no evidence for long-term adverse effects, however, and disturbances experienced during the first few exposures often disappear spontaneously. As an important precaution, patients with Bipolar I disorder—who are at risk for switching into full-blown manic episodes—need to be on a mood-stabilizing drug while using light therapy.

What should I do if I think I have SAD?

If your symptoms are mild—that is, if they don't interfere too much with your daily living, you may want to try light therapy as described above or experiment with adjusting the light in your surroundings with bright lamps and scheduling more time outdoors in winter.

If your depressive symptoms are severe enough to significantly affect your daily living, consult a mental health professional qualified to treat SAD. He or she can help you find the most appropriate treatment for you.

Chapter 49

Migraine Headaches

What is a migraine headache?

A migraine headache is a severe pain felt on one, and sometimes both, sides of the head. The pain is mostly in the front around the temples or behind one eye or ear. Besides pain, you may have nausea and vomiting, and be very sensitive to light and sound. Migraine can occur any time of the day, though it often starts in the morning. The pain can last a few hours or up to one or two days.

We don't know what causes migraine headaches, but some things are more common in people who have them:

- Most often, migraine affects people between the ages of fifteen and fifty-five.
- Many people have a family history of migraine.
- They are more common in women.
- Migraine often becomes less severe and frequent with age.

What causes migraine?

One theory about the cause of migraine is the blood flow theory, which focuses on blood vessel activity in the brain. Blood vessels either narrow or expand. Narrowing can constrict blood flow, causing

---

Excerpted from "Migraine Headaches," National Women's Health Information Center, November 2004. Revised by David A. Cooke, M.D., December 2008.

problems with sight or dizziness. When the blood vessels expand, they press on nerves nearby, which causes pain.

Another theory focuses on chemical changes in the brain. When chemicals in the brain that send messages from one cell to another, including the messages to blood vessels to get narrow or expand, are interrupted, migraines can occur.

More recently, genes have been linked to migraine. People who get migraines may inherit abnormal genes that control the functions of certain brain cells. And something the person's body is sensitive to in some way triggers the actual headaches.

Headache triggers can vary from person to person. Most migraines are not caused by a single factor or event. Your response to triggers can also vary from headache to headache. Many women with migraine tend to have attacks brought on by the following:

- Lack of food or sleep
- Bright light or loud noise
- Hormone changes during the menstrual cycle
- Stress and anxiety
- Weather changes
- Chocolate, alcohol, or nicotine
- Some foods and food additives, such as monosodium glutamate (MSG) or nitrates

To help pinpoint your headache triggers, it may be helpful to keep a headache "diary." Each time you have a migraine, write down the time of day, point in your menstrual cycle, where you are at the time, and what you were doing when the migraine started. Talk with your doctor about what sets off your headaches to help find the right treatment for you.

Are there different kinds of migraine?

Yes, there are many forms of migraine headache. But the two forms seen most often are classic and common migraine.

Classic migraine: With a classic migraine, a person has these visual symptoms (also called an "aura") ten to thirty minutes before an attack: sees flashing lights or zigzag lines or has blind spots or loses vision for a short time. The aura can include seeing or hearing strange things. It can even disturb the senses of smell, taste, or touch. Women have this form of migraine less often than men.

Common migraine: With a common migraine, a person does not have an aura, but does have the other migraine symptoms, such as nausea and vomiting.

How does a migraine headache differ from a tension headache?

While migraine headaches affect millions of people, they are still less common than tension headaches. Tension headaches cause a more steady pain over the entire head rather than throbbing pain in one spot. Most of the time, migraine attacks happen once in awhile, but tension headaches can occur as often as every day. While fatigue and stress can bring on both tension and migraine headaches, migraines can be triggered by certain foods, changes in the body's hormone levels, and even changes in the weather.

When should I seek help for my headaches?

Nearly half of the people in the United States who have migraine do not get diagnosed and treated. The National Headache Foundation suggests you talk to your doctor about your headaches if any of the following are true:

- You have several headaches per month and each lasts for several hours or days
- Your headaches disrupt your home, work, or school life
- You have nausea, vomiting, vision, or other sensory problems

What tests are used to find out if I have migraine?

If you think you get migraine headaches, talk with your doctor. Before your appointment, write down the following things:

- How often you have headaches
- Where the pain is
- How long the headaches last
- When the headaches happen, such as during your menstrual cycle
- Other symptoms, such as nausea or blind spots
- Any family history of migraine

Your doctor may also do an exam and ask more questions about your health history. This could include past head injury, sinus or dental problems, or medicine use. By just talking with your doctor, you may be able to give enough information to diagnose migraine.

You may get a blood test and other tests if your doctor thinks that something else could be causing your symptoms. Work with your doctor to decide on the best tests for you.

Are women more prone to migraine headaches?

Yes, migraine headaches are more common in women. In fact, about three out of four people who have migraines are women. They are most common in women between the ages of thirty-five and forty-five; this is often a time that women have more job, family, and social commitments. Women also tend to report higher levels of pain, longer headache time, and more symptoms, such as nausea and vomiting.

Hormones may also trigger migraine. Over half of women with migraine report having them right before, during, or after their period. Others get them for the first time when taking birth control pills. And some women start getting them when they enter menopause.

How is a woman's menstrual cycle related to migraine?

More than half of women with migraine have more headaches around or during their menstrual cycle. This is often called "menstrual migraine." But just a small fraction of these women only have migraine at this time. Most have migraine headaches at other times of the month as well.

How the menstrual cycle and migraine are linked is still unclear. We know that just before the cycle begins, levels of the female hormones, estrogen and progesterone, sharply go down. This drop in hormones may trigger a migraine, because estrogen controls chemicals in the brain that affect a woman's pain sensation.

Talk with your doctor if you think you have menstrual migraine. You may find that medicines, making lifestyle changes, and home treatment methods can prevent or reduce the pain.

Can using birth control pills make my migraines worse?

In some women, birth control pills improve migraine. They reduce the number of attacks and attacks may be less severe. But in others, birth control pills cause migraine.

For these women, migraine headaches seem to occur during the last week of the cycle when they take sugar pills, or the pills that don't have the hormones. The last seven pills in the monthly pack (if included) help remind you to take them daily. But without the hormones, this fall in estrogen may trigger migraine in some women.

Talk with your doctor if you think birth control pills cause your migraines or make them worse. Switching to another pill or dose or taking a type of pill that contains all "active" pills in the monthly pack, instead of skipping a week, may help. Lifestyle changes, such as getting on a regular sleep pattern and eating a healthful diet, can help too.

Can stress really cause migraines?

Yes, stress is the most common trigger of headache. Events like getting married, moving to a new home, or having a baby are all sources of stress. But studies have found that it is the day-to-day stresses, not these major life changes, that are most linked to headaches. Juggling our many roles, such as being a mother and wife, having a career, and financial pressures, can be daily stresses for women.

Learning to make time for yourself and finding healthy ways to deal with stress are important. Some things you can do to help prevent or reduce stress include the following:

- Eating a healthy diet
- Being active (at least thirty minutes most days of the week is best)
- Doing relaxation exercises
- Getting enough sleep

Also, it may be helpful to pinpoint which factors in your life cause stress. You may find that you can even avoid some of these stresses. And for other stresses that you can't control, try to think of things you can do ahead of time to help you cope with them.

How are migraines treated?

Even though migraine has no cure, you can work with your doctor to come up with a treatment plan that meets your needs. Make sure your plan has ways to treat the headache symptoms when they happen, as well as ways to help make your headaches less frequent or severe. It may include all or some of the following methods.

Lifestyle changes: Finding and avoiding things that cause headache is one way to reduce how often attacks happen and how painful they are. Your diet, the amount of stress in your life, and other lifestyle habits may add to getting migraines. Eating a healthful diet, quitting smoking, and reducing your alcohol intake may help improve your headaches. Learn stress reduction techniques and find other positive ways to cope with stress. Try to get on a regular sleep pattern.

Medicine: There are two ways to approach the treatment of migraine headache with drugs—prevent the attacks, or relieve the symptoms during the attacks. Many people with migraine use both forms of treatment. Some medicines used to help prevent attacks include drugs that were designed to treat epilepsy, high blood pressure, and depression. Commonly used preventative medications include beta blockers, calcium channel blockers, antidepressants, and several types of anti-seizure medications. Many people will respond well to one medication but not another, and it is common to need to try several different drugs before finding the best one for you.

To relieve symptoms during attacks, your doctor may start by telling you to take over-the-counter drugs such as aspirin, acetaminophen, or NSAIDs (nonsteroidal anti-inflammatory drugs) like ibuprofen. If these drugs don't work to give you relief, your doctor can prescribe types of drugs called ergotamines or triptans. Ergotamines narrow the blood vessels, which helps the migraine's throbbing pain. Triptans are drugs that relieve pain by both narrowing blood vessels and balancing the chemicals in the brain. They are often more effective than other drugs, but they can interact with other medications, and can also be quite expensive. Hormone therapy may help some women whose migraines seem to be linked to their menstrual cycle. Work with your doctor to choose the best medicine for you.

Alternative methods: Biofeedback has been shown to help some people with migraine. It involves learning to control how your body reacts to stress to reduce its effects. Other methods, such as acupuncture and relaxation, may help relieve stress. Counseling can also help if you think your migraines may be related to depression or anxiety. Small studies have suggested that certain vitamins and supplements such as coenzyme Q10 or riboflavin may be effective in preventing migraines. Talk with your doctor about these treatment methods.

I'm pregnant. Can my migraines still be treated?

Pregnancy can have variable effects on migraines. Some women have fewer migraines while pregnant, and some have them worsen. When you are pregnant, your doctor may advise against taking some medicines commonly used for migraines. Some of these drugs may cause birth defects and other problems. This includes over-the-counter medicines as well. Taking aspirin may increase your risk and the baby's risk of bleeding. Ergotamines and triptans can cause miscarriage, and must not be used during pregnancy. Talk with your doctor if migraine is a problem while you are pregnant or if you plan to become pregnant. Other home treatment methods can help, such as doing relaxation techniques and using cold packs.

Is taking medicine for migraine dangerous if I am breastfeeding?

Ask your doctor about what medicines, even over-the-counter medicines, are safe to take while breastfeeding. Some medicines can be passed through breast milk and can be harmful for your baby.

Can migraine be worse during menopause?

If your migraines are closely linked to your menstrual cycle, menopause may make them less severe. As you get older, nausea, vomiting, and pain may be less as well.

But for some women, menopause worsens migraine or triggers them to start. It is not clear why this happens. Hormone therapy, which is prescribed for some women during menopause, may be linked to migraines during this time.

What are some ways I can prevent migraine?

The best way to prevent migraine is to find out what events or lifestyle factors, such as stress or certain foods, set off your headaches. Try to avoid or limit these triggers as much as you can. Since migraine headaches are more common during stressful times, find healthy ways to cope with stress. Talk with your doctor about starting an exercise program or taking a class to learn relaxation skills.

If your doctor has prescribed medicine for you to help prevent migraine, take them exactly as prescribed. Ask what you should do if you miss a dose and how long should take the medicine. If you use headache medicines too often or more than what your doctor prescribes, the medicines can even start to cause a condition called "rebound headaches." With this condition, your medicines stop helping your pain and actually begin to cause headaches. Talk with your doctor if the amount of medicine you are prescribed is not helping your headaches, or if you are needing to take medicine more frequently.

Chapter 50

Osteoporosis

Osteoporosis, or porous bone, is a disease characterized by low bone mass and structural deterioration of bone tissue, leading to bone fragility and an increased risk of fractures of the hip, spine, and wrist. Men as well as women are affected by osteoporosis, a disease that can be prevented and treated.

What Is Bone?

Bone is living, growing tissue. It is made mostly of collagen, a protein that provides a soft framework, and calcium phosphate, a mineral that adds strength and hardens the framework.

This combination of collagen and calcium makes bone both flexible and strong, which in turn helps it to withstand stress. More than 99 percent of the body's calcium is contained in the bones and teeth. The remaining 1 percent is found in the blood.

Throughout your lifetime, old bone is removed (resorption) and new bone is added to the skeleton (formation). During childhood and teenage years, new bone is added faster than old bone is removed. As a result, bones become larger, heavier, and denser. Bone formation outpaces resorption until peak bone mass (maximum bone density and strength) is reached around age thirty. After that time, bone resorption slowly begins to exceed bone formation.

Excerpted from "Osteoporosis Overview," National Institute of Arthritis and Musculoskeletal and Skin Diseases, National Institutes of Health, December 2007.

For women, bone loss is fastest in the first few years after menopause, and it continues into the postmenopausal years. Osteoporosis—which mainly affects women but may also affect men—will develop when bone resorption occurs too quickly or when replacement occurs too slowly. Osteoporosis is more likely to develop if you did not reach optimal peak bone mass during your bone-building years.

Risk Factors

Certain risk factors are linked to the development of osteoporosis and contribute to an individual's likelihood of developing the disease. Many people with osteoporosis have several risk factors, but others who develop the disease have no known risk factors. There are some you cannot change and others you can.

Risk factors you cannot change include the following:

- **Gender:** Your chances of developing osteoporosis are greater if you are a woman. Women have less bone tissue and lose bone faster than men because of the changes that happen with menopause.
- **Age:** The older you are, the greater your risk of osteoporosis. Your bones become thinner and weaker as you age.
- **Body size:** Small, thin-boned women are at greater risk.
- **Ethnicity:** Caucasian and Asian women are at highest risk. African American and Hispanic women have a lower but significant risk.
- **Family history:** Fracture risk may be due, in part, to heredity. People whose parents have a history of fractures also seem to have reduced bone mass and may be at risk for fractures.

Risk factors you can change include the following:

- **Sex hormones:** Abnormal absence of menstrual periods (amenorrhea), low estrogen level (menopause), and low testosterone level in men can bring on osteoporosis.
- **Anorexia nervosa:** Characterized by an irrational fear of weight gain, this eating disorder increases your risk for osteoporosis.
- **Calcium and vitamin D intake:** A lifetime diet low in calcium and vitamin D makes you more prone to bone loss.

- **Medication use:** Long-term use of glucocorticoids and some anticonvulsants can lead to loss of bone density and fractures.
- **Lifestyle:** An inactive lifestyle or extended bed rest tends to weaken bones.
- **Cigarette smoking:** Cigarettes are bad for bones as well as the heart and lungs.
- **Alcohol intake:** Excessive consumption increases the risk of bone loss and fractures.

Prevention

To reach optimal peak bone mass and continue building new bone tissue as you age, there are several factors you should consider.

Calcium: An inadequate supply of calcium over a lifetime contributes to the development of osteoporosis. Many published studies show that low calcium intake appears to be associated with low bone mass, rapid bone loss, and high fracture rates. National nutrition surveys show that many people consume less than half the amount of calcium recommended to build and maintain healthy bones. Good sources of

Table 50.1. Recommended Calcium Intakes (mg/day) (Source: National Academy of Sciences [1997])

Ages	mg/day
Birth–6 months	210
6 months–1 year	270
1–3	500
4–8	800
9–13	1300
14–18	1300
19–30	1000
31–50	1000
51–70	1200
70 or older	1200
Pregnant or lactating	
14–18	1300
19–50	1000

calcium include low-fat dairy products, such as milk, yogurt, cheese, and ice cream; dark green, leafy vegetables, such as broccoli, collard greens, bok choy, and spinach; sardines and salmon with bones; tofu; almonds; and foods fortified with calcium, such as orange juice, cereals, and breads. Depending upon how much calcium you get each day from food, you may need to take a calcium supplement.

Calcium needs change during one's lifetime. The body's demand for calcium is greater during childhood and adolescence, when the skeleton is growing rapidly, and during pregnancy and breastfeeding. Postmenopausal women and older men also need to consume more calcium. Also, as you age, your body becomes less efficient at absorbing calcium and other nutrients. Older adults also are more likely to have chronic medical problems and to use medications that may impair calcium absorption.

Vitamin D: Vitamin D plays an important role in calcium absorption and in bone health. It is made in the skin through exposure to sunlight. While many people are able to obtain enough vitamin D naturally, studies show that vitamin D production decreases in the elderly, in people who are housebound, and for people in general during the winter. Depending on your situation, you may need to take vitamin D supplements to ensure a daily intake of between 400 to 800 international units (IU) of vitamin D. Massive doses are not recommended.

Exercise: Like muscle, bone is living tissue that responds to exercise by becoming stronger. Weight-bearing exercise is the best for your bones because it forces you to work against gravity. Examples include walking, hiking, jogging, stair climbing, weight training, tennis, and dancing.

Smoking: Smoking is bad for your bones as well as for your heart and lungs. Women who smoke have lower levels of estrogen compared to nonsmokers, and they often go through menopause earlier. Smokers also may absorb less calcium from their diets.

Alcohol: Regular consumption of two to three ounces a day of alcohol may be damaging to the skeleton, even in young women and men. Those who drink heavily are more prone to bone loss and fractures, because of both poor nutrition and increased risk of falling.

Medications that cause bone loss: The long-term use of glucocorticoids (medications prescribed for a wide range of diseases, including arthritis, asthma, Crohn disease, lupus, and other diseases of the lungs, kidneys, and liver) can lead to a loss of bone density and fractures. Bone loss can also result from long-term treatment with certain antiseizure drugs, such as phenytoin (Dilantin®) and barbiturates; gonadotropin-releasing hormone (GnRH) drugs used to treat endometriosis; excessive use of aluminum-containing antacids; certain cancer treatments; and excessive thyroid hormone. It is important to discuss the use of these drugs with your physician and not to stop or change your medication dose on your own.

Preventive medications: Various medications are available for preventing and treating osteoporosis.

Symptoms

Osteoporosis is often called the "silent disease" because bone loss occurs without symptoms. People may not know that they have osteoporosis until their bones become so weak that a sudden strain, bump, or fall causes a hip to fracture or a vertebra to collapse. Collapsed vertebrae may initially be felt or seen in the form of severe back pain, loss of height, or spinal deformities such as kyphosis (severely stooped posture).

Detection

Following a comprehensive medical assessment, your doctor may recommend that you have your bone mass measured. A bone mineral density (BMD) test is the best way to determine your bone health. BMD tests can identify osteoporosis, determine your risk for fractures (broken bones), and measure your response to osteoporosis treatment. The most widely recognized bone mineral density test is called a dual-energy x-ray absorptiometry or DXA test. It is painless—a bit like having an x-ray, but with much less exposure to radiation. It can measure bone density at your hip and spine. Bone density tests can do the following:

- Detect low bone density before a fracture occurs
- Confirm a diagnosis of osteoporosis if you already have one or more fractures
- Predict your chances of fracturing in the future
- Determine your rate of bone loss, or monitor the effects of treatment if the test is conducted at intervals of a year or more

Treatment

A comprehensive osteoporosis treatment program includes a focus on proper nutrition, exercise, and safety issues to prevent falls that may result in fractures. In addition, your physician may prescribe a medication to slow or stop bone loss, increase bone density, and reduce fracture risk.

Nutrition

The foods we eat contain a variety of vitamins, minerals, and other important nutrients that help keep our bodies healthy. All of these nutrients are needed in balanced proportion. In particular, calcium and vitamin D are needed for strong bones, and for your heart, muscles, and nerves to function properly.

Exercise

Exercise is an important component of an osteoporosis prevention and treatment program. Exercise not only improves your bone health, but it increases muscle strength, coordination, and balance, and leads to better overall health. While exercise is good for someone with osteoporosis, it should not put any sudden or excessive strain on your bones. As extra insurance against fractures, your doctor can recommend specific exercises to strengthen and support your back.

Therapeutic Medications

Currently, alendronate, raloxifene, risedronate, and ibandronate are approved by the U.S. Food and Drug Administration (FDA) for preventing and treating postmenopausal osteoporosis. Teriparatide is approved for treating the disease in postmenopausal women and men at high risk for fracture. Estrogen/hormone therapy (ET/HT) is approved for preventing postmenopausal osteoporosis, and calcitonin is approved for treatment.

Bisphosphonates: Alendronate (Fosamax®), risedronate (Actonel®), and ibandronate (Boniva®) are medications from the class of drugs called bisphosphonates. Like estrogen and raloxifene, these bisphosphonates are approved for both prevention and treatment of postmenopausal osteoporosis. Another bisphosphonate, zoledronic acid (Reclast®), is approved for the treatment of postmenopausal osteoporosis. Alendronate is also approved to treat bone loss that results from glucocorticoid medications like prednisone or cortisone and is approved for treating osteoporosis in men. Risedronate is approved to prevent and treat glucocorticoid-induced osteoporosis and to treat osteoporosis in men. Alendronate, risedronate, and zoledronic acid have been shown to increase bone mass and reduce the incidence of spine, hip, and other fractures. Ibandronate has been shown to reduce the incidence of spine fractures.

Raloxifene: Raloxifene (Evista®) is approved for the prevention and treatment of postmenopausal osteoporosis. It is from a class of drugs called estrogen agonists/antagonists, commonly referred to as selective estrogen receptor modulators (SERMs). Raloxifene appears to prevent bone loss in the spine, hip, and total body. It has beneficial effects on bone mass and bone turnover and can reduce the risk of vertebral fractures.

Calcitonin: Calcitonin (Miacalcin®, Fortical®) is a naturally occurring hormone involved in calcium regulation and bone metabolism. In women who are at least 5 years past menopause, calcitonin slows bone loss, increases spinal bone density, and may relieve the pain associated with bone fractures. Calcitonin reduces the risk of spinal fractures and may reduce hip fracture risk as well. Studies on fracture reduction are ongoing.

Teriparatide: Teriparatide (Forteo®) is an injectable form of human parathyroid hormone. It is approved for postmenopausal women and men with osteoporosis who are at high risk for having a fracture. Unlike the other drugs used in osteoporosis, teriparatide acts by stimulating new bone formation in both the spine and the hip. It also reduces the risk of vertebral and nonvertebral fractures in postmenopausal women. In men, teriparatide reduces the risk of vertebral fractures. However, it is not known whether teriparatide reduces the risk of nonvertebral fractures.

Estrogen/hormone therapy: Estrogen/hormone therapy (ET/HT) has been shown to reduce bone loss, increase bone density in both the spine and hip, and reduce the risk of spine and hip fractures in postmenopausal women. ET/HT is approved for preventing postmenopausal osteoporosis and is most commonly administered in the form of a pill or skin patch. When estrogen—also known as estrogen therapy or ET—is taken alone, it can increase a woman's risk of developing cancer of the uterine lining (endometrial cancer). To eliminate this risk, physicians prescribe the hormone progestin—also known as hormone therapy or HT—in combination with estrogen for those women who have not had a hysterectomy.

The Women's Health Initiative (WHI), a large government-funded research study, recently demonstrated that the drug Prempro® (estrogen combined with progestin), which is used in hormone therapy, is associated with a modest increase in the risk of breast cancer, stroke, and heart attack. The WHI also demonstrated that in patients who had a hysterectomy, estrogen therapy alone was associated with an increase in the risk of stroke, but not of breast cancer or cardiovascular disease. A large study from the National Cancer Institute indicated that long-term use of estrogen therapy may be associated with an increased risk of ovarian cancer.

Estrogen therapy is approved for treatment of menopausal symptoms but should be prescribed for the shortest period of time possible. When used solely for the prevention of postmenopausal osteoporosis, any ET/HT regimen should only be considered for women at significant risk of osteoporosis, and nonestrogen medications should be carefully considered first.

Fall Prevention

Preventing falls is a special concern for men and women with osteoporosis. Falls can increase the likelihood of fracturing a bone in the hip, wrist, spine, or other part of the skeleton. In addition to the environmental factors listed below, falls can also be caused by impaired vision and/or balance, chronic diseases that affect mental or physical functioning, and certain medications, such as sedatives and antidepressants. It is important that individuals with osteoporosis be aware of any physical changes that affect their balance or gait, and that they discuss these changes with their health care provider. Here are some tips to help eliminate the environmental factors that lead to falls.

Outdoors

- Use a cane or walker for added stability.
- Wear rubber-soled shoes for traction.
- Walk on grass when sidewalks are slippery.
- In winter, carry salt or kitty litter to sprinkle on slippery sidewalks.

- Be careful on highly polished floors that become slick and dangerous when wet.
- Use plastic or carpet runners when possible.

Indoors

- Keep rooms free of clutter, especially on floors.
- Keep floor surfaces smooth but not slippery.
- Wear supportive, low-heeled shoes even at home.
- Avoid walking in socks, stockings, or slippers.
- Be sure carpets and area rugs have skid-proof backing or are tacked to the floor.
- Be sure stairwells are well lit and that stairs have handrails on both sides.
- Install grab bars on bathroom walls near tub, shower, and toilet.
- Use a rubber bath mat in shower or tub.
- Keep a flashlight with fresh batteries beside your bed.
- If using a step stool for hard-to-reach areas, use a sturdy one with a handrail and wide steps.
- Add ceiling fixtures to rooms lit by lamps.
- Consider purchasing a cordless phone so that you don't have to rush to answer the phone when it rings, or so that you can call for help if you do fall.

Chapter 51

Thyroid Disorders

Chapter Contents

Section 51.1

Goiter

What is a goiter?

The term "goiter" simply refers to the abnormal enlargement of the thyroid gland. It is important to know that the presence of a goiter does not necessarily mean that the thyroid gland is malfunctioning. A goiter can occur in a gland that is producing too much hormone (hyperthyroidism), too little hormone (hypothyroidism), or the correct amount of hormone (euthyroidism). A goiter indicates there is a condition present which is causing the thyroid to grow abnormally.

What causes a goiter?

One of the most common causes of goiter formation worldwide is iodine deficiency. While this was a very frequent cause of goiter in the United States many years ago, it is no longer commonly observed. The primary activity of the thyroid gland is to concentrate iodine from the blood to make thyroid hormone. The gland cannot make enough thyroid hormone if it does not have enough iodine. Therefore, with iodine deficiency the individual will become hypothyroid. Consequently, the pituitary gland in the brain senses the thyroid hormone level is too low and sends a signal to the thyroid. This signal is called thyroid stimulating hormone (TSH). As the name implies, this hormone stimulates the thyroid to produce thyroid hormone and to grow in size. This abnormal growth in size produces what is termed a "goiter." Thus, iodine deficiency is one cause of goiter development. Wherever iodine deficiency is common, goiter will be common. It remains a common cause of goiters in other parts of the world.

Hashimoto thyroiditis is a more common cause of goiter formation in the United States. This is an autoimmune condition in which there is destruction of the thyroid gland by one's own immune system. As the gland becomes more damaged, it is less able to make adequate supplies of thyroid hormone. The pituitary gland senses a low thyroid hormone level and secretes more TSH to stimulate the thyroid. This stimulation causes the thyroid to grow, which may produce a goiter.

Another common cause of goiter is Graves disease. In this case, one's immune system produces a protein, called thyroid stimulating immunoglobulin (TSI). As with TSH, TSI stimulates the thyroid gland to enlarge, producing a goiter. However, TSI also stimulates the thyroid to make too much thyroid hormone (causes hyperthyroidism). Since the pituitary senses too much thyroid hormone, it stops secreting TSH. In spite of this the thyroid gland continues to grow and make thyroid hormone. Therefore, Graves disease produces a goiter and hyperthyroidism.

Multinodular goiters are another common cause of goiters. Individuals with this disorder have one or more nodules within the gland which cause thyroid enlargement. This is often detected as a nodular feeling gland on physical exam. Patients can present with a single large nodule with smaller nodules in the gland, or may show as multiple nodules when first detected. Unlike the other goiters discussed, the cause of this type of goiter is not well understood.

In addition to the common causes of goiter, there are many other less common causes. Some of these are due to genetic defects, others are related to injury or infections in the thyroid, and some are due to tumors (both cancerous and benign tumors).

How do you diagnose a goiter?

As mentioned earlier, the diagnosis of a goiter is usually made at the time of a physical examination when an enlargement of the thyroid is found. However, the presence of a goiter indicates there is an abnormality of the thyroid gland. Therefore, it is important to determine the cause of the goiter. As a first step, you will likely have thyroid function tests to determine if your thyroid is underactive or overactive. Any subsequent tests performed will be dependent upon the results of the thyroid function tests.

If the thyroid is diffusely enlarged and you are hyperthyroid, your doctor will likely proceed with tests to help diagnose Graves disease. If you are hypothyroid, you may have Hashimoto thyroiditis and you may get additional blood tests to confirm this diagnosis. Other tests used to help diagnose the cause of the goiter may include a radioactive iodine scan, thyroid ultrasound, or a fine needle aspiration biopsy.

How is a goiter treated?

The treatment will depend upon the cause of the goiter. If the goiter was due to a deficiency of iodine in the diet (not common in the United States), you will be given iodine supplementation by mouth. This will lead to a reduction in the size of the goiter, but often the goiter will not completely resolve.

If the goiter is due to Hashimoto thyroiditis, and you are hypothyroid, you will be given thyroid hormone supplement as a daily pill. This treatment will restore your thyroid hormone levels to normal, but does not usually make the goiter go completely away. While the goiter may get smaller, sometimes there is too much scar tissue in the gland to allow it to get much smaller. However, thyroid hormone treatment will usually prevent it from getting any larger.

If the goiter is due to hyperthyroidism, the treatment will depend upon the cause of the hyperthyroidism. For some causes of hyperthyroidism, the treatment may lead to a disappearance of the goiter. For example, treatment of Graves disease with radioactive iodine usually leads to a decrease or disappearance of the goiter.

Many goiters, such as the multinodular goiter, are associated with normal levels of thyroid hormone in the blood. These goiters usually do not require any specific treatment after the appropriate diagnosis is made. If no specific treatment is suggested, you may be warned that you are at risk for becoming hypothyroid or hyperthyroid in the future. However, if there are problems associated with the size of the thyroid per se, such as the goiter getting so large that it constricts the airway, your doctor may suggest that the goiter be treated by surgical removal.

Section 51.2

Hyperthyroidism

What is hyperthyroidism?

The term hyperthyroidism refers to any condition in which there is too much thyroid hormone in the body. In other words, the thyroid gland is overactive.

What are the symptoms of hyperthyroidism?

Thyroid hormone generally controls the pace of all of the processes in the body. This pace is called your metabolism. If there is too much thyroid hormone, every function of the body tends to speed up. It is not surprising then that some of the symptoms of hyperthyroidism are nervousness, irritability, increased perspiration, heart racing, hand tremors, anxiety, difficulty sleeping, thinning of your skin, fine brittle hair, and muscular weakness—especially in the upper arms and thighs. You may have more frequent bowel movements, but diarrhea is uncommon. You may lose weight despite a good appetite and, for women, menstrual flow may lighten and menstrual periods may occur less often.

Hyperthyroidism usually begins slowly. At first, the symptoms may be mistaken for simple nervousness due to stress. If you have been trying to lose weight by dieting, you may be pleased with your success until the hyperthyroidism, which has quickened the weight loss, causes other problems.

In Graves disease, which is the most common form of hyperthyroidism, the eyes may look enlarged because the upper lids are elevated. Sometimes, one or both eyes may bulge. Some patients have swelling of the front of the neck from an enlarged thyroid gland (a goiter).

What causes hyperthyroidism?

The most common cause (in more than 70 percent of people) is overproduction of thyroid hormone by the entire thyroid gland. This condition is also known as Graves disease. Graves disease is caused by antibodies in the blood that stimulate the thyroid to grow and secrete too much thyroid hormone. This type of hyperthyroidism tends to run in families, and it occurs more often in young women. Little is known about why specific individuals get this disease. Another type of hyperthyroidism is characterized by one or more nodules or lumps in the thyroid that may gradually grow and increase their activity so that the total output of thyroid hormone into the blood is greater than normal. This condition is known as toxic nodular or multinodular goiter. Also, people may temporarily have symptoms of hyperthyroidism if they have a condition called thyroiditis. This condition is caused by a problem with the immune system or a viral infection that causes the gland to leak thyroid hormone. It can also be caused by taking too much thyroid hormone in tablet form.

How is hyperthyroidism diagnosed?

If your physician suspects that you have hyperthyroidism, diagnosis is usually a simple matter. A physical examination usually detects an enlarged thyroid gland and a rapid pulse. The physician will also look for moist, smooth skin and a tremor of your fingertips. Your reflexes are likely to be fast, and your eyes may have some abnormalities if you have Graves disease.

The diagnosis of hyperthyroidism will be confirmed by laboratory tests that measure the amount of thyroid hormones— thyroxine (T4) and triiodothyronine (T3)—and thyroid-stimulating hormone (TSH) in your blood. A high level of thyroid hormone in the blood plus a low level of TSH is common with an overactive thyroid gland. If blood tests show that your thyroid is overactive, your doctor may want to obtain a picture of your thyroid (a thyroid scan). The scan will find out if your entire thyroid gland is overactive or whether you have a toxic nodular goiter or thyroiditis (thyroid inflammation). A test that measures the ability of the gland to collect iodine may be done at the same time.

How is hyperthyroidism treated?

No single treatment is best for all patients with hyperthyroidism. Your doctor's choice of treatment will be influenced by your age, the type of hyperthyroidism that you have, the severity of your hyperthyroidism, and other medical conditions that may be affecting your health. It may be a good idea to consult with a physician who is experienced in the treatment of hyperthyroid patients. If you are unconvinced or unclear about any thyroid treatment plan, a second opinion is a good idea.

Antithyroid drugs: Drugs known as antithyroid agents—methimazole (Tapazole®) or propylthiouracil (PTU)—may be prescribed if your doctor chooses to treat the hyperthyroidism by blocking the thyroid gland's ability to make new thyroid hormone. These drugs work well to control the overactive thyroid, bring prompt control of hyperthyroidism, and do not cause permanent damage to the thyroid gland. In about 20 to 30 percent of patients with Graves disease, treatment with antithyroid drugs for a period of twelve to eighteen months will result in prolonged remission of the disease. For patients with toxic nodular or multinodular goiter, antithyroid drugs are used in preparation for either radioiodine treatment or surgery. Antithyroid drugs cause allergic reactions in about 5 percent of patients who take them. Common minor reactions are red skin rashes, hives, and occasionally fever and joint pains. A rarer (occurring in one of five hundred patients) but more serious side effect is a decrease in the number of white blood cells. Such a decrease can lower your resistance to infection. Very rarely, these white blood cells disappear completely, producing a condition known as agranulocytosis, a potentially fatal problem if a serious infection occurs. If you are taking one of these drugs and get an infection such as a fever or sore throat, you should stop the drug immediately and have a white blood cell count that day. Even if the drug has lowered your white blood cell count, the count will return to normal if the drug is stopped immediately. But if you continue to take one of these drugs in spite of a low white blood cell count, there is a risk of a more serious, even life-threatening infection. Liver damage is another very rare side effect. You should stop the drug and call your doctor if you develop yellow eyes, dark urine, severe fatigue, or abdominal pain.

Radioactive iodine: Another way to treat hyperthyroidism is to damage or destroy the thyroid cells that make thyroid hormone. Because these cells need iodine to make thyroid hormone, they will take up any form of iodine in your blood stream, whether it is radioactive or not. The radioactive iodine used in this treatment is administered by mouth, usually in a small capsule that is taken just once. Once swallowed, the radioiodine gets into your blood stream and quickly is taken up by the overactive thyroid cells. The radioiodine that is not taken up by the thyroid cells disappears from the body within days.

It is either eliminated in the urine or transformed by radioactive decay into a nonradioactive state. Over a period of several weeks to several months (during which time drug treatment may be used to control hyperthyroid symptoms), radioactive iodine damages the cells that have taken it up. The result is that the thyroid or thyroid nodules shrink in size, and the level of thyroid hormone in the blood returns to normal. Sometimes patients will remain hyperthyroid, but usually to a lesser degree than before. For them, a second radioiodine treatment can be given if needed. More often, hypothyroidism (an underactive thyroid) occurs after a few months. In fact, most patients treated with radioactive iodine will become hypothyroid after a period of several months to many years. Hypothyroidism can easily be treated with a thyroid hormone supplement taken once a day.

Radioactive iodine has been used to treat patients for hyperthyroidism for over sixty years. Because of concern that the radioactive iodine might somehow damage other cells in the body, produce cancer, or have other long-term unwanted effects such as infertility or birth defects, the physicians who first used radioiodine treatments were careful to treat only adults and to observe them carefully for the rest of their lives. Fortunately, no complications from radioiodine treatment have become apparent over many decades of careful follow-up of patients. As a result, in the United States more than 70 percent of adults who develop hyperthyroidism are treated with radioactive iodine. More and more children are also being treated with radioiodine.

Surgery: Your hyperthyroidism can be permanently cured by surgical removal of most of your thyroid gland. This procedure is best performed by a surgeon who has much experience in thyroid surgery. An operation could be risky unless your hyperthyroidism is first controlled by an antithyroid drug (see above) or a beta-blocking drug (see below). Usually for some days before surgery, your surgeon may want you to take drops of nonradioactive iodine—either Lugol iodine or supersaturated potassium iodide (SSKI). This extra iodine reduces the blood supply to the thyroid gland and thus makes the surgery easier and safer. Although any surgery is risky, major complications of thyroid surgery occur in less than 1 percent of patients operated on by an experienced thyroid surgeon. These complications include damage to the parathyroid glands that surround the thyroid and control your body's calcium levels (causing problems with low calcium levels) and damage to the nerves that control your vocal cords (causing you to have a hoarse voice).

After your thyroid gland is removed, the source of your hyperthyroidism is gone and you will likely become hypothyroid. As with hypothyroidism that develops after radioiodine treatment, your thyroid hormone levels can be restored to normal by treatment once a day with a thyroid hormone supplement.

Beta-blockers: No matter which of these three methods of treatment you have for your hyperthyroidism, your physician may prescribe a class of drugs known as the beta adrenergic blocking agents that block the action of thyroid hormone on your body. They usually make you feel better within hours, even though they do not change the high levels of thyroid hormone in your blood. These drugs may be extremely helpful in slowing down your heart rate and reducing the symptoms of palpitations, shakes, and nervousness until one of the other forms of treatment has a chance to take effect. Propranolol (Inderal®) was the first of these drugs to be developed. Some physicians now prefer related, but longer-acting beta-blocking drugs such as atenolol (Tenormin®), metoprolol (Lopressor®) and nadolol (Corgard®), and Inderal-LA® because of their more convenient once- or twice-a-day dosage.

Other family members at risk: Because hyperthyroidism, especially Graves disease, may run in families, examinations of the members of your family may reveal other individuals with thyroid problems.

Section 51.3

Hypothyroidism

What Is Hypothyroidism?

Hypothyroidism is an underactive thyroid gland. Hypothyroidism means that the thyroid gland can't make enough thyroid hormone to keep the body running normally. People are hypothyroid if they have too little thyroid hormone in the blood. Common causes are autoimmune disease, surgical removal of the thyroid, and radiation treatment.

Symptoms

What Are the Symptoms?

When thyroid hormone levels are too low, the body's cells can't get enough thyroid hormone and the body's processes start slowing down. As the body slows, you may notice that you feel colder, you tire more easily, your skin is getting drier, you're becoming forgetful and depressed, and you've started getting constipated. Because the symptoms are so variable, the only way to know for sure whether you have hypothyroidism is with blood tests.

Keeping Other People Informed

Tell your family members. Because thyroid disease runs in families, you should explain your hypothyroidism to your relatives and encourage them to get regular TSH tests. Tell your other doctors and your pharmacist about your hypothyroidism and the drug and dose with which it is being treated. If you start seeing a new doctor, tell the doctor that you have hypothyroidism and you need your TSH tested every year. If you are seeing an endocrinologist, ask that copies of your reports be sent to your primary care doctor.

What Can You Expect Over the Long Term?

There is no cure for hypothyroidism, and most patients have it for life. There are exceptions: many patients with viral thyroiditis have their thyroid function return to normal, as do some patients with thyroiditis after pregnancy.

Hypothyroidism may become more or less severe, and your dose of thyroxine may need to change over time. You have to make a lifetime commitment to treatment. But if you take your pills every day and work with your doctor to get and keep your thyroxine dose right, you should be able to keep your hypothyroidism completely controlled throughout your life. Your symptoms should disappear and the serious effects of low thyroid hormone should stop getting worse and should actually improve. If you keep your hypothyroidism well controlled, it will not shorten your life span.

Causes

What Causes Hypothyroidism?

There can be many reasons why the cells in the thyroid gland can't make enough thyroid hormone. Here are the major causes, from the most to the least common.

Autoimmune disease: In some people's bodies, the immune system that protects the body from invading infections can mistake thyroid gland cells and their enzymes for invaders and can attack them. Then there aren't enough thyroid cells and enzymes left to make enough thyroid hormone. This is more common in women than men. Autoimmune thyroiditis can begin suddenly or it can develop slowly over years. The most common forms are Hashimoto thyroiditis and atrophic thyroiditis.

Surgical removal of part or all of the thyroid gland: Some people with thyroid nodules, thyroid cancer, or Graves disease need to have part or all of their thyroid removed. If the whole thyroid is removed, people will definitely become hypothyroid. If part of the gland is left, it may be able to make enough thyroid hormone to keep blood levels normal.

Radiation treatment: Some people with Graves disease, nodular goiter, or thyroid cancer are treated with radioactive iodine (I-131) for the purpose of destroying their thyroid gland. Patients with Hodgkin disease, lymphoma, or cancers of the head or neck are treated with radiation. All these patients can lose part or all of their thyroid function.

Congenital hypothyroidism (hypothyroidism that a baby is born with): A few babies are born without a thyroid or with only a partly formed one. A few have part or all of their thyroid in the wrong place (ectopic thyroid). In some babies, the thyroid cells or their enzymes don't work right.

Thyroiditis: Thyroiditis is an inflammation of the thyroid gland, usually caused by an autoimmune attack or by a viral infection. Thyroiditis can make the thyroid dump its whole supply of stored thyroid hormone into the blood at once, causing brief *hyper*thyroidism (too much thyroid activity); then the thyroid becomes underactive.

Medicines: Medicines such as amiodarone, lithium, interferon alpha, and interleukin-2 can prevent the thyroid gland from being able to make hormone normally. These drugs are most likely to trigger hypothyroidism in patients who have a genetic tendency to autoimmune thyroid disease.

Too much or too little iodine: The thyroid gland must have iodine to make thyroid hormone. Iodine comes into the body in food and travels through the blood to the thyroid. Keeping thyroid hormone production in balance requires the right amount of iodine. Taking in too much iodine can cause or worsen hypothyroidism.

Damage to the pituitary gland: The pituitary, the "master gland," tells the thyroid how much hormone to make. When the pituitary is damaged by a tumor, radiation, or surgery, it may no longer be able to give the thyroid instructions, and the thyroid may stop making enough hormone.

Rare disorders that infiltrate the thyroid: In a few people, diseases deposit abnormal substances in the thyroid. For example, amyloidosis can deposit amyloid protein, sarcoidosis can deposit granulomas, and hemochromatosis can deposit iron.

Diagnosis

How Is Hypothyroidism Diagnosed?

The correct diagnosis of hypothyroidism depends on the following:

- **Symptoms:** Hypothyroidism doesn't have any characteristic symptoms. There are no symptoms that people with hypothyroidism always have but that no one with another disease ever has. One way to help figure out whether your complaints are symptoms of hypothyroidism is to think about whether you've always had a symptom (hypothyroidism is less likely) or whether the symptom is a change from the way you used to feel (hypothyroidism is more likely).
- **Medical and family history:** You should tell your doctor about changes in your health that suggest that your body is slowing down; if you've ever had thyroid surgery; if you've ever had radiation to your neck to treat cancer; if you're taking any of the medicines that can cause hypothyroidism— amiodarone, lithium, interferon alpha, interleukin- 2, and maybe thalidomide; and whether any of your family members have thyroid disease.
- **Physical exam:** The doctor will check your thyroid gland and look for changes such as dry skin, swelling, slower reflexes, and a slower heart rate.
- **Blood tests:** There are two blood tests that are used in the diagnosis of hypothyroidism:
    - *TSH (thyroid-stimulating hormone) test:* This is the most important and sensitive test for hypothyroidism. It measures how much of the thyroid hormone thyroxine (T4) the thyroid gland is being asked to make. An abnormally high TSH means hypothyroidism: the thyroid gland is being asked to make more T4 because there isn't enough T4 in the blood.
    - *T4 tests:* Most of the T4 in the blood is attached to a protein called thyroxine-binding globulin. The "bound" T4 can't get into body cells. Only about 1 to 2 percent of T4 in the blood is unattached ("free") and can get into cells. The free T4 and the free T4 index are both simple blood tests that measure how much unattached T4 is in the blood and available to get into cells.

Treatment

How Is Hypothyroidism Treated?

Thyroxine (T4) replacement: Hypothyroidism can't be cured. But in almost every patient, hypothyroidism can be completely controlled. It is treated by replacing the amount of hormone that your own thyroid can no longer make, to bring your T4 and TSH back to normal levels. So even if your thyroid gland can't work right, T4 replacement can restore your body's thyroid hormone levels and your body's function. Synthetic thyroxine pills contain hormone exactly like the T4 that the thyroid gland itself makes. All hypothyroid patients except those with severe myxedema can be treated as outpatients, not having to be admitted to the hospital.

Side effects and complications: The only dangers of thyroxine are caused by taking too little or too much. If you take too little, your hypothyroidism will continue. If you take too much, you'll develop the symptoms of hyperthyroidism—an overactive thyroid gland. The most common symptoms of too much thyroid hormone are fatigue but inability to sleep, greater appetite, nervousness, shakiness, feeling hot when other people are cold, and trouble exercising because of weak muscles, shortness of breath, and a racing, skipping heart. Patients who have hyperthyroid symptoms should have their TSH tested. If it is low, indicating too much thyroid hormone, their dose may need to be lowered.

Follow-up

You'll need to have your TSH checked about every six to ten weeks after a thyroxine dose change. You may need tests more often if you're pregnant or you're taking a medicine that interferes with your body's ability to use thyroxine. The goal of treatment is to get and keep your TSH in the normal range. Babies must get all their daily treatments and have their TSH levels checked as they grow, to prevent mental retardation and stunted growth. Once you've settled into a thyroxine dose, you can return for TSH tests only about once a year. You need to return sooner if any of the following apply to you:

- Your symptoms return or get worse.
- You want to change your thyroxine dose or brand, or change taking your pills with or without food.
- You gain or lose a lot of weight (as little as a ten-pound difference for those who weren't overweight to begin with).
- You start or stop taking a drug that can interfere with absorbing thyroxine, or you change your dose of such a drug.
- You're not taking all your thyroxine pills. Tell your doctor honestly how many pills you've missed.
- You want to try stopping thyroxine treatment. If ever you think you're doing well enough not to need thyroxine treatment any

longer, try it only under your doctor's close supervision. Rather than stopping your pills completely, you might ask your doctor to try lowering your dose. If your TSH goes up, you'll know that you need to continue treatment.

Section 51.4

Thyroid Nodules

What is a thyroid nodule?

The term thyroid nodule refers to any abnormal growth of thyroid cells into a lump within the thyroid. Although the vast majority of thyroid nodules are benign (noncancerous), a small proportion of thyroid nodules do contain thyroid cancer. Because of this possibility, the evaluation of a thyroid nodule is aimed at discovering a potential thyroid cancer.

What are the symptoms of a thyroid nodule?

Most thyroid nodules do not cause any symptoms. Your doctor usually discovers them during a routine physical examination, or you might notice a lump in your neck while looking in a mirror. If the nodule is made up of thyroid cells that actively produce thyroid hormone without regard to the body's need, a patient may complain of hyperthyroid symptoms. A few patients with thyroid nodules may complain of pain in the neck, jaw, or ear. If the nodule is large enough, it may cause difficulty swallowing or cause a "tickle in the throat" or shortness of breath if it is pressing on the windpipe. Rarely, hoarseness can be caused if the nodule irritates a nerve to the voice box.

What causes a thyroid nodule?

The thyroid nodule is the most common endocrine problem in the United States. The chances are one in ten that you or someone you know will develop a thyroid nodule. Although thyroid cancer is the most important cause of the thyroid nodule, fortunately it occurs in less than 10 percent of nodules. This means that about nine of ten nodules are benign (noncancerous). The most common types of noncancerous thyroid nodules are known as colloid nodules and follicular neoplasms. If a nodule produces thyroid hormone without regard to the body's need, it is called an autonomous nodule, and it can occasionally lead to hyperthyroidism. If the nodule is filled with fluid or blood, it is called a thyroid cyst.

We do not know what causes most noncancerous thyroid nodules to form. A patient with hypothyroidism may also have a thyroid nodule, particularly if the cause is the inflammation known as Hashimoto thyroiditis. Sometimes a lack of iodine in the diet can cause a thyroid gland to produce nodules. Some autonomous nodules have a genetic defect that causes them to grow.

How is the thyroid nodule diagnosed?

Since most patients with thyroid nodules do not have symptoms, most nodules are discovered during an examination of the neck for another reason, such as during a routine physical examination or when you are sick with a cold or flu. Once the nodule is discovered, your doctor will try to determine whether the lump is the only problem with your thyroid or whether the entire thyroid gland has been affected by a more general condition such as hyperthyroidism or hypothyroidism. Your physician will feel the thyroid to see whether the entire gland is enlarged, whether there is a single nodule present, or whether there are many lumps or nodules in your thyroid. The initial laboratory tests may include blood tests to measure the amount of thyroid hormone (thyroxine, or T4) and thyroid-stimulating hormone (TSH) in your blood to determine whether your thyroid is functioning normally. Most patients with thyroid nodules will also have normal thyroid function tests.

Rarely is it possible to determine whether a thyroid nodule is cancerous by physical examination and blood tests alone, and so the evaluation of the thyroid nodule often includes specialized tests such as a thyroid fine needle biopsy, a thyroid scan, and/or a thyroid ultrasound.

Thyroid fine needle biopsy: A fine needle biopsy of a thyroid nodule may sound frightening, but the needle used is very small and a local anesthetic can be used. This simple procedure is done in the doctor's office. It does not require any special preparation (no fasting), and patients usually return home or to work after the biopsy without any ill effects. For a fine needle biopsy, your doctor will use a very thin needle to withdraw cells from the thyroid nodule. Ordinarily, several samples will be taken from different parts of the nodule to give your doctor the best chance of finding cancerous cells if a tumor is present. The cells are then examined under a microscope by a pathologist.

The report of a thyroid fine needle biopsy will usually indicate one of the following findings:

- *The nodule is benign (noncancerous):* This result is obtained in 50 to 60 percent of biopsies and often indicates a colloid nodule. The risk of overlooking a cancer when the biopsy is benign is generally under three in one hundred and is even lower when the biopsy is reviewed by an experienced pathologist at a major medical center. Generally, these nodules need not be removed, but another biopsy may be required in the future, especially if they get bigger.
- *The nodule is malignant (cancerous):* This result is obtained in about 5 percent of biopsies and often indicates papillary cancer, one of the most common thyroid cancers. All of these nodules should be removed surgically, preferably by an experienced thyroid surgeon.
- *The nodule is suspicious:* This result is obtained in about 10 percent of biopsies and indicates either a follicular adenoma (noncancerous) or a follicular cancer. Often, your doctor may want to obtain a thyroid scan to determine which nodules should be removed surgically.
- *The biopsy is nondiagnostic or inadequate:* This result is obtained in up to 20 percent of biopsies and indicates that not enough cells were obtained to make a diagnosis. This is a common result if the nodule is a cyst. These nodules may be removed surgically or be re-evaluated with second fine needle biopsy, depending on the clinical judgment of your doctor.

Thyroid scan: The thyroid scan uses a small amount of a radioactive substance, usually radioactive iodine, to obtain a picture of the thyroid gland. Because thyroid cancer cells do not take up radioactive iodine as easily as normal thyroid cells do, this test is used to determine the likelihood that a thyroid nodule contains a cancer. If done as the first test, the thyroid scan is used to determine those patients who most need a biopsy. The scan usually gives the following results:

- *The nodule is cold:* In other words, the nodule is not taking up radioactive iodine normally. This patient is referred for a fine needle biopsy of the nodule.
- *The nodule is functioning:* Its uptake of radioactive iodine is similar to that of normal cells. A biopsy is not needed right away since the likelihood of cancer is very low.
- *The nodule is hot:* Its uptake of radioactive iodine is greater than that of normal cells. The likelihood of cancer is extremely rare, and so biopsy is usually not necessary.

If the fine needle biopsy was done as the first test, then a scan is usually ordered to evaluate a suspicious biopsy result. In this case, patients with a "cold" nodule result should have their nodule removed. Patients with "functioning" or "hot" nodules on a scan and a suspicious biopsy can be watched, and surgery is not immediately necessary.

Thyroid ultrasound: The thyroid ultrasound uses high-frequency sound waves to obtain a picture of the thyroid. This very sensitive test can easily determine if a nodule is solid or cystic, and it can determine the precise size of the nodule. The thyroid ultrasound can be used to keep an eye on thyroid nodules that are not removed by surgery to determine if they are growing or shrinking. Some ultrasound characteristics of a nodule are more frequent in thyroid cancer than in noncancerous nodules. Even so, the thyroid ultrasound alone is rarely able to determine if a nodule is a thyroid cancer. The thyroid ultrasound also can be used to assist the placement of the needle within the nodule during a fine needle biopsy, especially if the nodule is hard to feel. Finally, the thyroid ultrasound can identify nodules that are very small and cannot be felt during a physical examination. The clinical importance of these very small nodules is uncertain; however, the ultrasound provides a means by which an accurate fine needle biopsy can be performed if your doctor thinks a biopsy is needed.

How are thyroid nodules treated?

All thyroid nodules that are found to contain a thyroid cancer, or that are highly suspicious of containing a cancer, should be removed surgically by an experienced thyroid surgeon. Most thyroid cancers are curable and rarely cause life-threatening problems. Any thyroid nodule not removed needs to be watched closely, with an examination of the nodule every six to twelve months. This follow-up may involve a physical examination by a doctor or a thyroid ultrasound or both. Occasionally, your doctor may want to try to shrink your nodule by treating you with thyroid hormone at doses slightly higher than your body needs (called suppression therapy). Whether you are on thyroid hormone suppression therapy or not, a repeat fine needle biopsy may be indicated if the nodule gets bigger. Also, even if the biopsy is benign, surgery may be recommended for removal of a nodule that is getting bigger.

Section 51.5

Thyroiditis

What is thyroiditis?

Thyroiditis includes a group of individual disorders that all cause thyroidal inflammation. As a result, there may be many different clinical presentations, from hypothyroidism to an enlarged thyroid (goiter) to symptoms similar to hyperthyroidism.

What causes thyroiditis?

Thyroiditis is caused by an attack on the thyroid, causing inflammation and damage to the thyroid cells. Antibodies that attack the thyroid cause most types of thyroiditis. Thyroiditis can also be caused by an infection, such as a virus or bacteria, or certain drugs.

What are the clinical symptoms of thyroiditis?

There are no symptoms unique to thyroiditis. If the thyroiditis causes slow and chronic thyroid cell damage and destruction, leading to a fall in thyroid hormone levels in the blood, the symptoms would be those of hypothyroidism. If the thyroiditis causes rapid thyroid cell damage and destruction, the thyroid hormone that is stored in the gland leaks out, increasing thyroid hormone levels in the blood, and produces symptoms of thyrotoxicosis, which are similar to hyperthyroidism. Pain in the thyroid can be seen in patients with subacute thyroiditis.

What are the types and clinical course of thyroiditis?

Hashimoto thyroiditis: Patients usually present with hypothyroidism, which is usually permanent.

Subacute, painless and postpartum thyroiditis: These disorders follow the same general clinical course of thyrotoxicosis followed by hypothyroidism. The thyrotoxic phase usually lasts for one to three months and is associated with symptoms including anxiety, insomnia, palpitations (fast heart rate), fatigue, weight loss, and irritability. Thyroidal pain in subacute thyroiditis follows the thyrotoxic phase. The hypothyroid phase typically occurs one to three months after the thyrotoxic phase and may last up to nine to twelve months. Typical symptoms include fatigue, weight gain, constipation, dry skin, depression, and poor exercise tolerance. Most patients (80–95 percent) will have return of their thyroid function to normal within twelve to eighteen months of the onset of symptoms.

Drug-induced and radiation thyroiditis: Both thyrotoxicosis and hypothyroidism may be seen. The thyrotoxicosis is usually short-lived. Drug-induced hypothyroidism often resolves with the cessation of the drug, while the hypothyroidism related to radiation thyroiditis is usually permanent.

Acute/infectious thyroiditis: Symptoms range from thyroidal pain, systemic illness, painless enlargement of the thyroid, and hypothyroidism. The symptoms usually resolve once the infection resolves.

How is thyroiditis treated?

Treatment depends on the type of thyroiditis and the clinical presentation.

Thyrotoxicosis: Beta-blockers to decrease palpitations and reduce shakes and tremors may be helpful. Antithyroid medications are not used for the thyrotoxic phase of thyroiditis of any kind since the thyroid is not overactive.

Hypothyroidism: Treatment is initiated with thyroid hormone replacement for hypothyroidism due to Hashimoto thyroiditis. If thyroid hormone therapy is begun in patients with subacute, painless and postpartum thyroiditis, treatment should be continued for approximately six to twelve months and then tapered to see if thyroid hormone is required permanently.

Thyroidal pain: The pain associated with subacute thyroiditis usually can be managed with mild anti-inflammatory medications such as aspirin or ibuprofen. Occasionally, the pain can be severe and require steroid therapy with prednisone.

Chapter 52

Urinary Tract Disorders

Chapter Contents

Section 52.1

Interstitial Cystitis (Painful Bladder Syndrome)

Reprinted from "Interstitial Cystitis (Painful Bladder Syndrome)," National Women's Health Information Center, March 2007.

What is interstitial cystitis (IC)?

IC is a chronic bladder problem that can cause pain and other symptoms. People with IC can have an inflamed and irritated bladder. This can lead to the following:

- Scarring and stiffening of the bladder
- Less bladder capacity
- Bleeding in the bladder

More than seven hundred thousand Americans have IC. IC often shows up between the ages of thirty and forty. Women are ten times more likely to have IC than men.

Some people with IC feel only mild discomfort and some have severe pain. Severe cases of IC can keep people from doing their daily tasks, such as going to work or school.

What are the causes of IC?

No one knows what causes IC. Researchers are working to learn more about it and find treatments that will ease symptoms. Right now, there is no cure for IC.

Current research shows that a substance found in the urine of some people with IC may block the normal growth of the cells that line the inside wall of the bladder. Learning more about this substance may lead to a better understanding of the causes of IC.

It is thought that genes may play a role in some forms of IC. In a few cases, IC has affected a mother and daughter or two sisters. Still, it does not commonly run in families.

What are some symptoms and signs of IC?

The symptoms of IC vary from person to person. Also, one person can have symptoms of IC that change over time. People with IC may have an inflamed and irritated bladder. They may have mild discomfort, pressure, tenderness, or intense pain in the bladder and pelvic area. The pelvic area is between your navel (belly button) and your thigh. Symptoms also may include feeling like you need to urinate right away, often, or both.

Pain may get better or worse as the bladder fills with urine or as it empties. Women's symptoms often get worse during their periods. Pain during sex is common.

How can I tell if I have IC?

Your doctor can tell if you have IC if you have the symptoms above and by ruling out other diseases with similar symptoms.

The first step in diagnosing IC is to rule out other health problems that may be causing the symptoms. Symptoms of urinary tract infections, bladder cancer, endometriosis, sexually transmitted diseases (STDs), and kidney stones can be the same as those caused by IC. Tests on your urine, bladder, and urinary tract may be done. These can include the following:

- **Urine culture:** Looking at urine under a microscope can show if you have germs that show you have a urinary tract infection or an STD. Your doctor will insert a catheter, which is a thin tube to drain urine. Or you may be asked to give a urine sample using the "clean catch" method. For a clean catch, you will wash the genital area before collecting urine midstream in a sterile container.
- **Cystoscopy with or without bladder distention:** Your doctor may use a device called a cystoscope to see inside the bladder and rule out cancer. Further testing may include slowly stretching the bladder, called bladder distention, by filling it with liquid. This helps the doctor get a better look inside the bladder. This test can find bladder wall inflammation; bleeding or ulcers; a thick, stiff bladder wall; and total bladder capacity. This test is often done as an outpatient surgery.
- **Biopsy:** A biopsy is a tissue sample that your doctor looks at under a microscope. Samples of the bladder and urethra may be removed during a cystoscopy. A biopsy helps your doctor rule out bladder cancer.

Is there a cure for IC?

Doctors have not yet found a cure for IC. They cannot predict who will respond best to the different treatment options. Sometimes, symptoms may go away for no reason or after a change in diet or treatment plan. Even when symptoms do go away, they may return after days, weeks, months, or years.

How is IC treated?

There are treatments available to help ease symptoms. Although many of these options are still being studied, they have shown to help some women feel better. Some of these include the following:

- **Bladder distention:** The doctor slowly stretches the bladder by filling it with liquid. Doctors are not sure why, but this test eases pain for some patients.
- **Bladder instillation (a bladder wash or bath):** The bladder is filled with a liquid that is held for different periods of time before being emptied. The only drug approved to date by the U.S. Food and Drug Administration (FDA) for use in bladder instillation is dimethyl sulfoxide. Other drugs for this use are being studied.
- **Oral medicines:** These medicines include a prescription medicine called pentosan polysulfate sodium (Elmiron®), which can help ease symptoms in some patients. Because Elmiron has not been tested in pregnant women, it is not recommended for use during pregnancy, except in severe cases. Other oral medicines used include aspirin and ibuprofen, other stronger painkillers, antidepressants, and antihistamines.
- **Transcutaneous electrical nerve stimulation (TENS):** Wires send mild electric pulses to the bladder area. Scientists do not know exactly how TENS works, but it helps ease pain and urinary frequency in some people. Sacral nerve stimulation implants are being studied as another way to relieve IC symptoms.
- **Self-help strategies:** Bladder training, dietary changes, quitting smoking, reducing stress, and low-impact exercise have been shown to help some people.
- **Surgery:** If other treatments have failed and the pain is disabling, surgery may be an option. Surgery may or may not ease symptoms.

Keep in mind, these treatments do not cure IC. For some people, these treatments have helped ease their IC symptoms.

How does diet affect IC?

There is no proof of a link between diet and IC. Still, some people think alcohol, tomatoes, spices, chocolate, caffeinated and citrus drinks, and high-acid foods may irritate the bladder. Others notice that their symptoms get worse after eating or drinking products made with artificial sweeteners. If you think certain foods or drinks may be making your symptoms worse, try avoiding them. You can start eating or drinking these products again one at a time to see if any affect your symptoms.

I have IC and just found out I'm pregnant. Will it affect my baby?

Doctors do not have much information about pregnancy and IC. IC is not thought to affect fertility or the health of a fetus. Some women find that their IC symptoms get better during pregnancy. Others find their symptoms get worse.

Section 52.2

Urinary Incontinence

Excerpted from "Urinary Incontinence in Women," National Institute of Diabetes and Digestive and Kidney Diseases, National Institutes of Health, NIH Publication No. 08-4132, October 2007.

Millions of women experience involuntary loss of urine called urinary incontinence (UI). Some women may lose a few drops of urine while running or coughing. Others may feel a strong, sudden urge to urinate just before losing a large amount of urine. Many women experience both symptoms. UI can be slightly bothersome or totally debilitating. For some women, the risk of public embarrassment keeps them from enjoying many activities with their family and friends. Urine loss can also occur during sexual activity and cause tremendous emotional distress.

Women experience UI twice as often as men. Pregnancy and childbirth, menopause, and the structure of the female urinary tract account for this difference. But both women and men can become incontinent from neurologic injury, birth defects, stroke, multiple sclerosis, and physical problems associated with aging.

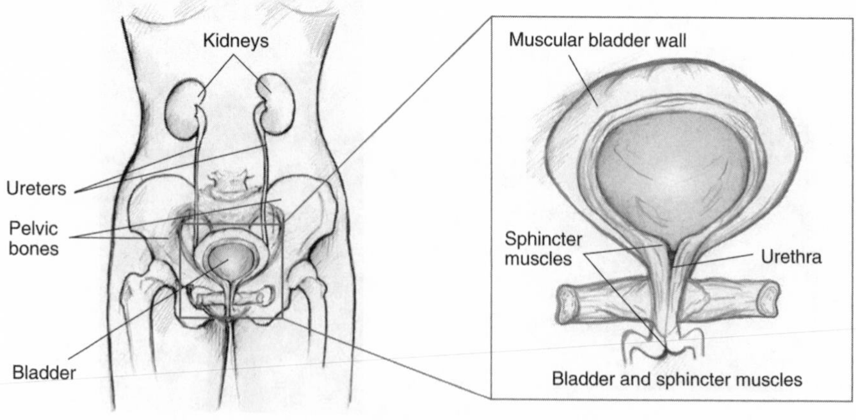

Figure 52.1. *Front view of bladder and sphincter muscles*

Older women experience UI more often than younger women. But incontinence is not inevitable with age. UI is a medical problem. Your doctor or nurse can help you find a solution. No single treatment works for everyone, but many women can find improvement without surgery.

Incontinence occurs because of problems with muscles and nerves that help to hold or release urine. The body stores urine—water and wastes removed by the kidneys—in the bladder, a balloon-like organ. The bladder connects to the urethra, the tube through which urine leaves the body.

During urination, muscles in the wall of the bladder contract, forcing urine out of the bladder and into the urethra. At the same time, sphincter muscles surrounding the urethra relax, letting urine pass out of the body. Incontinence will occur if your bladder muscles suddenly contract or the sphincter muscles are not strong enough to hold back urine. Urine may escape with less pressure than usual if the muscles are damaged, causing a change in the position of the bladder. Obesity, which is associated with increased abdominal pressure, can worsen incontinence. Fortunately, weight loss can reduce its severity.

What are the types of incontinence?

Stress incontinence: If coughing, laughing, sneezing, or other movements that put pressure on the bladder cause you to leak urine, you may have stress incontinence. Physical changes resulting from pregnancy, childbirth, and menopause often cause stress incontinence. This type of incontinence is common in women and, in many cases, can be treated.

Childbirth and other events can injure the scaffolding that helps support the bladder in women. Pelvic floor muscles, the vagina, and ligaments support your bladder (see Figure 52.2). If these structures weaken, your bladder can move downward, pushing slightly out of the bottom of the pelvis toward the vagina. This prevents muscles that ordinarily force the urethra shut from squeezing as tightly as they should. As a result, urine can leak into the urethra during moments of physical stress. Stress incontinence also occurs if the squeezing muscles weaken.

Stress incontinence can worsen during the week before your menstrual period. At that time, lowered estrogen levels might lead to lower muscular pressure around the urethra, increasing chances of leakage. The incidence of stress incontinence increases following menopause.

Urge incontinence: If you lose urine for no apparent reason after suddenly feeling the need or urge to urinate, you may have urge incontinence. A common cause of urge incontinence is inappropriate bladder contractions. Abnormal nerve signals might be the cause of these bladder spasms.

Urge incontinence can mean that your bladder empties during sleep, after drinking a small amount of water, or when you touch water or hear it running (as when washing dishes or hearing someone else taking a shower). Certain fluids and medications such as diuretics or emotional states such as anxiety can worsen this condition. Some medical conditions, such as hyperthyroidism and uncontrolled diabetes, can also lead to or worsen urge incontinence.

Involuntary actions of bladder muscles can occur because of damage to the nerves of the bladder, to the nervous system (spinal cord and brain), or to the muscles themselves. Multiple sclerosis, Parkinson disease, Alzheimer disease, stroke, and injury—including injury that occurs during surgery—all can harm bladder nerves or muscles.

Overactive bladder: Overactive bladder occurs when abnormal nerves send signals to the bladder at the wrong time, causing its

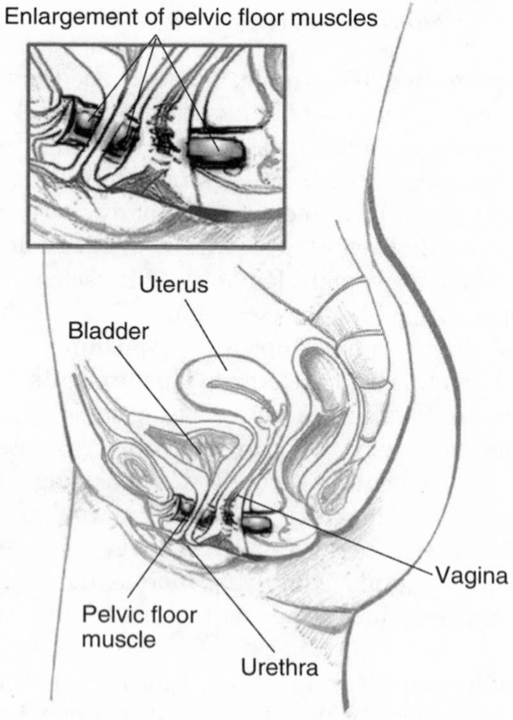

Figure 52.2. *Side view of female pelvic muscles*

muscles to squeeze without warning. Voiding up to seven times a day is normal for many women, but women with overactive bladder may find that they must urinate even more frequently.

Specifically, the symptoms of overactive bladder include the following:

- *Urinary frequency:* Bothersome urination eight or more times a day or two or more times at night
- *Urinary urgency:* The sudden, strong need to urinate immediately
- *Urge incontinence:* Leakage or gushing of urine that follows a sudden, strong urge
- *Nocturia:* Awaking at night to urinate

Functional incontinence: People with medical problems that interfere with thinking, moving, or communicating may have trouble reaching a toilet. A person with Alzheimer disease, for example, may not think well enough to plan a timely trip to a restroom. A person in a wheelchair may have a hard time getting to a toilet in time. Functional incontinence is the result of these physical and medical conditions. Conditions such as arthritis often develop with age and account for some of the incontinence of elderly women in nursing homes.

Overflow incontinence: Overflow incontinence happens when the bladder doesn't empty properly, causing it to spill over. Your doctor can check for this problem. Weak bladder muscles or a blocked urethra can cause this type of incontinence. Nerve damage from diabetes or other diseases can lead to weak bladder muscles; tumors and urinary stones can block the urethra. Overflow incontinence is rare in women.

Other types of incontinence: Stress and urge incontinence often occur together in women. Combinations of incontinence—and this combination in particular—are sometimes referred to as mixed incontinence. Most women don't have pure stress or urge incontinence, and many studies show that mixed incontinence is the most common type of urine loss in women.

Transient incontinence is a temporary version of incontinence. Medications, urinary tract infections, mental impairment, and restricted mobility can all trigger transient incontinence. Severe constipation can cause transient incontinence when the impacted stool pushes against the urinary tract and obstructs outflow. A cold can trigger incontinence, which resolves once the coughing spells cease.

How is incontinence evaluated?

The first step toward relief is to see a doctor who has experience treating incontinence to learn what type you have. A urologist specializes in the urinary tract, and some urologists further specialize in the female urinary tract. Gynecologists and obstetricians specialize in the female reproductive tract and childbirth. A urogynecologist focuses on urinary and associated pelvic problems in women. Family practitioners and internists see patients for all kinds of health conditions. Any of these doctors may be able to help you. In addition, some nurses and other health care providers often provide rehabilitation services and teach behavioral therapies such as fluid management and pelvic floor strengthening.

To diagnose the problem, your doctor will first ask about symptoms and medical history. Your pattern of voiding and urine leakage may suggest the type of incontinence you have. Thus, many specialists begin with having you fill out a bladder diary over several days. These diaries can reveal obvious factors that can help define the problem—including straining and discomfort, fluid intake, use of drugs, recent surgery, and illness. Often you can begin treatment at the first medical visit.

Your doctor may instruct you to keep a diary for a day or more—sometimes up to a week—to record when you void. This diary should note the times you urinate and the amounts of urine you produce. To measure your urine, you can use a special pan that fits over the toilet rim. You can also use the bladder diary to record your fluid intake, episodes of urine leakage, and estimated amounts of leakage.

If your diary and medical history do not define the problem, they will at least suggest which tests you need.

Your doctor will physically examine you for signs of medical conditions causing incontinence, including treatable blockages from bowel or pelvic growths. In addition, weakness of the pelvic floor leading to incontinence may cause a condition called prolapse, where the vagina or bladder begins to protrude out of your body. This condition is also important to diagnose at the time of an evaluation.

Your doctor may measure your bladder capacity. The doctor may also measure the residual urine for evidence of poorly functioning bladder muscles. To do this, you will urinate into a measuring pan, after which the nurse or doctor will measure any urine remaining in the bladder. Your doctor may also recommend other tests:

- **Bladder stress test:** You cough vigorously as the doctor watches for loss of urine from the urinary opening.

- **Urinalysis and urine culture:** Laboratory technicians test your urine for evidence of infection, urinary stones, or other contributing causes.
- **Ultrasound:** This test uses sound waves to create an image of the kidneys, ureters, bladder, and urethra.
- **Cystoscopy:** The doctor inserts a thin tube with a tiny camera in the urethra to see inside the urethra and bladder.
- **Urodynamics:** Various techniques measure pressure in the bladder and the flow of urine.

How is incontinence treated?

Behavioral remedies—bladder retraining and Kegel exercises: By looking at your bladder diary, the doctor may see a pattern and suggest making it a point to use the bathroom at regular timed intervals, a habit called timed voiding. As you gain control, you can extend the time between scheduled trips to the bathroom. Behavioral treatment also includes Kegel exercises to strengthen the muscles that help hold in urine.

How to do Kegel exercises: The first step is to find the right muscles. One way to find them is to imagine that you are sitting on a marble and want to pick up the marble with your vagina. Imagine sucking or drawing the marble into your vagina.

Try not to squeeze other muscles at the same time. Be careful not to tighten your stomach, legs, or buttocks. Squeezing the wrong muscles can put more pressure on your bladder control muscles. Just squeeze the pelvic muscles. Don't hold your breath. Do not practice while urinating.

Repeat, but don't overdo it. At first, find a quiet spot to practice—your bathroom or bedroom—so you can concentrate. Pull in the pelvic muscles and hold for a count of three. Then relax for a count of three. Work up to three sets of 10 repeats. Start doing your pelvic muscle exercises lying down. This is the easiest position to do them in because the muscles do not need to work against gravity. When your muscles get stronger, do your exercises sitting or standing. Working against gravity is like adding more weight.

Be patient. Don't give up. It takes just five minutes a day. You may not feel your bladder control improve for three to six weeks. Still, most people do notice an improvement after a few weeks.

Some people with nerve damage cannot tell whether they are doing Kegel exercises correctly. If you are not sure, ask your doctor or nurse to examine you while you try to do them. If it turns out that you are not squeezing the right muscles, you may still be able to learn proper Kegel exercises by doing special training with biofeedback, electrical stimulation, or both.

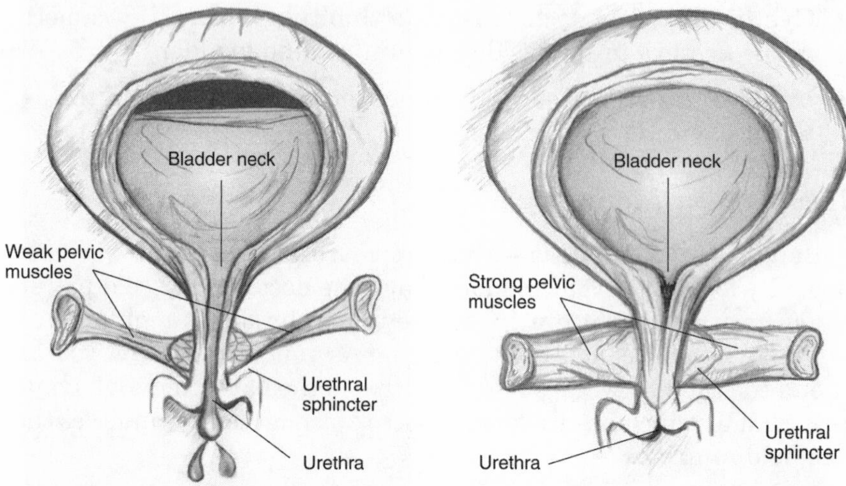

Figure 52.3. *Front view of bladder. Weak pelvic muscles allow urine leakage (left). Strong pelvic muscles keep the urethra closed (right).*

Medicines for overactive bladder: If you have an overactive bladder, your doctor may prescribe a medicine to block the nerve signals that cause frequent urination and urgency.

Several medicines from a class of drugs called anticholinergics can help relax bladder muscles and prevent bladder spasms. Their most common side effect is dry mouth, although larger doses may cause blurred vision, constipation, a faster heartbeat, and flushing. Other side effects include drowsiness, confusion, or memory loss. If you have glaucoma, ask your ophthalmologist if these drugs are safe for you.

Some medicines can affect the nerves and muscles of the urinary tract in different ways. Pills to treat swelling (edema) or high blood pressure may increase your urine output and contribute to bladder control problems. Talk with your doctor; you may find that taking an alternative to a medicine you already take may solve the problem without adding another prescription.

Scientists are studying other drugs and injections that have not yet received U.S. Food and Drug Administration (FDA) approval for incontinence to see if they are effective treatments for people who were unsuccessful with behavioral therapy or pills.

Biofeedback: Biofeedback uses measuring devices to help you become aware of your body's functioning. By using electronic devices or diaries to track when your bladder and urethral muscles contract, you can gain control over these muscles. Biofeedback can supplement pelvic muscle exercises and electrical stimulation to relieve stress and urge incontinence.

Neuromodulation: For urge incontinence not responding to behavioral treatments or drugs, stimulation of nerves to the bladder leaving the spine can be effective in some patients. Neuromodulation is the name of this therapy. The FDA has approved a device called InterStim® for this purpose. Your doctor will need to test to determine if this device would be helpful to you. The doctor applies an external stimulator to determine if neuromodulation works in you. If you have a 50 percent reduction in symptoms, a surgeon will implant the device. Although neuromodulation can be effective, it is not for everyone. The therapy is expensive, involving surgery with possible surgical revisions and replacement.

Vaginal devices for stress incontinence: One of the reasons for stress incontinence may be weak pelvic muscles, the muscles that hold the bladder in place and hold urine inside. A pessary is a stiff ring that a doctor or nurse inserts into the vagina, where it presses against the wall of the vagina and the nearby urethra. The pressure helps reposition the urethra, leading to less stress leakage. If you use a pessary, you should watch for possible vaginal and urinary tract infections and see your doctor regularly.

Injections for stress incontinence: A variety of bulking agents, such as collagen and carbon spheres, are available for injection near the urinary sphincter. The doctor injects the bulking agent into tissues around the bladder neck and urethra to make the tissues thicker and close the bladder opening to reduce stress incontinence. After using local anesthesia or sedation, a doctor can inject the material in about half an hour. Over time, the body may slowly eliminate certain bulking agents, so you will need repeat injections. Before you receive an injection, a doctor may perform a skin test to determine whether you could have an allergic reaction to the material. Scientists are testing newer agents, including your own muscle cells, to see if they are effective in treating stress incontinence. Your doctor will discuss which bulking agent may be best for you.

Surgery for stress incontinence: In some women, the bladder can move out of its normal position, especially following childbirth. Surgeons have developed different techniques for supporting the bladder back to its normal position. The three main types of surgery are retropubic suspension and two types of sling procedures.

Retropubic suspension uses surgical threads called sutures to support the bladder neck. The most common retropubic suspension procedure is called the Burch procedure. In this operation, the surgeon makes an incision in the abdomen a few inches below the navel and then secures the threads to strong ligaments within the pelvis to support the urethral sphincter. This common procedure is often done at the time of an abdominal procedure such as a hysterectomy.

Sling procedures are performed through a vaginal incision. The traditional sling procedure uses a strip of your own tissue called fascia to cradle the bladder neck. Some slings may consist of natural tissue or man-made material. The surgeon attaches both ends of the sling to the pubic bone or ties them in front of the abdomen just above the pubic bone.

Midurethral slings are newer procedures that you can have on an outpatient basis. These procedures use synthetic mesh materials that the surgeon places midway along the urethra. The two general types of midurethral slings are retropubic slings, such as the transvaginal

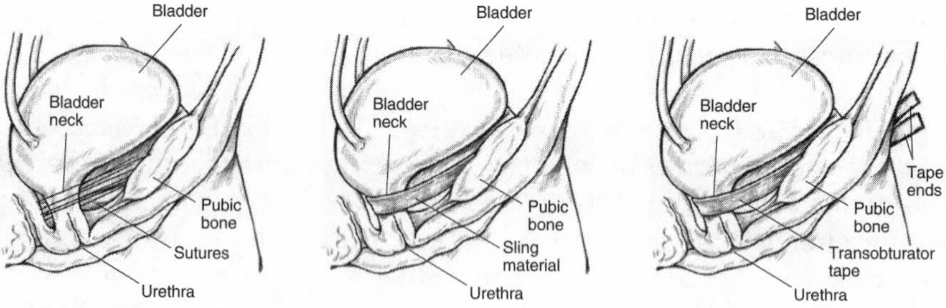

Figure 52.4. *Side view. Supporting sutures in place following retropubic or transvaginal suspension (left). Sling in place, secured to the pubic bone (center). The ends of the transobturator tape supporting the urethra are pulled through incisions in the groin to achieve the right amount of support (right). The tape ends are removed when the incisions are closed.*

tapes (TVT), and transobturator slings (TOT). The surgeon makes small incisions behind the pubic bone or just by the sides of the vaginal opening as well as a small incision in the vagina. The surgeon uses specially designed needles to position a synthetic tape under the urethra. The surgeon pulls the ends of the tape through the incisions and adjusts them to provide the right amount of support to the urethra.

If you have pelvic prolapse, your surgeon may recommend an anti-incontinence procedure with a prolapse repair and possibly a hysterectomy.

Recent women's health studies performed with the Urinary Incontinence Treatment Network (UITN) compared the suspension and sling procedures and found that, two years after surgery, about two-thirds of women with a sling and about half of women with a suspension were cured of stress incontinence. Women with a sling, however, had more urinary tract infections, voiding problems, and urge incontinence than women with a suspension. Overall, 86 percent of women with a sling and 78 percent of women with a suspension said they were satisfied with their results.

Talk with your doctor about whether surgery will help your condition and what type of surgery is best for you. The procedure you choose may depend on your own preferences or on your surgeon's experience. Ask what you should expect after the procedure. You may also wish to talk with someone who has recently had the procedure. Surgeons have described more than two hundred procedures for stress incontinence, so no single surgery stands out as best.

Catheterization: If you are incontinent because your bladder never empties completely—overflow incontinence—or your bladder cannot empty because of poor muscle tone, past surgery, or spinal cord injury, you might use a catheter to empty your bladder. A catheter is a tube that you can learn to insert through the urethra into the bladder to drain urine. You may use a catheter once in a while or on a constant basis, in which case the tube connects to a bag that you can attach to your leg. If you use an indwelling—long-term—catheter, you should watch for possible urinary tract infections.

Other helpful hints: Many women manage urinary incontinence with menstrual pads that catch slight leakage during activities such as exercising. Also, many people find they can reduce incontinence by restricting certain liquids, such as coffee, tea, and alcohol.

Finally, many women are afraid to mention their problem. They may have urinary incontinence that can improve with treatment but remain silent sufferers and resort to wearing absorbent undergarments, or diapers. This practice is unfortunate, because diapering can lead to diminished self-esteem, as well as skin irritation and sores. If you are relying on diapers to manage your incontinence, you and your family should discuss with your doctor the possible effectiveness of treatments such as timed voiding and pelvic muscle exercises.

Section 52.3

Urinary Tract Infections

"Facts about Urinary Tract Infections," reprinted courtesy of the Illinois Department of Public Health (www.idph.state.il.us). The text of this document is available online at http://www.idph.state.il.us/about/womenshealth/factsheets/uti.htm; accessed May 12, 2008.

What are the causes of urinary tract infections?

Normal urine is sterile. It contains fluids, salts, and waste products, but it is free of bacteria, viruses, and fungi. An infection occurs when microorganisms, usually bacteria from the digestive tract, cling to the opening of the urethra and begin to multiply. Most infections arise from one type of bacteria, *Escherichia coli* (*E. coli*), which normally lives in the colon.

In most cases, bacteria first begin growing in the urethra. An infection limited to the urethra is called urethritis. From there bacteria often move on to the bladder, causing a bladder infection (cystitis). If the infection is not treated promptly, bacteria may then go up the ureters to infect the kidneys (pyelonephritis).

The urinary system is structured in a way that helps ward off infection. The ureters and bladder normally prevent urine from backing up toward the kidneys, and the flow of urine from the bladder helps wash bacteria out of the body. In men, the prostate gland produces secretions that slow bacterial growth. In both sexes, immune defenses also prevent infection. Despite these safeguards, infections still occur.

Are women at a higher risk for urinary tract infections (UTIs)?

Some people are more prone to getting a UTI than others. Any abnormality of the urinary tract that obstructs the flow of urine (a kidney stone, for example) sets the stage for an infection. An enlarged prostate gland also can slow the flow of urine, thus raising the risk of infection. Scientists are not sure why women have more urinary infections than men. One factor may be that a woman's urethra is short, allowing bacteria quick access to the bladder. Also, a woman's urethral opening is near sources of bacteria from the anus and vagina. For many women, sexual intercourse seems to trigger an infection, although the reasons for this linkage are unclear. One woman in five develops a UTI during her lifetime.

According to several studies, women who use a diaphragm are more likely to develop a UTI than women who use other forms of birth control. Recently, researchers found that women whose partners use a condom with spermicidal foam also tend to have growth of *E. coli* bacteria in the vagina, which may increase the risk of a UTI.

Infections in pregnancy: Pregnant women seem no more prone to UTIs than other women. However, when a UTI does occur, it is more likely to travel to the kidneys. According to some reports, about 2 to 4 percent of pregnant women develop a urinary infection. Scientists think that hormonal changes and shifts in the position of the urinary tract during pregnancy make it easier for bacteria to travel up the ureters to the kidneys. For this reason, many doctors recommend periodic testing of urine.

What are the symptoms of UTI?

Not everyone with a UTI has symptoms, but most people have at least one. Symptoms may include a frequent urge to urinate and a painful, burning feeling in the area of the bladder or urethra during urination. It is not unusual to feel bad all over—tired, shaky, washed out—and to feel pain even when not urinating. Often, women feel an uncomfortable pressure above the pubic bone, and some men experience a fullness in the rectum. It is common for a person with a urinary infection to complain that, despite the urge to urinate, only a small amount of urine is passed. The urine itself may look milky or cloudy, even reddish if blood is present. A fever may mean that the infection has reached the kidneys. Other symptoms of a kidney infection include pain in the back or side below the ribs, nausea or vomiting.

How is UTI diagnosed?

To find out whether you have a UTI, your doctor will test a sample of urine for pus and bacteria. You will be asked to give a "clean catch" urine sample by washing the genital area and collecting a "midstream" sample of urine in a sterile container. This method of collecting urine helps prevent bacteria around the genital area from getting into the sample and confusing the test results.

How is UTI treated?

UTIs are treated with antibacterial drugs. The choice of drug and length of treatment depends on the patient's history and the urine tests that identify the offending bacteria. The sensitivity test is especially useful in helping the doctor select the most effective drug. Often a UTI can be cured with one or two days of treatment if the infection is not complicated by an obstruction or nervous system disorder. Still, many doctors ask their patients to take antibiotics for a week or two to ensure that the infection has been cured.

Part Six

Additional Help and Information

Chapter 53

Glossary of Terms Related to Women's Health

alveoli cells: Tiny glands in the breast that produce milk.

amniotic fluid: Clear, slightly yellowish liquid that surrounds the unborn baby (fetus) during pregnancy. It is contained in the amniotic sac.

amniotic sac: During pregnancy, the amniotic sac is formed within the uterus and encloses the fetus.

aneurysm: A thin or weak spot in an artery that balloons out and can burst.

angina: A recurring pain or discomfort in the chest that happens when some part of the heart does not receive enough blood. It is a common symptom of coronary heart disease.

anorexia nervosa: An eating disorder caused by a person having a distorted body image and not consuming the appropriate calorie intake resulting in severe weight loss.

anovulation: Absence of ovulation.

anxiety disorder: Serious medical illness that fills people's lives with anxiety and fear. Some anxiety disorders include panic disorder, obsessive-compulsive disorder, post-traumatic stress disorder, social

---

Excerpted from "Glossary," Women's Health Information Center; available online at http://www.womenshealth.gov/glossary; accessed May 12, 2008.

phobia (or social anxiety disorder), specific phobias, and generalized anxiety disorder.

areola: The dark-colored skin on the breast that surrounds the nipple.

arthritis: Swelling, redness, heat and pain of the joints. There are over one hundred types of arthritis.

assisted reproductive technology: Technology that involves procedures that handle a woman's eggs and a man's sperm to help infertile couples conceive a child.

atherosclerosis: A disease in which fatty material is deposited on the wall of the arteries. This fatty material causes the arteries to become narrow and it eventually restricts blood flow.

autoimmune disease: Disease caused by an immune response against foreign substances in the tissues of one's own body.

bacterial vaginosis: The most common vaginal infection in women of childbearing age, which happens when the normal bacteria (germs) in the vagina get out of balance, such as from douching or from sexual contact.

binge eating disorder: An eating disorder caused by a person being unable to control the need to overeat.

biopsy: Removal of a small piece of tissue for testing or examination under a microscope.

body mass index: A measure of body fat based on a person's height and weight.

bulimia nervosa: An eating disorder caused by a person consuming an extreme amount of food all at once followed by self-induced vomiting or other purging.

cancer: A group of diseases in which abnormal cells divide without control. Cancer cells can invade nearby tissues and can spread through the bloodstream and lymphatic system to other parts of the body.

cardiovascular diseases: Disease of the heart and blood vessels.

cervix: The lower, narrow part of the uterus (womb). The cervix forms a canal that opens into the vagina, which leads to the outside of the body.

cesarean (C-section): Procedure where the baby is delivered through an abdominal incision.

chlamydia: A common sexually transmitted disease (STD).

chorionic villus sampling (CVS): If necessary this test is performed between ten and twelve weeks of pregnancy and can indicate the same chromosomal abnormalities and genetic disorders as amniocentesis can. It also can detect the baby's sex and risk of spina bifida.

chronic fatigue syndrome (CFS): A complex disorder characterized by extreme fatigue that lasts six months or longer, and does not improve with rest or is worsened by physical or mental activity.

colonoscopy: A diagnostic procedure in which a flexible tube with a light source in inserted into the colon (large intestine or large bowel) through the anus to view all sections of the colon for abnormalities.

colposcopy: Procedure that uses a special microscope (called a colposcope) to look into the vagina and to look very closely at the cervix.

Crohn disease: An ongoing condition that causes inflammation of the digestive tract, also called the GI tract. It can affect any part of the GI tract—from the mouth to the anus. It often affects the lower part of the small intestine, causing pain and diarrhea.

depression: Term used to describe an emotional state involving sadness, lack of energy and low self-esteem.

diabetes: A disease in which blood glucose (blood sugar) levels are above normal.

dialysis: A treatment used when kidneys fail. It filters the blood to rid the body of harmful wastes, salt, and extra water.

diaphragm: Birth control device made of a thin flexible disk, usually made of rubber, that is designed to cover the cervix to prevent the entry of sperm during sexual intercourse.

dietary fiber: Coarse fibrous substances found in grains, fruits, and vegetables. Dietary fiber is generally not digested but helps move food through the digestive tract.

diuretics: A type of medication sometimes called "water pills" because they work in the kidney and flush excess water and sodium from the body.

ductules: Small milk ducts in the breast leading to the mammary or lactiferous ducts.

eating disorder: Eating disorders, such as anorexia nervosa, bulimia nervosa, and binge-eating disorder, involve serious problems with eating. This could include an extreme decrease of food or severe overeating, as well as feelings of distress and concern about body shape or weight.

ectopic pregnancy: A pregnancy that is not in the uterus. It happens when a fertilized egg settles and grows in a place other than the inner lining of the uterus. Most happen in the fallopian tube, but can happen in the ovary, cervix, or abdominal cavity.

endometriosis: A condition in which tissue that normally lines the uterus grows in other areas of the body, usually inside the abdominal cavity, but acts as if it were inside the uterus.

endoscopy: A diagnostic procedure in which a thin, flexible tube is introduced through the mouth or rectum to view parts of the digestive tract.

epidural: During labor a woman may be offered an epidural, where a needle is inserted into the epidural space at the end of the spine, to numb the lower body and reduce pain.

episiotomy: A procedure where an incision is made in the perineum (area between the vagina and the anus) to make the vaginal opening larger in order to prevent the area from tearing during delivery.

estrogen: A group of female hormones that are responsible for the development of breasts and other secondary sex characteristics in women. Estrogen is produced by the ovaries and other body tissues.

fallopian tubes: Part of the female reproductive system, these tubes carry eggs from the ovaries to the uterus (or womb).

follicle: Each month, an egg develops inside the ovary in a fluid filled pocket called a follicle. This follicle releases the egg into the fallopian tube.

follicle-stimulating hormone (FSH): A hormone produced by the pituitary gland. In women, it helps control the menstrual cycle and the production of eggs by the ovaries.

goiter: Enlargement of the thyroid gland that is not associated with inflammation or cancer.

gonorrhea: A sexually transmitted disease that often has no symptoms. Untreated gonorrhea can cause serious and permanent health problems like pelvic inflammatory disease (PID).

hormone: Substance produced by one tissue and conveyed by the bloodstream to another to effect a function of the body, such as growth or metabolism.

hysterectomy: Surgery to remove the uterus.

infertility: A condition in which a couple has problems conceiving, or getting pregnant, after one year of regular sexual intercourse without using any birth control methods.

inflammatory bowel disease: Long-lasting problems that cause irritation and ulcers in the gastrointestinal tract. The most common disorders are ulcerative colitis and Crohn disease.

interstitial cystitis: A long-lasting condition also known as painful bladder syndrome or frequency-urgency-dysuria syndrome. The wall of the bladder becomes inflamed or irritated, which affects the amount of urine the bladder can hold and causes scarring, stiffening, and bleeding in the bladder.

intrauterine device: A small device that is placed inside a woman's uterus by a health care provider, which prevents pregnancy by changing the environment of the uterus (or womb).

inverted nipple: A nipple that retracts, rather than protrudes when the areola is compressed.

lactation: Breastfeeding, or the secretion of breast milk.

luteinizing hormone: A hormone that triggers ovulation and stimulates the corpus luteum (empty follicle) to make progesterone.

mammary ducts: Ducts in the breast that carry milk to the lactiferous sinuses and the nipple.

mastitis: A condition that occurs mostly in breastfeeding women, causing a hard spot on the breast that can be sore or uncomfortable. It is caused by infection from bacteria that enters the breast through a break or crack in the skin on the nipple or by a plugged milk duct.

menopausal hormone therapy (MHT): Replaces the hormones that a woman's ovaries stop making at the time of menopause, easing symptoms like hot flashes and vaginal dryness.

menopause: The transition in a woman's life when production of the hormone estrogen in her body falls permanently to very low levels, the ovaries stop producing eggs, and menstrual periods stop for good.

menstrual cycle: A recurring cycle in which the lining of the uterus thickens in preparation for pregnancy and then is shed if pregnancy does not occur.

miscarriage: An unplanned loss of a pregnancy. Also called a spontaneous abortion.

osteoporosis: A bone disease that is characterized by progressive loss of bone density and thinning of bone tissue, causing bones to break easily.

ovaries: Part of a woman's reproductive system, the ovaries produce her eggs.

ovulation: The release of a single egg from a follicle that developed in the ovary. It usually occurs regularly, around day fourteen of a twenty-eight-day menstrual cycle.

oxytocin: A hormone that increases during pregnancy and acts on the breast to help produce the milk-ejection reflex. Oxytocin also causes uterine contractions.

panic disorder: An anxiety disorder in which a person suffers from sudden attacks of fear and panic.

Pap test: This test finds changes on the cervix. To do a Pap test, the doctor uses a small brush to take cells from the cervix.

pelvic exam: During this exam, the doctor or nurse practitioner looks for redness, swelling, discharge, or sores on the outside and inside of the vagina. A Pap test tests for cell changes on the cervix. The doctor or nurse practitioner will also put two fingers inside the vagina and press on the abdomen with the other hand to check for cysts or growths on the ovaries and uterus. STD tests may also be done.

pelvic inflammatory disease (PID): An infection of the female reproductive organs that are above the cervix, such as the fallopian tubes and ovaries. It is the most common and serious problem caused by sexually transmitted diseases (STDs).

perinatal depression: Depression that occurs during pregnancy or within a year after delivery.

peripartum depression: Depression after pregnancy.

phobias: An anxiety disorder in which a person suffers from an unusual amount of fear of a certain activity or situation.

placenta: During pregnancy, a temporary organ joining the mother and fetus. The placenta transfers oxygen and nutrients from the mother to the fetus, and permits the release of carbon dioxide and waste products from the fetus.

postpartum depression (PPD): A serious condition that requires treatment from a health care provider. With this condition, feelings of the baby blues (feeling sad, anxious, afraid, or confused after having a baby) do not go away or get worse.

pre-term labor: Labor that occurs before thirty-seven completed weeks of pregnancy.

preeclampsia: Also known as toxemia, it is a condition that can occur in a woman in the second half of her pregnancy that can cause serious problems for both her and the baby. It causes high blood pressure, protein in the urine, blood changes and other problems.

progesterone: A female hormone produced by the ovaries. Progesterone, along with estrogen, prepares the uterus (womb) for a possible pregnancy each month and supports the fertilized egg if conception occurs. Progesterone also helps prepare the breasts for milk production and breastfeeding.

progestin: A hormone that works by causing changes in the uterus.

prolactin: A hormone that increases during pregnancy and breastfeeding. It stimulates the human breast to produce milk. Prolactin also helps inhibit ovulation.

puberty: Time when the body is changing from the body of a child to the body of an adult. This process begins earlier in girls than in boys, usually between ages eight and thirteen, and lasts two to four years.

purging: Forcing oneself to vomit.

radiation: Treatment using radiation to destroy cancer cells.

sexually transmitted diseases (STDs): Diseases that are spread by sexual activity.

spermicides: Chemical jellies, foams, creams, or suppositories, inserted into the vagina prior to intercourse that kill sperm.

stillbirth: When a fetus dies during birth, or when the fetus dies during the late stages of pregnancy when it would have been otherwise expected to survive.

stroke: Stoppage of blood flow to an area of the brain, causing permanent damage to nerve cells in that region.

syphilis: A sexually transmitted disease which may or may not have symptoms. If left untreated, syphilis can permanently damage the brain, nerves, eyes, heart, blood vessels, liver, bones, and joints.

systemic lupus erythematosus: An autoimmune disease that can cause inflammation and damage to the joints, skin, kidneys, heart, lungs, blood vessels, and brain.

thyroid: A small gland in the neck that makes and stores hormones that help regulate heart rate, blood pressure, body temperature, and the rate at which food is converted into energy.

transient ischemic attack (TIA): A "mini-stroke" where there is a short-term reduction in blood flow to the brain usually resulting in temporary stoke symptoms.

trichomoniasis: A very common STD in both women and men that is caused by a parasite that is passed from one person to another during sexual contact.

triple screen: Blood test that indicates if there's an increased risk of a birth defect, or a condition like Down syndrome, in the fetus. This test can also show twins.

ultrasound: A painless, harmless test that uses sound waves to produce images of the organs and structures of the body on a screen. Also called sonography.

umbilical cord: Connected to the placenta and provides the transfer of nutrients and waste between the woman and the fetus.

urinary tract infection: An infection anywhere in the urinary tract, or organs that collect and store urine and release it from your body (the kidneys, ureters, bladder, and urethra).

uterine fibroids: Common, benign (noncancerous) tumors that grow in the muscle of the uterus, or womb.

uterus: A woman's womb, or the hollow, pear-shaped organ located in a woman's lower abdomen between the bladder and the rectum.

vagina: The muscular canal that extends from the cervix to the outside of the body. Its walls are lined with mucus membranes and tiny glands that make vaginal secretions.

vulva: Opening to the vagina.

yeast infections: A common infection in women caused by an overgrowth of the fungus *Candida*. It is normal to have some yeast in your vagina, but sometimes it can overgrow because of hormonal changes in your body, such as during pregnancy, or from taking certain medications, such as antibiotics.

Chapter 54

Directory of Women's Health Resources

General

American Academy of Family Physicians
Phone: 913-906-6000
Website: http://www.aafp.org

Centers for Disease Control and Prevention
Toll-Free: 800-232-4636
Website: http://www.cdc.gov

Food and Drug Administration (FDA)
Toll-Free: 888-463-6332
Website: www.fda.gov

National Institute on Aging
Building 31, Room 5C27
31 Center Drive, MSC 2292
Bethesda, MD 20892
Phone: 301-496-1752
Fax: 301-496-1072
TTY: 1-800-222-4225
Website: http://www.nia.nih.gov

National Women's Health Information Center
Office on Women's Health
200 Independence Ave., S.W., Room 712E
Washington, DC 20201
Toll-Free: 800-994-9662
TDD: 888-220-5446
Phone: 202-690-7650
Fax: 202-205-2631
Website: http://www.4woman.gov

The information in this chapter was compiled from various sources deemed accurate. All contact information was verified and updated in January 2009. Inclusion does not imply endorsement. This list is intended to serve as a starting point for information gathering; it is not comprehensive.

The Nemours Foundation
Phone: 302-651-4046
Website: http://www.nemours.org

Cancer

American Cancer Society
Toll-Free: 800-ACS-2345 (800-227-2345)
Website: http://www.cancer.org

Gynecologic Cancer Foundation
Toll-Free: 800-444-4441
Website: http://www.thegcf.org

Susan G. Komen Breast Cancer Foundation
Toll-Free: 800-462-9273
Website: http://www.komen.org

National Breast and Cervical Cancer Early Detection Program
Website: http://www.cdc.gov/cancer/nbccedp/index.htm

National Cancer Institute
Toll-Free: 800-422-6237
Website: http://www.cancer.gov

National Ovarian Cancer Coalition
2501 Oak Lawn Avenue
Suite 435
Dallas, TX 75219
Toll-Free: 888-OVARIAN
Website: http://www.ovarian.org

National Skin Cancer Prevention Education Program
Website: http://www.cdc.gov/cancer/nscpep/index.htm

Skin Cancer Foundation
Phone: 212-725-5176
Website: http://www.skincancer.org

Diabetes

American Diabetes Association
Toll-Free: 800-342-2383
Website: www.diabetes.org

National Diabetes Education Program
Toll-Free: 800-438-5383
Website: http://ndep.nih.gov

National Diabetes Information Clearinghouse, National Institute of Diabetes and Digestive and Kidney Diseases
Toll-Free: 800-860-8747
Website: http://www.niddk.nih.gov

Eating Disorders

Academy for Eating Disorders
Phone: 847-498-4274
Website: http://www.aedweb.org

National Association of Anorexia Nervosa and Associated Disorders
Phone: 847-831-3438
Website: http://www.anad.org

National Eating Disorders Association
Toll-Free: 800-931-2237
Website: http://www.nationaleatingdisorders.org

Gastrointestinal Disorders

American College of Gastroenterology
Phone: 301-263-9000
Website: www.acg.gi.org

American Gastroenterological Association
Phone: 301-654-2055
Website: www.gastro.org

Crohn's and Colitis Foundation of America, Inc.
Toll-Free: 800-932-2423
Phone: 212-685-3440
Website: www.ccfa.org

International Foundation for Functional Gastrointestinal Disorders
Toll-Free: 888-964-2001
Website: http://www.iffgd.org

National Digestive Diseases Information Clearinghouse
2 Information Way Bethesda, MD 20892-3570
E-mail: nddic@info.niddk.nih.gov

Heart Disease

Act In Time to Heart Attack Signs Campaign
National Heart Attack Alert Program
National Heart, Lung, and Blood Institute (NHLBI)
Phone: 301-592-8573
Website: http://www.nhlbi.nih.gov/actintime

American Heart Association
Toll-Free: 800-242-8721
Website: http://www.americanheart.org

The Heart Truth
National Awareness Campaign for Women about Heart Disease
National Heart, Lung, and Blood Institute (NHLBI)
Website: http://www.nhlbi.nih.gov/health/hearttruth

National Cholesterol Education Program
National Heart, Lung, and Blood Institute (NHLBI)
Phone: 301-592-8573
Website: http://www.nhlbi.nih.gov/about/ncep

National Heart, Lung, and Blood Institute (NHLBI)
Phone: 301-592-8573
Website: http://www.nhlbi.nih.gov

National High Blood Pressure Education Program
National Heart, Lung, and Blood Institute (NHLBI)
Website: http://www.nhlbi.nih.gov/about/nhbpep

WomenHeart
Phone: 202-728-7199
Website: www.womenheart.org

Gynecological Concerns

American College of Obstetricians and Gynecologists
409 12th St., S.W.
Washington, DC 20024-218
Phone: 202-638-5577
Website: http://www.acog.org

Endometriosis Association
8585 N. 76th Place
Milwaukee, WI 53223
Phone: 414-355-2200
Fax: 414-355-6065
Website: http://www.endometriosisassn.org

Endometriosis Research Center
630 Ibis Drive
Delray Beach, FL 33444
Toll Free: 800-239-7280
Phone: 561-274-7442
Fax: 561-274-0931
Website: http://www.endocenter.org

National Uterine Fibroids Foundation
Phone: 719-633-3454
Website: http://www.nuff.org
E-mail: info@nuff.org

Polycystic Ovarian Syndrome Association, Inc. (PCOSA)
Website: http://www.pcosupport.org

Infertility

American Society for Reproductive Medicine (ASRM)
Phone: 205-978-5000
Website: http://www.asrm.org

Center for Applied Reproductive Science (CARS)
Phone: 423-461-8880
Website: http://www.ivf-et.com

InterNational Council on Infertility Information Dissemination, Inc. (INCIID)
Phone: 703-379-9178
Website: http://www.inciid.org

Resolve: The National Infertility Association
Toll-Free: 703-556-7172
Website: http://www.resolve.org

Lesbian Health

Gay and Lesbian Medical Association (GLMA)
Phone: 415-255-4547
Website: http://www.glma.org

Lesbian Health Research Center, Institute for Health and Aging
Phone: 415-502-5209
Website: http://www.lesbianhealthinfo.org

Lesbian STD Web Site, University of Washington
Website: http://depts.washington.edu/wswstd

Mautner Project
Phone: 202-332-5536
Website: http://www.mautnerproject.org

National Center for Lesbian Rights
Phone: 415-392-6257
Website: http://www.nclrights.org

Lupus

Alliance for Lupus Research
Phone: 212-218-2840
Website: www.lupusresearch.org

American Autoimmune Related Diseases Association, Inc.
Phone: 586-776-3900
Website: www.aarda.org

American College of Rheumatology
Phone: 404-633-3777
Website: www.rheumatology.org

Arthritis Foundation
Toll-Free: 800-283-7800
Website: www.arthritis.org

Lupus Foundation of America
Toll-Free: 800-558-0121
Website: www.lupus.org

SLE Foundation
Phone: 212-685-4118
Website: www.lupusny.org

Menopause

The Hormone Foundation
Toll-Free: 800-467-6663
Website: http://www.hormone.org

International Premature Ovarian Failure Association
P.O. Box 23643
Alexandria, VA 22304
Website: http://www.POFsupport.org
E-mail: info@pofsupport.org

National Institute on Aging (NIA)
Toll-Free: 800-222-2225
Website: http://www.nih.gov/nia

North American Menopause Society (NAMS)
Toll-Free: 800-774-5342
Website: http://www.menopause.org

Mental Health

American Institute of Stress
Phone: 914-963-1200
Website: http://www.stress.org

American Psychiatric Association
Phone: 703-907-7300
Website: http://www.psych.org

American Psychological Association
Toll-Free: 800-374-2721
Website: http://www.apa.org

Anxiety Disorders Association of America
Phone: 240-485-1001
Website: http://www.adaa.org

National Alliance for the Mentally Ill
Toll-Free: 800-950-6264
Website: http://www.nami.org

National Center for Post Traumatic Stress Disorder
Phone: 802-296-5132
Website: http://www.ncptsd.org

National Institute of Mental Health
Phone: 301-443-4513
Website: http://www.nimh.nih.gov

National Mental Health Association
Toll-Free: 800-969-6642
Website: http://www.nmha.org

National Mental Health Consumers' Self-Help Clearinghouse
Toll-Free: 800-553-4539
Website: http://www.mhselfhelp.org

National Mental Health Information Center
Toll-Free: 800-789-2647
Website: http://www.mentalhealth.org

Postpartum Education for Parents
Phone: 805-564-3888
Website: http://www.sbpep.org

Postpartum Support International
Phone: 805-967-7636
Website: http://www.postpartum.net

Osteoporosis

National Institute of Arthritis and Musculoskeletal and Skin Diseases
Phone: 301-495-4484
Website: http://www.nih.gov/niams

National Institute on Aging
Toll-Free: 800-222-2225
Website: http://www.nih.gov/nia

National Osteoporosis Foundation
Phone: 877-868-4520
Website: http://www.nof.org

Osteoporosis and Related Bone Diseases National Resource Center
Toll-Free: 800-624-2663
Website: http://www.osteo.org

Plastic Surgery

American Academy of Facial Plastic and Reconstructive Surgery
310 S. Henry Street
Alexandria, VA 22314
Phone: 703-299-9291
Website: http://www.aafprs.org
E-mail: info@aafprs.org

American Society for Aesthetic Plastic Surgery
11081 Winners Circle
Los Alamitos, CA 90720-2813
Toll-Free: 888-ASAPS-11 (272-7711)
Website: http://www.surgery.org

American Society of Plastic Surgeons
444 E. Algonquin Rd.
Arlington Heights, IL 60005
Phone: 847-228-9900
Website: http://www.plasticsurgery.org

Pregnancy

American College of Obstetricians and Gynecologists
409 12th St., S.W.
Washington, DC 20090-6920
Phone: 202-638-5577
Website: http://www.acog.org

American Pregnancy Association
1425 Greenway Drive, Suite 440
Irving, TX 75038
Phone: 972-550-0140
Fax: 972-550-0800
Website: http://www.americanpregnancy.org
E-mail: questions@americanpregnancy.org

March of Dimes
Toll-Free: 888-663-4637
Phone: 914-428-7100
Website: http://www.modimes.org

Smart Moms, Healthy Babies
Website: http://www.smartmoms.org

Promoting Wellness

American Council on Exercise
Toll-Free: 800-825-3636
Website: http://www.acefitness.org

American Dietetic Association
Toll-Free: 800-877-1600
Website: http://www.eatright.org

American Obesity Association
Toll-Free: 301-563-6526
Website: http://www.obesity.org

Food and Nutrition Information Center
Phone: 301-504-5414
Website: http://www.nal.usda.gov/fnic

International Food Information Council
Phone: 202-296-6540
Website: http://www.ific.org

President's Council on Physical Fitness and Sports
Phone: 202-690-9000
Website: http://www.fitness.gov

Steps to a HealthierUS
Website: http://www.healthierus.gov

United States Department of Agriculture
Center for Nutrition Policy and Promotion
Phone: (703) 605-4266
Website: http://www.usda.gov/cnpp

Weight Control Information Network
Phone: 877-946-4627
Website: http://win.niddk.nih.gov

Sexually Transmitted Diseases

American Social Health Association
Toll-Free: 800-783-9877
Website: http://www.ashastd.org

National Center for HIV, STD and TB Prevention
Website: http://www.cdc.gov/std

National Institute of Allergy and Infectious Diseases (NIAID)
Phone: 301-496-5717
Website: http://www.niaid.nih.gov

Planned Parenthood Federation of America
Toll-Free: 800-230-PLAN (7526)
Website: http://www.plannedparenthood.org

Urological Concerns

American Urological Association Foundation
Toll-Free: 800-242-2383
Website: www.auafoundation.org

American Urogynecologic Society
Phone: 202-367-1167
Website: http://www.augs.org

Interstitial Cystitis Association
Toll-Free: 800-HELP ICA (800-435-7422)
Website: www.ichelp.org

National Association for Continence
Toll-Free: 800-252-3337
Website: http://www.nafc.org

National Kidney and Urologic Diseases Information Clearinghouse
Toll-Free: 800-891-5390
Website: http://kidney.niddk.nih.gov

Varicose Veins and Spider Veins

American Academy of Dermatology
Toll-Free: 888-462-DERM (3376)
Phone: 847-330-0230
Website: http://www.aad.org

American College of Phlebology
Phone: 510-346-6800
Website: http://www.phlebology.org

American Society for Dermatologic Surgery
Phone: 847-956-0900
Website: http://www.asds-net.org

Index

Index

Page numbers followed by 'n' indicate a footnote. Page numbers in *italics* indicate a table or illustration.

A

B

C

D

E

F

G

H

K

L

M

N

O

P

Q

R

S

T

U

V

W

X

Y

Z

Health Reference Series

Complete Catalog

List price $93 per volume. School and library price $84 per volume.

Adolescent Health Sourcebook, 2nd Edition

Basic Consumer Health Information about the Physical, Mental, and Emotional Growth and Development of Adolescents, Including Medical Care, Nutritional and Physical Activity Requirements, Puberty, Sexual Activity, Acne, Tanning, Body Piercing, Common Physical Illnesses and Disorders, Eating Disorders, Attention Deficit Hyperactivity Disorder, Depression, Bullying, Hazing, and Adolescent Injuries Related to Sports, Driving, and Work

Along with Substance Abuse Information about Nicotine, Alcohol, and Drug Use, a Glossary, and Directory of Additional Resources

Edited by Joyce Brennfleck Shannon. 655 pages. 2007. 978-0-7808-0943-7.

"A particularly good resource for both parents and teens. The concise presentation of the material in brief and well-organized chapters creates an easy volume to browse."

—*School Library Journal, Jun '07*

"I don't believe there are any other books written in such easy to understand language that encompass such a breadth of topics. This is a complete revision of the book and is an excellent resource for parents and teens."

—*Doody's Review Service, 2007*

Adult Health Concerns Sourcebook

Basic Consumer Health Information about Medical and Mental Concerns of Adults, Including Facts about Choosing Healthcare Providers, Navigating Insurance Options, Maintaining Wellness, Preventing Cancer, Heart Disease, Stroke, Diabetes, and Osteoporosis, and Understanding Aging-Related Health Concerns, Including Menopause, Cognitive Changes, and Changes in the Coronary and Vascular Systems

Along with Tips on Caring for Aging Parents and Dealing with Health-Related Work and Travel Issues, a Glossary, and a Directory of Resources for Additional Help and Information

Edited by Sandra J. Judd. 648 pages. 2008. 978-0-7808-0999-4.

"Provides a thorough list of topics that are important to adult health and for caregivers."

—*CHOICE, Nov '08*

"Written in easy-to-understand language . . . the content is well-organized and is intended to aid adults in making health care-related decisions."

—*AORN Journal, Dec '08*

AIDS Sourcebook, 4th Edition

Basic Consumer Health Information about Human Immunodeficiency Virus (HIV) and Acquired Immunodeficiency Syndrome (AIDS), Featuring Updated Statistics and Facts about Risks, Prevention, Screening, Diagnosis, Treatments, Side Effects, and Complications, and Including a Section about the Impact of HIV/AIDS on the Health of Women, Children, and Adolescents

Along with Tips on Managing Life with AIDS, Reports on Current Research Initiatives and Clinical Trials, a Glossary of Related Terms, and Resource Directories for Further Help and Information

Edited by Ivy L. Alexander. 680 pages. 2008. 978-0-7808-0997-0.

SEE ALSO *Contagious Diseases Sourcebook, 2nd Edition*

Alcoholism Sourcebook, 2nd Edition

Basic Consumer Health Information about Alcohol Use, Abuse, and Dependence, Featuring Facts about the Physical, Mental, and Social Health Effects of Alcohol Addiction, Including Alcoholic Liver Disease, Pancreatic Disease, Cardiovascular Disease, Neurological Disorders, and the Effects of Drinking during Pregnancy

Along with Information about Alcohol Treatment, Medications, and Recovery Programs, in Addition to Tips for Reducing the Prevalence of Underage Drinking, Statistics about Alcohol Use, a Glossary of Related Terms, and Directories of Resources for More Help and Information

Edited by Amy L. Sutton. 625 pages. 2007. 978-0-7808-0942-0.

"A comprehensive look at the adverse effects of alcohol on people of all ages . . . It serves to whet the reader's appetite to continue learning using other resources. It is practical, easy to read, and enlightening, and is the first book a lay person should consult to learn about alcoholism."

—*Doody's Review Service, 2007*

"Should be a basic acquisition for any serious public or college-level library including health reference titles for general-interest readers."

—*California Bookwatch, Feb '07*

SEE ALSO *Drug Abuse Sourcebook, 2nd Edition*

Allergies Sourcebook, 3rd Edition

Basic Consumer Health Information about Allergic Disorders, Such as Anaphylaxis, Hives, Eczema, Rhinitis, Sinusitis, and Conjunctivitis, and Their Triggers, Including Pollen, Mold, Dust Mites, Animal Dander, Insects, Chemicals, Food, Food Additives, and Medications

Along with Advice about the Diagnosis and Treatment of Allergy Symptoms, a Glossary of Related Terms, a Directory of Resources for Help and Information, and Suggestions for Additional Reading

Edited by Amy L. Sutton. 588 pages. 2007. 978-0-7808-0950-5.

SEE ALSO *Asthma Sourcebook, 2nd Edition*

Alzheimer Disease Sourcebook, 4th Edition

Basic Consumer Health Information about Alzheimer Disease, Other Dementias, and Related Disorders, Including Multi-Infarct Dementia, Dementia with Lewy Bodies, Frontotemporal Dementia (Pick Disease), Wernicke-Korsakoff Syndrome (Alcohol-Related Dementia), AIDS Dementia Complex, Huntington Disease, Creutzfeldt-Jacob Disease, and Delirium

Along with Information about Coping with Memory Loss and Forgetfulness, Maintaining Skills, and Long-Term Planning for People with Dementia, and Suggestions Addressing Common Caregiver Concerns, Updated Information about Current Research Efforts, a Glossary of Related Terms, and Directories of Sources for Additional Help and Information

Edited by Karen Bellenir. 603 pages. 2008. 978-0-7808-1001-3.

"An invaluable resource for persons who have received a diagnosis, for caregivers, and for family members dealing with this insidious disease. It is recommended for public, community college, and ready-reference sections in academic libraries."

—*ARBAonline, Jul '08*

SEE ALSO *Brain Disorders Sourcebook, 2nd Edition*

Arthritis Sourcebook, 2nd Edition

Basic Consumer Health Information about Osteoarthritis, Rheumatoid Arthritis, Other Rheumatic Disorders, Infectious Forms of Arthritis, and Diseases with Symptoms Linked to Arthritis, Featuring Facts about Diagnosis, Pain Management, and Surgical Therapies

Along with Coping Strategies, Research Updates, a Glossary, and Resources for Additional Help and Information

Edited by Amy L. Sutton. 567 pages. 2004. 978-0-7808-0667-2.

"This easy-to-read volume is recommended for consumer health collections within public or academic libraries."

—*E-Streams, May '05*

"As expected, this updated edition continues the excellent reputation of this series in providing sound, usable health information. . . . Highly recommended."

—*American Reference Books Annual, 2005*

Asthma Sourcebook, 2nd Edition

Basic Consumer Health Information about the Causes, Symptoms, Diagnosis, and Treatment of Asthma in Infants, Children, Teenagers, and Adults, Including Facts about Different Types of Asthma, Common Co-Occurring Conditions, Asthma Management Plans, Triggers, Medications, and Medication Delivery Devices

Along with Asthma Statistics, Research Updates, a Glossary, a Directory of Asthma-Related Resources, and More

Edited by Karen Bellenir. 581 pages. 2006. 978-0-7808-0866-9.

Attention Deficit Disorder Sourcebook

Basic Consumer Health Information about Attention Deficit/Hyperactivity Disorder in Children and Adults, Including Facts about Causes, Symptoms, Diagnostic Criteria, and Treatment Options Such as Medications, Behavior Therapy, Coaching, and Homeopathy

Along with Reports on Current Research Initiatives, Legal Issues, and Government Regulations, and Featuring a Glossary of Related Terms, Internet Resources, and a List of Additional Reading Material

Edited by Dawn D. Matthews. 447 pages. 2002. 978-0-7808-0624-5.

"Recommended reference source."

—*Booklist, Jan '03*

SEE ALSO *Learning Disabilities Sourcebook, 3rd Edition*

Autism and Pervasive Developmental Disorders Sourcebook

Basic Consumer Health Information about Autism Spectrum and Pervasive Developmental Disorders, Such as Classical Autism, Asperger Syndrome, Rett Syndrome, and Childhood Disintegrative Disorder, Including Information about Related Genetic Disorders and Medical Problems and Facts about Causes, Screening Methods, Diagnostic Criteria, Treatments and Interventions, and Family and Education Issues

Along with a Glossary of Related Terms, Tips for Evaluating the Validity of Health Claims, and a Directory of Resources for Additional Help and Information

Edited by Sandra J. Judd. 603 pages. 2007. 978-0-7808-0953-6.

"Recommended for public libraries"

—*SciTech Book News, Mar '08*

SEE ALSO *Learning Disabilities Sourcebook, 3rd Edition*

Back and Neck Disorders Sourcebook, 2nd Edition

Basic Consumer Health Information about Spinal Pain, Spinal Cord Injuries, and Related Disorders, Such as Degenerative Disk Disease, Osteoarthritis, Scoliosis, Sciatica, Spina Bifida, and Spinal Stenosis, and Featuring Facts about Maintaining Spinal Health, Self-Care, Pain Management, Rehabilitative Care, Chiropractic Care, Spinal Surgeries, and Complementary Therapies

Along with Suggestions for Preventing Back and Neck Pain, a Glossary of Related Terms, and a Directory of Resources

Edited by Amy L. Sutton. 607 pages. 2004. 978-0-7808-0738-9.

"Recommended. ...An easy to use, comprehensive medical reference book."

—*E-Streams, Sep '05*

"For anyone who has back or neck problems, this book is ideal. Its easy-to-understand language and variety of topics makes this sourcebook a worthwhile read. The price...is reasonable for the amount of information contained in the book"

—*Occupational Therapy in Health Care, 2007*

Blood and Circulatory Disorders Sourcebook, 2nd Edition

Basic Consumer Health Information about the Blood and Circulatory System and Related Disorders, Such as Anemia and Other Hemoglobin Diseases, Cancer of the Blood and Associated Bone Marrow Disorders, Clotting and Bleeding Problems, and Conditions That Affect the Veins, Blood Vessels, and Arteries, Including Facts about the Donation and Transplantation of Bone Marrow, Stem Cells, and Blood and Tips for Keeping the Blood and Circulatory System Healthy

Along with a Glossary of Related Terms and Resources for Additional Help and Information

Edited by Amy L. Sutton. 634 pages. 2005. 978-0-7808-0746-4.

"Highly recommended pick for basic consumer health reference holdings at all levels."

—*The Bookwatch, Aug '05*

Brain Disorders Sourcebook, 2nd Edition

Basic Consumer Health Information about Acquired and Traumatic Brain Injuries, Infections of the Brain, Epilepsy and Seizure Disorders, Cerebral Palsy, and Degenerative Neurological Disorders, Including Amyotrophic Lateral Sclerosis (ALS), Dementias, Multiple Sclerosis, and More

Along with Information on the Brain's Structure and Function, Treatment and Rehabilitation Options, Reports on Current Research Initiatives, a Glossary of Terms Related to Brain Disorders and Injuries, and a Directory of Sources for Further Help and Information

Edited by Sandra J. Judd. 600 pages. 2005. 978-0-7808-0744-0.

"This easy-to-read volume provides up-to-date health information... Recommended for consumer health collections within public or academic libraries."

—*E-Streams, Feb '06*

SEE ALSO *Alzheimer Disease Sourcebook, 4th Edition*

Breast Cancer Sourcebook, 3rd Edition

Basic Consumer Health Information about Breast Health and Breast Cancer, Including Facts about Environmental, Genetic, and Other Risk Factors, Prevention Efforts, Screening and Diagnostic Methods, Surgical Treatment Options and Other Care Choices, Complementary and Alternative Therapies, and Post-Treatment Concerns

Along with Statistical Data, News about Research Advances, a Glossary of Related Terms, and Directories of Resources for Additional Information and Support

Edited by Karen Bellenir. 606 pages. 2009. 978-0-7808-1030-3.

SEE ALSO *Cancer Sourcebook for Women, 3rd Edition, Women's Health Concerns Sourcebook, 3rd Edition*

Breastfeeding Sourcebook

Basic Consumer Health Information about the Benefits of Breastmilk, Preparing to Breastfeed, Breastfeeding as a Baby Grows, Nutrition, and More, Including Information on Special Situations and Concerns Such as Mastitis, Illness, Medications, Allergies, Multiple Births, Prematurity, Special Needs, and Adoption

Along with a Glossary and Resources for Additional Help and Information

Edited by Jenni Lynn Colson. 367 pages. 2002. 978-0-7808-0332-9.

SEE ALSO *Pregnancy and Birth Sourcebook, 2nd Edition*

Burns Sourcebook

Basic Consumer Health Information about Various Types of Burns and Scalds, Including Flame, Heat, Cold, Electrical, Chemical, and Sun Burns

Along with Information on Short-Term and Long-Term Treatments, Tissue Reconstruction, Plastic Surgery, Prevention Suggestions, and First Aid

Edited by Allan R. Cook. 604 pages. 1999. 978-0-7808-0204-9.

"This is an exceptional addition to the series and is highly recommended for all consumer health collections, hospital libraries, and academic medical centers."

—*E-Streams, Mar '00*

"This key reference guide is an invaluable addition to all health care and public libraries in confronting this ongoing health issue."

—*American Reference Books Annual, 2000*

SEE ALSO *Dermatological Disorders Sourcebook, 2nd Edition*

Cancer Sourcebook, 5th Edition

Basic Consumer Health Information about Major Forms and Stages of Cancer, Featuring Facts about Head and Neck Cancers, Lung Cancers, Gastrointestinal Cancers, Genitourinary Cancers, Lymphomas, Blood Cell Cancers, Endocrine Cancers, Skin Cancers, Bone Cancers, Metastatic Cancers, and More

Along with Facts about Cancer Treatments, Cancer Risks and Prevention, a Glossary of Related Terms, Statistical Data, and a Directory of Resources for Additional Information

Edited by Karen Bellenir. 1105 pages. 2007. 978-0-7808-0947-5.

"The 5th, updated edition of *Cancer Sourcebook* should be in every public and health lending library collection... An unparalleled discussion essential for any health collections considering an all-in-one basic general reference."

—*California Bookwatch, Aug '07*

SEE ALSO *Breast Cancer Sourcebook, 3rd Edition, Cancer Sourcebook for Women, 3rd Edition, Cancer Survivorship Sourcebook, Leukemia Sourcebook*

Cancer Sourcebook for Women, 3rd Edition

Basic Consumer Health Information about Leading Causes of Cancer in Women, Featuring Facts about Gynecologic Cancers and Related Concerns, Such as Breast Cancer, Cervical Cancer, Endometrial Cancer, Uterine Sarcoma, Vaginal Cancer, Vulvar Cancer, and Common Non-Cancerous Gynecologic Conditions, in Addition to Facts about Lung Cancer, Colorectal Cancer, and Thyroid Cancer in Women

Along with Information about Cancer Risk Factors, Screening and Prevention, Treatment Options, and Tips on Coping with Life after Cancer Treatment, a Glossary of Cancer Terms, and a Directory of Resources for Additional Help and Information

Edited by Amy L. Sutton. 687 pages. 2006. 978-0-7808-0867-6.

"This excellent book provides the general public with information compiled in a way that will help them to gain the knowledge they need. 4 Stars!"

—*Doody's Review Service, Dec '06*

"An indispensable reference for health consumers and cancer patients. Recommended for public libraries and academic libraries with a medical department."

—*E-Streams, Sep '08*

Cancer Survivorship Sourcebook

Basic Consumer Health Information about the Physical, Educational, Emotional, Social, and Financial Needs of Cancer Patients from Diagnosis, through Cancer Treatment, and Beyond, Including Facts about Researching Specific Types of Cancer and Learning about Clinical Trials and Treatment Options, and Featuring Tips for Coping with the Side Effects of Cancer Treatments and Adjusting to Life after Cancer Treatment Concludes

Along with Suggestions for Caregivers, Friends, and Family Members of Cancer Patients, a Glossary of Cancer Care Terms, and Directories of Related Resources

Edited by Karen Bellenir. 633 pages. 2007. 978-0-7808-0985-7.

"Well organized and comprehensive in coverage, the book speaks to issues encountered both during and after cancer treatment. Recommended for consumer health and public libraries."

—*Library Journal, Aug 1 '07*

"*Cancer Survivorship Sourcebook* will be useful to anyone who has a friend or loved one with a cancer diagnosis."

—*American Reference Books Annual, 2008*

SEE ALSO *Cancer Sourcebook, 5th Edition*

Cardiovascular Diseases and Disorders Sourcebook, 3rd Edition

Basic Consumer Health Information about Heart and Vascular Diseases and Disorders, Such as Angina, Heart Attacks, Arrhythmias, Cardiomyopathy, Valve Disease, Atherosclerosis, and Aneurysms, with Information about Managing Cardiovascular Risk Factors and Maintaining Heart Health, Medications and Procedures Used to Treat Cardiovascular Disorders, and Concerns of Special Significance to Women

Along with Reports on Current Research Initiatives, a Glossary of Related Medical Terms, and a Directory of Sources for Further Help and Information

Edited by Sandra J. Judd. 687 pages. 2005. 978-0-7808-0739-6.

"This updated sourcebook is still the best first stop for comprehensive introductory information on cardiovascular diseases."

—*American Reference Books Annual, 2006*

"Recommended for public libraries and libraries supporting health care professionals."

—*E-Streams, Sep '05*

Caregiving Sourcebook

Basic Consumer Health Information for Caregivers, Including a Profile of Caregivers, Caregiving Responsibilities and Concerns, Tips for Specific Conditions, Care Environments, and the Effects of Caregiving

Along with Facts about Legal Issues, Financial Information, and Future Planning, a Glossary, and a Listing of Additional Resources

Edited by Joyce Brennfleck Shannon. 583 pages. 2001. 978-0-7808-0331-2.

"Essential for most collections."

—*Library Journal, Apr 1 '02*

"An ideal addition to the reference collection of any public library. Health sciences information professionals may also want to acquire the *Caregiving Sourcebook* for their hospital or academic library for use as a ready reference tool by health care workers interested in aging and caregiving."

—*E-Streams, Jan '02*

Child Abuse Sourcebook, 2nd Edition

Basic Consumer Health Information about the Physical, Sexual, and Emotional Abuse of Children, Neglect, Münchhausen Syndrome by Proxy (MSBP), and Shaken Baby Syndrome, and Featuring Facts about Withholding Medical Care, Corporal Punishment, Child Maltreatment in Youth Sports, and Parental Substance Abuse

Along with Information about Child Protective Services, Foster Care, Adoption, Parenting Challenges, Abuse Prevention Programs, and Intervention, Treatment, and Recovery Guidelines, a Glossary of Related Terms, and Resources for Additional Help and Information

Edited by Joyce Brennfleck Shannon. 600 pages. 2009. 978-0-7808-1037-2.

SEE ALSO *Domestic Violence Sourcebook, 3rd Edition*

Childhood Diseases and Disorders Sourcebook, 2nd Edition

Basic Consumer Health Information about the Physical, Mental, and Developmental Health of Pre-Adolescent Children, Including Facts about Infectious Diseases, Asthma, Allergies, Diabetes, and Other Acute and Chronic Conditions Affecting the Gastrointestinal Tract, Ears, Nose, Throat, Liver, Kidneys, Heart, Blood, Brain, Muscles, Bones, and Skin

Along with Reports on Recommended Childhood Vaccinations, Wellness Guidelines, a Glossary of Related Medical Terms, and a List of Resources for Parents

Edited by Sandra J. Judd. 694 pages. 2009. 978-0-7808-1031-0.

SEE ALSO *Healthy Children Sourcebook*

Colds, Flu and Other Common Ailments Sourcebook

Basic Consumer Health Information about Common Ailments and Injuries, Including Colds, Coughs, the Flu, Sinus Problems, Headaches, Fever, Nausea and Vomiting, Menstrual Cramps, Diarrhea, Constipation, Hemorrhoids, Back Pain, Dandruff, Dry and Itchy Skin, Cuts, Scrapes, Sprains, Bruises, and More

Along with Information about Prevention, Self-Care, Choosing a Doctor, Over-the-Counter Medications, Folk Remedies, and Alternative Therapies, and Including a Glossary of Important Terms and a Directory of Resources for Further Help and Information

Edited by Chad T. Kimball. 622 pages. 2001. 978-0-7808-0435-7.

"A good starting point for research on common illnesses. It will be a useful addition to public and consumer health library collections."

—*American Reference Books Annual, 2002*

"Will prove valuable to any library seeking to maintain a current, comprehensive reference collection of health resources. . . Excellent reference."

—*The Bookwatch, Aug '01*

Communication Disorders Sourcebook

Basic Information about Deafness and Hearing Loss, Speech and Language Disorders, Voice Disorders, Balance and Vestibular Disorders, and Disorders of Smell, Taste, and Touch

Edited by Linda M. Ross. 533 pages. 1996. 978-0-7808-0077-9.

"This is skillfully edited and is a welcome resource for the layperson. It should be found in every public and medical library."

—*Booklist Health Sciences Supplement, Oct '97*

Complementary and Alternative Medicine Sourcebook, 3rd Edition

Basic Consumer Health Information about Complementary and Alternative Medical Therapies, Including Acupuncture, Ayurveda, Traditional Chinese Medicine, Herbal Medicine, Homeopathy, Naturopathy, Biofeedback, Hypnotherapy, Yoga, Art Therapy, Aromatherapy, Clinical Nutrition, Vitamin and Mineral Supplements, Chiropractic, Massage, Reflexology, Crystal Therapy, Therapeutic Touch, and More

Along with Facts about Alternative and Complementary Treatments for Specific Conditions Such as Cancer, Diabetes, Osteoarthritis, Chronic Pain, Menopause, Gastrointestinal Disorders, Headaches, and Mental Illness, a Glossary, and a Resource List for Additional Help and Information

Edited by Sandra J. Judd. 630 pages. 2006. 978-0-7808-0864-5.

"A 'must' reference for any serious healthcare collection. Public library holdings, too, will welcome it as a popular reference."

—*California Bookwatch, Oct '06*

"Both basic and informative at the same time. . . a useful resource for health care professionals as well as consumers interested in learning more information about CAM therapies."

—*AORN Journal, Jan '08*

"A quality, indexed, referenced guideline for many alternative practices that are quite popular around the world...It is neatly organized to find facts quickly, is peer-reviewed, and stays current with the most recent advances."

—*Journal of Dental Hygiene, Jul '07*

Congenital Disorders Sourcebook, 2nd Edition

Basic Consumer Health Information about Nonhereditary Birth Defects and Disorders Related to Prematurity, Gestational Injuries, Congenital Infections, and Birth Complications, Including Heart Defects, Hydrocephalus, Spina Bifida, Cleft Lip and Palate, Cerebral Palsy, and More

Along with Facts about the Prevention of Birth Defects, Fetal Surgery and Other Treatment Options, Research Initiatives, a Glossary of Related Terms, and Resources for Additional Information and Support

Edited by Sandra J. Judd. 619 pages. 2007. 978-0-7808-0945-1.

"Congenital Disorders Sourcebook provides an excellent, non-technical overview of many aspects of pregnancy with the focus on congenital disorders."

—*American Reference Books Annual, 2008*

"An excellent readable reference aimed at the lay public for difficult to understand medical problems. An excellent starting point for the interested parent or family member who may then be motivated to seek more information."

—*Doody's Review Service, 2007*

SEE ALSO *Pregnancy and Birth Sourcebook, 2nd Edition*

Contagious Diseases Sourcebook, 2nd Edition

Basic Consumer Health Information about Diseases Spread from Person to Person through Direct Physical Contact, Airborne Transmissions, Sexual Contact, or Contact with Blood or Other Body Fluids, Including Pneumococcal, Staphylococcal, and Streptococcal Diseases, Colds, Influenza, Lice, Measles, Mumps, Tuberculosis, and Others

Along with Facts about Self-Care and Over-the-Counter Medications, Antibiotics and Drug Resistance, Disease Prevention, Vaccines, and Bioterrorism, a Glossary, and a Directory of Resources for More Information

Edited by Joyce Brennfleck Shannon. 600 pages. 2009. 978-0-7808-1075-4.

SEE ALSO *AIDS Sourcebook, 4th Edition, Hepatitis Sourcebook*

Cosmetic and Reconstructive Surgery Sourcebook, 2nd Edition

Basic Consumer Information about Plastic Surgery and Non-Surgical Appearance-Enhancing Procedures, Including Facts about Botulinum Toxin, Collagen Replacement, Dermabrasion,

Chemical Peels, Eyelid Surgery, Nose Reshaping, Lip Augmentation, Liposuction, Breast Enlargement and Reduction, Tummy Tucking, and Other Skin, Hair, Facial, and Body Shaping Procedures

Along with Information about Reconstructive Procedures for Congenital Disorders, Disfiguring Diseases, Burns, and Traumatic Injuries, a Glossary of Related Terms, and a Directory of Additional Resources

Edited by Karen Bellenir. 483 pages. 2007. 978-0-7808-0951-2.

"A practical guide for health care consumers and health care workers. . . . This easy-to-read reference guide would be useful for novice and veteran health care consumers, surgical technology students, nursing students, and perioperative nurses new to plastic and reconstructive surgery. It also may be helpful for medical-surgical nurses as a guide for patient teaching in their practices."

—*AORN Journal, Aug '08*

SEE ALSO *Surgery Sourcebook, 2nd Edition*

Death and Dying Sourcebook, 2nd Edition

Basic Consumer Health Information about End-of-Life Care and Related Perspectives and Ethical Issues, Including End-of-Life Symptoms and Treatments, Pain Management, Quality-of-Life Concerns, the Use of Life Support, Patients' Rights and Privacy Issues, Advance Directives, Physician-Assisted Suicide, Caregiving, Organ and Tissue Donation, Autopsies, Funeral Arrangements, and Grief

Along with Statistical Data, Information about the Leading Causes of Death, a Glossary, and Directories of Support Groups and Other Resources

Edited by Joyce Brennfleck Shannon. 626 pages. 2006. 978-0-7808-0871-3.

Dental Care and Oral Health Sourcebook, 3rd Edition

Basic Consumer Health Information about Dental Care and Oral Health Throughout the Lifespan, Including Facts about Cavities, Bad Breath, Cold and Canker Sores, Dry Mouth, Toothaches, Gum Disease, Malocclusion, Temporomandibular Joint and Muscle Disorders, Oral Cancers, and Dental Emergencies

Along with Information about Mouth Hygiene, Crowns, Bridges, Implants, and Fillings, Surgical, Orthodontic, and Cosmetic Dental Procedures, Pain Management, Health Conditions that Impact Oral Care, a Glossary of Related Terms, and a Directory of Additional Resources

Edited by Amy L. Sutton. 619 pages. 2008. 978-0-7808-1032-7.

Depression Sourcebook, 2nd Edition

Basic Consumer Health Information about Unipolar Depression, Bipolar Disorder, Dysthymia, Seasonal Affective Disorder, Postpartum Depression, and Other Depressive Disorders, Including Facts about Populations at Special Risk, Coexisting Medical Conditions, Symptoms, Treatment Options, and Suicide Prevention

Along with Statistical Data, a Glossary of Related Terms, and a Directory of Resources for Additional Help and Information

Edited by Sandra J. Judd. 646 pages. 2008. 978-0-7808-1003-7.

"Recommended for public libraries."

—*ARBAonline, Nov '08*

SEE ALSO *Mental Health Disorders Sourcebook, 4th Edition*

Dermatological Disorders Sourcebook, 2nd Edition

Basic Consumer Health Information about Conditions and Disorders Affecting the Skin, Hair, and Nails, Such as Acne, Rosacea, Rashes, Dermatitis, Pigmentation Disorders, Birthmarks, Skin Cancer, Skin Injuries, Psoriasis, Scleroderma, and Hair Loss, Including Facts about Medications and Treatments for Dermatological Disorders and Tips for Maintaining Healthy Skin, Hair, and Nails

Along with Information about How Aging Affects the Skin, a Glossary of Related Terms, and a Directory of Resources for Additional Help and Information

Edited by Amy L. Sutton. 617 pages. 2006. 978-0-7808-0795-2.

"Helpfully brings together. . . sources in one convenient place, saving the user hours of research time."
—*American Reference Books Annual, 2006*

SEE ALSO *Burns Sourcebook*

Diabetes Sourcebook, 4th Edition

Basic Consumer Health Information about Type 1 and Type 2 Diabetes Mellitus, Gestational Diabetes, Monogenic Forms of Diabetes, and Insulin Resistance, with Guidelines for Lifestyle Modifications and the Medical Management of Diabetes, Including Facts about Insulin, Insulin Delivery Devices, Oral Diabetes Medications, Self-Monitoring of Blood Glucose, Meal Planning, Physical Activity Recommendations, Foot Care, and Treatment Options for People with Kidney Failure

Along with a Section about Diabetes Complications and Co-Occurring Conditions, a Glossary of Related Terms, and Directories of Resources for Additional Help and Information

Edited by Karen Bellenir. 627 pages. 2008. 978-0-7808-1005-1.

"Completely and comprehensively covering almost everything a student or physician would need to know.... well worth the investment."
—*Internet Bookwatch, Dec '08*

SEE ALSO *Endocrine and Metabolic Disorders Sourcebook, 2nd Edition*

Diet and Nutrition Sourcebook, 3rd Edition

Basic Consumer Health Information about Dietary Guidelines and the Food Guidance System, Recommended Daily Nutrient Intakes, Serving Proportions, Weight Control, Vitamins and Supplements, Nutrition Issues for Different Life Stages and Lifestyles, and the Needs of People with Specific Medical Concerns, Including Cancer, Celiac Disease, Diabetes, Eating Disorders, Food Allergies, and Cardiovascular Disease

Along with Facts about Federal Nutrition Support Programs, a Glossary of Nutrition and Dietary Terms, and Directories of Additional Resources for More Information about Nutrition

Edited by Joyce Brennfleck Shannon. 605 pages. 2006. 978-0-7808-0800-3.

"A valuable resource tool for any individual."
—*Journal of Dental Hygiene, Apr '07*

"From different recommended eating habits to reduce disease and common ailments to nutrition advice for those with specific conditions, *Diet and Nutrition Sourcebook* is especially important because so much is changing in this area, and so rapidly."
—*California Bookwatch, Jun '06*

SEE ALSO *Digestive Diseases and Disorders Sourcebook, Eating Disorders Sourcebook, 2nd Edition, Gastrointestinal Diseases and Disorders Sourcebook, 2nd Edition, Vegetarian Sourcebook*

Digestive Diseases and Disorders Sourcebook

Basic Consumer Health Information about Diseases and Disorders that Impact the Upper and Lower Digestive System, Including Celiac Disease, Constipation, Crohn's Disease, Cyclic Vomiting Syndrome, Diarrhea, Diverticulosis and Diverticulitis, Gallstones, Heartburn, Hemorrhoids, Hernias, Indigestion (Dyspepsia), Irritable Bowel Syndrome, Lactose Intolerance, Ulcers, and More

Along with Information about Medications and Other Treatments, Tips for Maintaining a Healthy Digestive Tract, a Glossary, and Directory of Digestive Diseases Organizations

Edited by Karen Bellenir. 323 pages. 2000. 978-0-7808-0327-5.

"An excellent addition to all public or patient-research libraries."
—*American Reference Books Annual, 2001*

"Recommended reference source."
—*Booklist, May '00*

SEE ALSO *Diet and Nutrition Sourcebook, 3rd Edition, Gastrointestinal Diseases and Disorders Sourcebook, 2nd Edition*

Disabilities Sourcebook

Basic Consumer Health Information about Physical and Psychiatric Disabilities, Including Descriptions of Major Causes of Disability, Assistive and Adaptive Aids, Workplace Issues, and Accessibility Concerns

Along with Information about the Americans with Disabilities Act, a Glossary, and Resources for Additional Help and Information

Edited by Dawn D. Matthews. 602 pages. 2000. 978-0-7808-0389-3.

"A must for libraries with a consumer health section."

—*American Reference Books Annual, 2002*

"A much needed addition to the Omnigraphics *Health Reference Series*. A current reference work to provide people with disabilities, their families, caregivers or those who work with them, a broad range of information in one volume, has not been available until now. . . . It is recommended for all public and academic library reference collections."

—*E-Streams, May '01*

"An excellent source book in easy-to-read format covering many current topics; highly recommended for all libraries."

—*CHOICE, Jan '01*

Disease Management Sourcebook

Basic Consumer Health Information about Coping with Chronic and Serious Illnesses, Navigating the Health Care System, Communicating with Health Care Providers, Assessing Health Care Quality, and Making Informed Health Care Decisions, Including Facts about Second Opinions, Hospitalization, Surgery, and Medications

Along with a Section about Children with Chronic Conditions, Information about Legal, Financial, and Insurance Issues, a Glossary of Related Terms, and Directories of Additional Resources

Edited by Joyce Brennfleck Shannon. 621 pages. 2008. 978-0-7808-1002-0.

"Consumers need to know how to manage their health care the same way they manage anything else in their lives. The text is very readable and is written for the layperson and consumer. The cost is not prohibitive. This book should be in all collections of health care libraries and public libraries."

—*ARBAonline, Jul '08*

"The information is very current, and the selection of font and layout make the book easy to read. A hardback that will stand up to much usage, this is an excellent resource for consumers. . . . Recommended. General readers."

—*CHOICE, Nov '08*

"Intended for lay readers, this resource clarifies the many confusing and overwhelming details associated with chronic disease care. Meticulous and clearly explained, the book even includes diagrams intended to ease comprehension of over-the-counter medication labels. An essential guide to navigating the health-care rapids."

—*Library Journal, Aug '08*

Domestic Violence Sourcebook, 3rd Edition

Basic Consumer Health Information about Warning Signs, Risk Factors, and Health Consequences of Intimate Partner Violence, Sexual Violence and Rape, Stalking, Human Trafficking, Child Maltreatment, Teen Dating Violence, and Elder Abuse

Along with Facts about Victims and Perpetrators, Strategies for Violence Prevention, and Emergency Interventions, Safety Plans, and Financial and Legal Tips for Victims, a Glossary of Related Terms, and Directories of Resources for Additional Information and Support

Edited by Joyce Brennfleck Shannon. 600 pages. 2009. 978-0-7808-1038-9.

SEE ALSO *Child Abuse Sourcebook, 2nd Edition*

Drug Abuse Sourcebook, 2nd Edition

Basic Consumer Health Information about Illicit Substances of Abuse and the Misuse of Prescription and Over-the-Counter Medications, Including Depressants, Hallucinogens, Inhalants, Marijuana, Stimulants, and Anabolic Steroids

Along with Facts about Related Health Risks, Treatment Programs, Prevention Programs, a Glossary of Abuse and Addiction Terms, a Glossary of Drug-Related Street Terms, and a Directory of Resources for More Information

Edited by Catherine Ginther. 581 pages. 2004. 978-0-7808-0740-2.

"Commendable for organizing useful, normally scattered government and association-produced data into a logical sequence."

—*American Reference Books Annual, 2006*

"An excellent library reference."
—*The Bookwatch, May '05*

SEE ALSO *Alcoholism Sourcebook, 2nd Edition*

Ear, Nose, and Throat Disorders Sourcebook, 2nd Edition

Basic Consumer Health Information about Disorders of the Ears, Hearing Loss, Vestibular Disorders, Nasal and Sinus Problems, Throat and Vocal Cord Disorders, and Otolaryngologic Cancers, Including Facts about Ear Infections and Injuries, Genetic and Congenital Deafness, Sensorineural Hearing Disorders, Tinnitus, Vertigo, Ménière Disease, Rhinitis, Sinusitis, Snoring, Sore Throats, Hoarseness, and More

Along with Reports on Current Research Initiatives, a Glossary of Related Medical Terms, and a Directory of Sources for Further Help and Information

Edited by Sandra J. Judd. 631 pages. 2007. 978-0-7808-0872-0.

"A resource book for the general public that provides comprehensive coverage of basic up-to-date medical information about the causes, symptoms, diagnosis, and treatment of diseases and disorders that affect the ears, nose, sinuses, throat, and voice. . . . The majority of information is presented in question and answer format, much like questions a patient might ask of a health care provider. An extensive index facilitates the reader's ability to easily access information on any specific topic."
—*Journal of Dental Hygiene, Oct '07*

"A handy compilation of information on common and some not so common ailments of the ears, nose, and throat."
—*Doody's Review Service, 2007*

Eating Disorders Sourcebook, 2nd Edition

Basic Consumer Health Information about Anorexia Nervosa, Bulimia, Binge Eating, Compulsive Exercise, Female Athlete Triad, and Other Eating Disorders, Including Facts about Body Image and Other Cultural and Age-Related Risk Factors, Prevention Efforts, Adverse Health Effects, Treatment Options, and the Recovery Process

Along with Guidelines for Healthy Weight Control, a Glossary, and Directories of Additional Resources

Edited by Joyce Brennfleck Shannon. 557 pages. 2007. 978-0-7808-0948-2.

"Recommended for the reference collection of large public libraries."
—*American Reference Books Annual, 2008*

"A basic health reference any health or general library needs."
—*Internet Bookwatch, Jun '07*

SEE ALSO *Diet and Nutrition Sourcebook, 3rd Edition, Mental Health Disorders Sourcebook, 4th Edition*

Emergency Medical Services Sourcebook

Basic Consumer Health Information about Preventing, Preparing for, and Managing Emergency Situations, When and Who to Call for Help, What to Expect in the Emergency Room, the Emergency Medical Team, Patient Issues, and Current Topics in Emergency Medicine

Along with Statistical Data, a Glossary, and Sources of Additional Help and Information

Edited by Jenni Lynn Colson. 472 pages. 2002. 978-0-7808-0420-3.

"Handy and convenient for home, public, school, and college libraries. Recommended."
—*CHOICE, Apr '03*

"This reference can provide the consumer with answers to most questions about emergency care in the United States, or it will direct them to a resource where the answer can be found."
—*American Reference Books Annual, 2003*

SEE ALSO *Injury and Trauma Sourcebook*

Endocrine and Metabolic Disorders Sourcebook, 2nd Edition

Basic Consumer Health Information about Hormonal and Metabolic Disorders that Affect the Body's Growth, Development, and Functioning, Including Disorders of the Pancreas, Ovaries and Testes, and Pituitary, Thyroid, Parathyroid, and Adrenal Glands, with Facts about Growth Disorders, Addison Disease, Cushing Syndrome, Conn Syndrome, Diabetic Disorders, Multiple Endocrine Neoplasia, Inborn Errors of Metabolism, and More

Along with Information about Endocrine Functioning, Diagnostic and Screening Tests, a Glossary of Related Terms, and Directories of Additional Resources

Edited by Joyce Brennfleck Shannon. 597 pages. 2007. 978-0-7808-0952-9.

SEE ALSO *Diabetes Sourcebook, 4th Edition*

Environmental Health Sourcebook, 2nd Edition

Basic Consumer Health Information about the Environment and Its Effect on Human Health, Including the Effects of Air Pollution, Water Pollution, Hazardous Chemicals, Food Hazards, Radiation Hazards, Biological Agents, Household Hazards, Such as Radon, Asbestos, Carbon Monoxide, and Mold, and Information about Associated Diseases and Disorders, Including Cancer, Allergies, Respiratory Problems, and Skin Disorders

Along with Information about Environmental Concerns for Specific Populations, a Glossary of Related Terms, and Resources for Further Help and Information

Edited by Dawn D. Matthews. 650 pages. 2003. 978-0-7808-0632-0.

"Recommended for teenage and adult students and readers, and for public and academic libraries, as well as any library focusing on consumer health."

—*E-Streams, May '04*

"This recently updated edition continues the level of quality and the reputation of the numerous other volumes in Omnigraphics' *Health Reference Series.*"

—*American Reference Books Annual, 2004*

Ethnic Diseases Sourcebook

Basic Consumer Health Information for Ethnic and Racial Minority Groups in the United States, Including General Health Indicators and Behaviors, Ethnic Diseases, Genetic Testing, the Impact of Chronic Diseases, Women's Health, Mental Health Issues, and Preventive Health Care Services

Along with a Glossary and a Listing of Additional Resources

Edited by Joyce Brennfleck Shannon. 648 pages. 2001. 978-0-7808-0336-7.

"Not many books have been written on this topic to date, and the *Ethnic Diseases Sourcebook* is a strong addition to the list. It will be an important introductory resource for health consumers, students, health care personnel, and social scientists. It is recommended for public, academic, and large hospital libraries."

—*American Reference Books Annual, 2002*

"Will prove valuable to any library seeking to maintain a current, comprehensive reference collection of health resources. . . . An excellent source of health information about genetic disorders which affect particular ethnic and racial minorities in the U.S."

—*The Bookwatch, Aug '01*

Eye Care Sourcebook, 3rd Edition

Basic Consumer Health Information about Eye Care and Eye Disorders, Including Facts about the Diagnosis, Prevention, and Treatment of Refractive Disorders, Cataracts, Glaucoma, Macular Degeneration, and Problems Affecting the Cornea, Retina, and Lacrimal Glands

Along with Advice about Preventing Eye Injuries and Tips for Living with Low Vision or Blindness, a Glossary of Related Terms, and Directories of Resources for More Help and Information

Edited by Amy L. Sutton. 646 pages. 2008. 978-0-7808-1000-6.

Family Planning Sourcebook

Basic Consumer Health Information about Planning for Pregnancy and Contraception, Including Traditional Methods, Barrier Methods, Hormonal Methods, Permanent Methods, Future Methods, Emergency Contraception, and Birth Control Choices for Women at Each Stage of Life

Along with Statistics, a Glossary, and Sources of Additional Information

Edited by Amy Marcaccio Keyzer. 503 pages. 2001. 978-0-7808-0379-4.

"Recommended for public, health, and undergraduate libraries as part of the circulating collection."

—*E-Streams, Mar '02*

"Will prove valuable to any library seeking to maintain a current, comprehensive reference collection of health resources. . . . Excellent reference."

—*The Bookwatch, Aug '01*

SEE ALSO *Pregnancy and Birth Sourcebook, 2nd Edition*

Fitness and Exercise Sourcebook, 3rd Edition

Basic Consumer Health Information about the Physical and Mental Benefits of Fitness, Including Cardiorespiratory Endurance, Muscular Strength, Muscular Endurance, and Flexibility, with Facts about Sports Nutrition and Exercise-Related Injuries and Tips about Physical Activity and Exercises for People of All Ages and for People with Health Concerns

Along with Advice on Selecting and Using Exercise Equipment, Maintaining Exercise Motivation, a Glossary of Related Terms, and a Directory of Resources for More Help and Information

Edited by Amy L. Sutton. 635 pages. 2007. 978-0-7808-0946-8.

"Updates the consumer information on the physical and mental benefits of physical activity throughout the lifespan offered in earlier editions. . . . Recommended. All readers; all levels."

—*CHOICE, Oct '07*

"An exceptionally well-rounded coverage perfect for any concerned about developing and understanding a fitness program."

—*California Bookwatch, Jun '07*

SEE ALSO *Sports Injuries Sourcebook, 3rd Edition*

Food Safety Sourcebook

Basic Consumer Health Information about the Safe Handling of Meat, Poultry, Seafood, Eggs, Fruit Juices, and Other Food Items, and Facts about Pesticides, Drinking Water, Food Safety Overseas, and the Onset, Duration, and Symptoms of Foodborne Illnesses, Including Types of Pathogenic Bacteria, Parasitic Protozoa, Worms, Viruses, and Natural Toxins

Along with the Role of the Consumer, the Food Handler, and the Government in Food Safety; a Glossary, and Resources for Additional Help and Information

Edited by Dawn D. Matthews. 327 pages. 1999. 978-0-7808-0326-8.

"Recommended reference source."

—*Booklist, May '00*

"This book takes the complex issues of food safety and foodborne pathogens and presents them in an easily understood manner. [It does] an excellent job of covering a large and often confusing topic."

— *American Reference Books Annual, 2000*

Forensic Medicine Sourcebook

Basic Consumer Information for the Layperson about Forensic Medicine, Including Crime Scene Investigation, Evidence Collection and Analysis, Expert Testimony, Computer-Aided Criminal Identification, Digital Imaging in the Courtroom, DNA Profiling, Accident Reconstruction, Autopsies, Ballistics, Drugs and Explosives Detection, Latent Fingerprints, Product Tampering, and Questioned Document Examination

Along with Statistical Data, a Glossary of Forensics Terminology, and Listings of Sources for Further Help and Information

Edited by Annemarie S. Muth. 574 pages. 1999. 978-0-7808-0232-2.

"Given the expected widespread interest in its content and its easy to read style, this book is recommended for most public and all college and university libraries."

—*E-Streams, Feb '01*

"A wealth of information, useful statistics, references are up-to-date and extremely complete. This wonderful collection of data will help students who are interested in a career in any type of forensic field. It is a great resource for attorneys who need information about types of expert witnesses needed in a particular case. It also offers useful information for fiction and nonfiction writers whose work involves a crime. A fascinating compilation. All levels."

—*CHOICE, Jan '00*

"There are several items that make this book attractive to consumers who are seeking certain forensic data. . . . This is a useful current

source for those seeking general forensic medical answers."

—*American Reference Books Annual, 2000*

Gastrointestinal Diseases and Disorders Sourcebook, 2nd Edition

Basic Consumer Health Information about the Upper and Lower Gastrointestinal (GI) Tract, Including the Esophagus, Stomach, Intestines, Rectum, Liver, and Pancreas, with Facts about Gastroesophageal Reflux Disease, Gastritis, Hernias, Ulcers, Celiac Disease, Diverticulitis, Irritable Bowel Syndrome, Hemorrhoids, Gastrointestinal Cancers, and Other Diseases and Disorders Related to the Digestive Process

Along with Information about Commonly Used Diagnostic and Surgical Procedures, Statistics, Reports on Current Research Initiatives and Clinical Trials, a Glossary, and Resources for Additional Help and Information

Edited by Sandra J. Judd. 654 pages. 2006. 978-0-7808-0798-3.

"The text is designed for the general reader seeking information on prevention, disease warning signs, diagnostic and therapeutic questions. . . . It is an excellent resource for the general reader to conveniently locate credible, coordinated and indexed information. . . . The sourcebook will prove very helpful for patients, caregivers and should be available in every physician waiting room."

—*Doody's Review Service, 2006*

SEE ALSO *Diet and Nutrition Sourcebook, 3rd Edition, Digestive Diseases and Disorders Sourcebook*

Genetic Disorders Sourcebook, 4th Edition

Basic Consumer Health Information about Hereditary Diseases and Disorders, Including Facts about the Human Genome, Genetic Inheritance Patterns, Disorders Associated with Specific Genes, Such as Sickle Cell Disease, Hemophilia, and Cystic Fibrosis, Chromosome Disorders, Such as Down Syndrome, Fragile X Syndrome, and Turner Syndrome, and Complex Diseases and Disorders Resulting from the Interaction of Environmental and Genetic Factors, Such as Allergies, Cancer, and Obesity

Along with Facts about Genetic Testing, Suggestions for Parents of Children with Special Needs, Reports on Current Research Initiatives, a Glossary of Genetic Terminology, and Resources for Additional Help and Information

Edited by Sandra J. Judd. 600 pages. 2009. 978-0-7808-1076-1.

Head Trauma Sourcebook

Basic Information for the Layperson about Open-Head and Closed-Head Injuries, Treatment Advances, Recovery, and Rehabilitation

Along with Reports on Current Research Initiatives

Edited by Karen Bellenir. 414 pages. 1997. 978-0-7808-0208-7.

Headache Sourcebook

Basic Consumer Health Information about Migraine, Tension, Cluster, Rebound and Other Types of Headaches, with Facts about the Cause and Prevention of Headaches, the Effects of Stress and the Environment, Headaches during Pregnancy and Menopause, and Childhood Headaches

Along with a Glossary and Other Resources for Additional Help and Information

Edited by Dawn D. Matthews. 342 pages. 2002. 978-0-7808-0337-4.

"Highly recommended for academic and medical reference collections."

—*Library Bookwatch, Sep '02*

SEE ALSO *Pain Sourcebook, 3rd Edition*

Healthy Aging Sourcebook

Basic Consumer Health Information about Maintaining Health through the Aging Process, Including Advice on Nutrition, Exercise, and Sleep, Help in Making Decisions about Midlife Issues and Retirement, and Guidance Concerning Practical and Informed Choices in Health Consumerism

Along with Data Concerning the Theories of Aging, Different Experiences in Aging by Minority Groups, and Facts about Aging Now and Aging in the Future; and Featuring a Glossary, a Guide to Consumer Help, Additional Suggested Reading, and Practical Resource Directory

Edited by Jenifer Swanson. 537 pages. 1999. 978-0-7808-0390-9.

"Recommended reference source."

—*Booklist, Feb '00*

SEE ALSO *Physical and Mental Issues in Aging Sourcebook*

Healthy Children Sourcebook

Basic Consumer Health Information about the Physical and Mental Development of Children between the Ages of 3 and 12, Including Routine Health Care, Preventative Health Services, Safety and First Aid, Healthy Sleep, Dental Care, Nutrition, and Fitness, and Featuring Parenting Tips on Such Topics as Bedwetting, Choosing Day Care, Monitoring TV and Other Media, and Establishing a Foundation for Substance Abuse Prevention

Along with a Glossary of Commonly Used Pediatric Terms and Resources for Additional Help and Information.

Edited by Chad T. Kimball. 624 pages. 2003. 978-0-7808-0247-6.

"Should be required reading for parents and teachers."

—*E-Streams, Jun '04*

"It is hard to imagine that any other single resource exists that would provide such a comprehensive guide of timely information on health promotion and disease prevention for children aged 3 to 12."

—*American Reference Books Annual, 2004*

"This easy-to-read volume is a tremendous resource."

—*AORN Journal, May '05*

SEE ALSO *Childhood Diseases and Disorders Sourcebook, 2nd Edition*

Healthy Heart Sourcebook for Women

Basic Consumer Health Information about Cardiac Issues Specific to Women, Including Facts about Major Risk Factors and Prevention, Treatment and Control Strategies, and Important Dietary Issues

Along with a Special Section Regarding the Pros and Cons of Hormone Replacement Therapy and Its Impact on Heart Health, and Additional Help, Including Recipes, a Glossary, and a Directory of Resources

Edited by Dawn D. Matthews. 321 pages. 2000. 978-0-7808-0329-9.

"A good reference source and recommended for all public, academic, medical, and hospital libraries."

—*Medical Reference Services Quarterly, Summer '01*

"Contains very important information about coronary artery disease that all women should know. The information is current and presented in an easy-to-read format. The book will make a good addition to any library."

—*American Medical Writers Association Journal, Summer '00*

SEE ALSO *Cardiovascular Diseases and Disorders Sourcebook, 3rd Edition, Women's Health Concerns Sourcebook, 3rd Edition*

Hepatitis Sourcebook

Basic Consumer Health Information about Hepatitis A, Hepatitis B, Hepatitis C, and Other Forms of Hepatitis, Including Autoimmune Hepatitis, Alcoholic Hepatitis, Nonalcoholic Steatohepatitis, and Toxic Hepatitis, with Facts about Risk Factors, Screening Methods, Diagnostic Tests, and Treatment Options

Along with Information on Liver Health, Tips for People Living with Chronic Hepatitis, Reports on Current Research Initiatives, a Glossary of Terms Related to Hepatitis, and a Directory of Sources for Further Help and Information

Edited by Sandra J. Judd. 570 pages. 2006. 978-0-7808-0749-5.

"The breadth of information found in this one book would not be readily found in another source. Highly recommended."

—*American Reference Books Annual, 2006*

SEE ALSO *Contagious Diseases Sourcebook*

Household Safety Sourcebook

Basic Consumer Health Information about Household Safety, Including Information about Poisons, Chemicals, Fire, and Water Hazards in the Home

Along with Advice about the Safe Use of Home Maintenance Equipment, Choosing Toys and Nursery Furniture, Holiday and Recreation Safety, a Glossary, and Resources for Further Help and Information

Edited by Dawn D. Matthews. 587 pages. 2002. 978-0-7808-0338-1.

"As a sourcebook on household safety this book meets its mark. It is encyclopedic in scope and covers a wide range of safety issues that are commonly seen in the home."

—*E-Streams, Jul '02*

Hypertension Sourcebook

Basic Consumer Health Information about the Causes, Diagnosis, and Treatment of High Blood Pressure, with Facts about Consequences, Complications, and Co-Occurring Disorders, Such as Coronary Heart Disease, Diabetes, Stroke, Kidney Disease, and Hypertensive Retinopathy, and Issues in Blood Pressure Control, Including Dietary Choices, Stress Management, and Medications

Along with Reports on Current Research Initiatives and Clinical Trials, a Glossary, and Resources for Additional Help and Information

Edited by Dawn D. Matthews and Karen Bellenir. 588 pages. 2004. 978-0-7808-0674-0.

"Academic, public, and medical libraries will want to add the *Hypertension Sourcebook* to their collections."

—*E-Streams, Aug '05*

"The strength of this source is the wide range of information given about hypertension."

—*American Reference Books Annual, 2005*

SEE ALSO *Stroke Sourcebook, 2nd Edition*

Immune System Disorders Sourcebook, 2nd Edition

Basic Consumer Health Information about Disorders of the Immune System, Including Immune System Function and Response, Diagnosis of Immune Disorders, Information about Inherited Immune Disease, Acquired Immune Disease, and Autoimmune Diseases, Including Primary Immune Deficiency, Acquired Immunodeficiency Syndrome (AIDS), Lupus, Multiple Sclerosis, Type 1 Diabetes, Rheumatoid Arthritis, and Graves' Disease

Along with Treatments, Tips for Coping with Immune Disorders, a Glossary, and a Directory of Additional Resources

Edited by Joyce Brennfleck Shannon. 643 pages. 2005. 978-0-7808-0748-8.

"Highly recommended for academic and public libraries."

—*American Reference Books Annual, 2006*

"The updated second edition is a 'must' for any consumer health library seeking a solid resource covering the treatments, symptoms, and options for immune disorder sufferers. . . . An excellent guide."

—*MBR Bookwatch, Jan '06*

SEE ALSO *AIDS Sourcebook, 4th Edition, Arthritis Sourcebook, 2nd Edition*

Infant and Toddler Health Sourcebook

Basic Consumer Health Information about the Physical and Mental Development of Newborns, Infants, and Toddlers, Including Neonatal Concerns, Nutrition Recommendations, Immunization Schedules, Common Pediatric Disorders, Assessments and Milestones, Safety Tips, and Advice for Parents and Other Caregivers

Along with a Glossary of Terms and Resource Listings for Additional Help

Edited by Jenifer Swanson. 570 pages. 2000. 978-0-7808-0246-9.

"As a reference for the general public, this would be useful in any library."

—*E-Streams, May '01*

"Recommended reference source."

—*Booklist, Feb '01*

Infectious Diseases Sourcebook

Basic Consumer Health Information about Non-Contagious Bacterial, Viral, Prion, Fungal, and Parasitic Diseases Spread by Food and Water, Insects and Animals, or Environmental Contact, Including Botulism, E. Coli, Encephalitis, Legionnaires' Disease, Lyme Disease, Malaria, Plague, Rabies, Salmonella, Tetanus, and Others, and Facts about Newly Emerging Diseases, Such as Hantavirus, Mad Cow Disease, Monkeypox, and West Nile Virus

Along with Information about Preventing Disease Transmission, the Threat of Bioterrorism, and Current Research Initiatives, with a Glossary and Directory of Resources for More Information

Edited by Karen Bellenir. 610 pages. 2004. 978-0-7808-0675-7.

"This reference continues the excellent tradition of the *Health Reference Series* in consolidating a wealth of information on a selected topic into a format that is easy to use and accessible to the general public."

—American Reference Books Annual, 2005

"Recommended for public and academic libraries."

—E-Streams, Jan '05

Injury and Trauma Sourcebook

Basic Consumer Health Information about the Impact of Injury, the Diagnosis and Treatment of Common and Traumatic Injuries, Emergency Care, and Specific Injuries Related to Home, Community, Workplace, Transportation, and Recreation

Along with Guidelines for Injury Prevention, a Glossary, and a Directory of Additional Resources

Edited by Joyce Brennfleck Shannon. 675 pages. 2002. 978-0-7808-0421-0.

"Practitioners should be aware of guides such as this in order to facilitate their use by patients and their families."

—Doody's Health Sciences Book Review Journal, Sep-Oct '02

"Recommended reference source."

—Booklist, Sep '02

"Highly recommended for academic and medical reference collections."

—Library Bookwatch, Sep '02

SEE ALSO *Emergency Medical Services Sourcebook, Sports Injuries Sourcebook, 3rd Edition*

Learning Disabilities Sourcebook, 3rd Edition

Basic Consumer Health Information about Dyslexia, Auditory and Visual Processing Disorders, Communication Disorders, Dyscalculia, Dysgraphia, and Other Conditions That Impede Learning, Including Attention Deficit/Hyperactivity Disorder, Autism Spectrum Disorders, Hearing and Visual Impairments, Chromosome-Based Disorders, and Brain Injury

Along with Facts about Brain Function, Assessment, Therapy and Remediation, Accommodations, Assistive Technology, Legal Protections, and Tips about Family Life, School Transitions, and Employment Strategies, a Glossary of Related Terms, and Directories of Additional Resources

Edited by Joyce Brennfleck Shannon. 613 pages. 2009. 978-0-7808-1039-6.

SEE ALSO *Attention Deficit Disorder Sourcebook, Autism and Pervasive Developmental Disorders Sourcebook*

Leukemia Sourcebook

Basic Consumer Health Information about Adult and Childhood Leukemias, Including Acute Lymphocytic Leukemia (ALL), Chronic Lymphocytic Leukemia (CLL), Acute Myelogenous Leukemia (AML), Chronic Myelogenous Leukemia (CML), and Hairy Cell Leukemia, and Treatments Such as Chemotherapy, Radiation Therapy, Peripheral Blood Stem Cell and Marrow Transplantation, and Immunotherapy

Along with Tips for Life During and After Treatment, a Glossary, and Directories of Additional Resources

Edited by Joyce Brennfleck Shannon. 564 pages. 2003. 978-0-7808-0627-6.

"Unlike other medical books for the layperson, . . . the language does not talk down to the reader. . . . This volume is highly recommended for all libraries."

—American Reference Books Annual, 2004

"A fine title which ranges from diagnosis to alternative treatments, staging, and tips for life during and after diagnosis."

—The Bookwatch, Dec '03

SEE ALSO *Cancer Sourcebook, 5th Edition*

Liver Disorders Sourcebook

Basic Consumer Health Information about the Liver and How It Works; Liver Diseases, Including Cancer, Cirrhosis, Hepatitis, and Toxic and Drug Related Diseases; Tips for Maintaining a Healthy Liver; Laboratory Tests, Radiology Tests, and Facts about Liver Transplantation

Along with a Section on Support Groups, a Glossary, and Resource Listings

Edited by Joyce Brennfleck Shannon. 580 pages. 2000. 978-0-7808-0383-1.

"This title is recommended for health sciences and public libraries with consumer health collections."

—*E-Streams, Oct '00*

"Recommended reference source."

—*Booklist, Jun '00*

SEE ALSO *Gastrointestinal Diseases and Disorders Sourcebook, 2nd Edition, Hepatitis Sourcebook*

Lung Disorders Sourcebook

Basic Consumer Health Information about Emphysema, Pneumonia, Tuberculosis, Asthma, Cystic Fibrosis, and Other Lung Disorders, Including Facts about Diagnostic Procedures, Treatment Strategies, Disease Prevention Efforts, and Such Risk Factors as Smoking, Air Pollution, and Exposure to Asbestos, Radon, and Other Agents

Along with a Glossary and Resources for Additional Help and Information

Edited by Dawn D. Matthews. 657 pages. 2002. 978-0-7808-0339-8.

"Highly recommended for academic and medical reference collections."

—*Library Bookwatch, Sep '02*

SEE ALSO *Respiratory Disorders Sourcebook, 2nd Edition*

Medical Tests Sourcebook, 3rd Edition

Basic Consumer Health Information about X-Rays, Blood Tests, Stool and Urine Tests, Biopsies, Mammography, Endoscopic Procedures, Ultrasound Exams, Computed Tomography, Magnetic Resonance Imaging (MRI), Nuclear Medicine, Genetic Testing, Home-Use Tests, and More

Along with Facts about Preventive Care and Screening Test Guidelines, Screening and Assessment Tests Associated with Such Specific Concerns as Cancer, Heart Disease, Allergies, Diabetes, Thyroid Disfunction, and Infertility, a Glossary of Related Terms, and a Directory of Resources for Additional Help and Information

Edited by Karen Bellenir. 627 pages. 2008. 978-0-7808-1040-2

"This volume has a wide scope that makes it useful . . . Can be a valuable reference guide."

—*ARBAonline, Nov '08*

Men's Health Concerns Sourcebook, 3rd Edition

Basic Consumer Health Information about Wellness in Men and Gender-Related Differences in Health, With Facts about Heart Disease, Cancer, Traumatic Injury, and Other Leading Causes of Death in Men, Reproductive Concerns, Sexual Dysfunction, Disorders of the Prostate, Penis, and Testes, Sex-Linked Genetic Disorders, and Other Medical and Mental Concerns of Men

Along with Statistical Data, a Glossary of Related Terms, and a Directory of Resources for Additional Information

Edited by Sandra J. Judd. 600 pages. 2009. 978-0-7808-1033-4.

SEE ALSO *Prostate and Urological Disorders Sourcebook*

Mental Health Disorders Sourcebook, 4th Edition

Basic Consumer Health Information about the Causes and Symptoms of Mental Health Problems, Including Depression, Bipolar Disorder, Anxiety Disorders, Posttraumatic Stress Disorder, Obsessive-Compulsive Disorder, Eating Disorders, Addictions, and Personality and Psychotic Disorders

Along with Information about Medications and Treatments, Mental Health Concerns in Children, Adolescents, and Adults, Tips on Living with Mental Health Disorders, a Glossary of Related Terms, and a Directory of Resources for Additional Help and Information

Edited by Amy L. Sutton. 600 pages. 2009. 978-0-7808-1041-9.

SEE ALSO *Depression Sourcebook, 2nd Edition, Stress-Related Disorders Sourcebook, 2nd Edition*

Mental Retardation Sourcebook

Basic Consumer Health Information about Mental Retardation and Its Causes, Including

Down Syndrome, Fetal Alcohol Syndrome, Fragile X Syndrome, Genetic Conditions, Injury, and Environmental Sources

Along with Preventive Strategies, Parenting Issues, Educational Implications, Health Care Needs, Employment and Economic Matters, Legal Issues, a Glossary, and a Resource Listing for Additional Help and Information

Edited by Joyce Brennfleck Shannon. 627 pages. 2000. 978-0-7808-0377-0.

"Public libraries will find the book useful for reference and as a beginning research point for students, parents, and caregivers."
—*American Reference Books Annual, 2001*

"The strength of this work is that it compiles many basic fact sheets and addresses for further information in one volume. It is intended and suitable for the general public."
—*E-Streams, Nov '00*

"An invaluable overview."
—*Reviewer's Bookwatch, Jul '00*

Movement Disorders Sourcebook, 2nd Edition

Basic Consumer Health Information about the Symptoms and Causes of Movement Disorders, Including Parkinson Disease, Amyotrophic Lateral Sclerosis, Cerebral Palsy, Muscular Dystrophy, Multiple Sclerosis, Myasthenia, Myoclonus, Spina Bifida, Dystonia, Essential Tremor, Choreatic Disorders, Huntington Disease, Tourette Syndrome, and Other Disorders That Cause Slowed, Absent, or Excessive Movements

Along with Information about Surgical and Nonsurgical Interventions, Physical Therapies, Strategies for Independent Living, a Glossary of Related Terms, and a Directory of Resources for Additional Help and Information

Edited by Amy L. Sutton. 600 pages. 2009. 978-0-7808-1034-1.

SEE ALSO *Multiple Sclerosis Sourcebook, Muscular Dystrophy Sourcebook*

Multiple Sclerosis Sourcebook

Basic Consumer Health Information about Multiple Sclerosis (MS) and Its Effects on Mobility, Vision, Bladder Function, Speech, Swallowing, and Cognition, Including Facts about Risk Factors, Causes, Diagnostic Procedures, Pain Management, Drug Treatments, and Physical and Occupational Therapies

Along with Guidelines for Nutrition and Exercise, Tips on Choosing Assistive Equipment, Information about Disability, Work, Financial, and Legal Issues, a Glossary of Related Terms, and a Directory of Additional Resources

Edited by Joyce Brennfleck Shannon. 553 pages. 2007. 978-0-7808-0998-7.

SEE ALSO *Movement Disorders Sourcebook, 2nd Edition*

Muscular Dystrophy Sourcebook

Basic Consumer Health Information about Congenital, Childhood-Onset, and Adult-Onset Forms of Muscular Dystrophy, Such as Duchenne, Becker, Emery-Dreifuss, Distal, Limb-Girdle, Facioscapulohumeral (FSHD), Myotonic, and Ophthalmoplegic Muscular Dystrophies, Including Facts about Diagnostic Tests, Medical and Physical Therapies, Management of Co-Occurring Conditions, and Parenting Guidelines

Along with Practical Tips for Home Care, a Glossary, and Directories of Additional Resources

Edited by Joyce Brennfleck Shannon. 552 pages. 2004. 978-0-7808-0676-4.

"This book is highly recommended for public and academic libraries as well as health care offices that support the information needs of patients and their families."
—*E-Streams, Apr '05*

"Excellent reference."
—*The Bookwatch, Jan '05*

SEE ALSO *Movement Disorders Sourcebook, 2nd Edition*

Obesity Sourcebook

Basic Consumer Health Information about Diseases and Other Problems Associated with Obesity, and Including Facts about Risk Factors, Prevention Issues, and Management Approaches

Along with Statistical and Demographic Data, Information about Special Populations,

Research Updates, a Glossary, and Source Listings for Further Help and Information

Edited by Wilma Caldwell and Chad T. Kimball. 360 pages. 2001. 978-0-7808-0333-6.

"The book synthesizes the reliable medical literature on obesity into one easy-to-read and useful resource for the general public."
—*American Reference Books Annual, 2002*

"Well suited for the health reference collection of a public library or an academic health science library that serves the general population."
—*E-Streams, Sep '01*

Osteoporosis Sourcebook

Basic Consumer Health Information about Primary and Secondary Osteoporosis and Juvenile Osteoporosis and Related Conditions, Including Fibrous Dysplasia, Gaucher Disease, Hyperthyroidism, Hypophosphatasia, Myeloma, Osteopetrosis, Osteogenesis Imperfecta, and Paget's Disease

Along with Information about Risk Factors, Treatments, Traditional and Non-Traditional Pain Management, a Glossary of Related Terms, and a Directory of Resources

Edited by Allan R. Cook. 568 pages. 2001. 978-0-7808-0239-1.

"This resource is recommended as a great reference source for public, health, and academic libraries, and is another triumph for the editors of Omnigraphics."
—*American Reference Books Annual, 2002*

"Will prove valuable to any library seeking to maintain a current, comprehensive reference collection of health resources. . . . From prevention to treatment and associated conditions, this provides an excellent survey."
—*The Bookwatch, Aug '01*

SEE ALSO *Healthy Aging Sourcebook, Women's Health Concerns Sourcebook, 3rd Edition*

Pain Sourcebook, 3rd Edition

Basic Consumer Health Information about Acute and Chronic Pain, Including Nerve Pain, Bone Pain, Muscle Pain, Cancer Pain, and Disorders Characterized by Pain, Such as Arthritis, Temporomandibular Muscle and Joint (TMJ) Disorder, Carpal Tunnel Syndrome, Headaches, Heartburn, Sciatica, and Shingles, and Facts about Diagnostic Tests and Treatment Options for Pain, Including Over-the-Counter and Prescription Drugs, Physical Rehabilitation, Injection and Infusion Therapies, Implantable Technologies, and Complementary Medicine

Along with Tips for Living with Pain, a Glossary of Related Terms, and a Directory of Additional Resources

Edited by Joyce Brennfleck Shannon. 644 pages. 2008. 978-0-7808-1006-8.

"Excellent for ready-reference users and can be used for beginning students in health fields . . . appropriate for the consumer health collection in both public and academic libraries."
—*ARBAonline, Nov '08*

Pediatric Cancer Sourcebook

Basic Consumer Health Information about Leukemias, Brain Tumors, Sarcomas, Lymphomas, and Other Cancers in Infants, Children, and Adolescents, Including Descriptions of Cancers, Treatments, and Coping Strategies

Along with Suggestions for Parents, Caregivers, and Concerned Relatives, a Glossary of Cancer Terms, and Resource Listings

Edited by Edward J. Prucha. 575 pages. 1999. 978-0-7808-0245-2.

"An excellent source of information. Recommended for public, hospital, and health science libraries with consumer health collections."
—*E-Streams, Jun '00*

"A valuable addition to all libraries specializing in health services and many public libraries."
—*American Reference Books Annual, 2000*

SEE ALSO *Childhood Diseases and Disorders Sourcebook, 2nd Edition, Healthy Children Sourcebook*

Physical and Mental Issues in Aging Sourcebook

Basic Consumer Health Information on Physical and Mental Disorders Associated with the Aging Process, Including Concerns about Cardiovascular Disease, Pulmonary Disease, Oral Health, Digestive Disorders, Musculoskeletal and Skin Disorders, Metabolic

Changes, Sexual and Reproductive Issues, and Changes in Vision, Hearing, and Other Senses

Along with Data about Longevity and Causes of Death, Information on Acute and Chronic Pain, Descriptions of Mental Concerns, a Glossary of Terms, and Resource Listings for Additional Help

Edited by Jenifer Swanson. 660 pages. 1999. 978-0-7808-0233-9.

"This is a treasure of health information for the layperson."
—*CHOICE Health Sciences Supplement, May '00*

"Recommended for public libraries."
—*American Reference Books Annual, 2000*

SEE ALSO *Healthy Aging Sourcebook*

Podiatry Sourcebook, 2nd Edition

Basic Consumer Health Information about Disorders, Diseases, and Deformities that Affect the Foot and Ankle, Including Sprains, Corns, Calluses, Bunions, Plantar Warts, Plantar Fasciitis, Neuromas, Clubfoot, Flat Feet, Achilles Tendonitis, and Much More

Along with Information about Selecting a Foot Care Specialist, Foot Fitness, Shoes and Socks, Diagnostic Tests and Corrective Procedures, Financial Assistance for Corrective Devices, a Glossary of Related Terms, and a Directory of Resources for Additional Help and Information

Edited by Ivy L. Alexander. 516 pages. 2007. 978-0-7808-0944-4.

"An excellent resource. . . . Although there have been various types of 'foot books' published in the past, none are as comprehensive as this one. 5 Stars (out of 5)!"
—*Doody's Review Service, 2007*

"Perfect for both health libraries and general-interest lending collections."
—*Internet Bookwatch, Jul '07*

Pregnancy and Birth Sourcebook, 3rd Edition

Basic Consumer Health Information about Pregnancy and Fetal Development, Including Facts about Fertility and Conception, Physical and Emotional Changes during Pregnancy, Prenatal Care and Diagnostic Tests, High-Risk Pregnancies and Complications, Labor, Delivery, and the Postpartum Period

Along with Tips on Maintaining Health and Wellness during Pregnancy and Caring for Newborn Infants, a Glossary of Related Terms, and Directories of Resources for Additional Help and Information

Edited by Amy L. Sutton. 600 pages. 2009. 978-0-7808-1074-7.

SEE ALSO *Breastfeeding Sourcebook, Congenital Disorders Sourcebook, 2nd Edition, Family Planning Sourcebook, Women's Health Concerns Sourcebook, 3rd Edition*

Prostate and Urological Disorders Sourcebook

Basic Consumer Health Information about Urogenital and Sexual Disorders in Men, Including Prostate and Other Andrological Cancers, Prostatitis, Benign Prostatic Hyperplasia, Testicular and Penile Trauma, Cryptorchidism, Peyronie Disease, Erectile Dysfunction, and Male Factor Infertility, and Facts about Commonly Used Tests and Procedures, Such as Prostatectomy, Vasectomy, Vasectomy Reversal, Penile Implants, and Semen Analysis

Along with a Glossary of Andrological Terms and a Directory of Resources for Additional Information

Edited by Karen Bellenir. 604 pages. 2006. 978-0-7808-0797-6.

"Certain to be a popular pick among library reference holdings. . . . No prior knowledge is assumed for any of the conditions or terms herein, making it a most accessible general-interest reference."
—*California Bookwatch, Apr '06*

SEE ALSO *Men's Health Concerns Sourcebook, 3rd Edition, Urinary Tract and Kidney Diseases and Disorders Sourcebook, 2nd Edition*

Prostate Cancer Sourcebook

Basic Consumer Health Information about Prostate Cancer, Including Information about the Associated Risk Factors, Detection, Diagnosis, and Treatment of Prostate Cancer

Along with Information on Non-Malignant Prostate Conditions, and Featuring a Section

Listing Support and Treatment Centers and a Glossary of Related Terms

Edited by Dawn D. Matthews. 340 pages. 2001. 978-0-7808-0324-4.

"Recommended reference source."
—*Booklist, Jan '02*

"A valuable resource for health care consumers seeking information on the subject. . . . All text is written in a clear, easy-to-understand language that avoids technical jargon. Any library that collects consumer health resources would strengthen their collection with the addition of the *Prostate Cancer Sourcebook.*"
—*American Reference Books Annual, 2002*

SEE ALSO *Cancer Sourcebook, 5th Edition, Men's Health Concerns Sourcebook, 3rd Edition*

Rehabilitation Sourcebook

Basic Consumer Health Information about Rehabilitation for People Recovering from Heart Surgery, Spinal Cord Injury, Stroke, Orthopedic Impairments, Amputation, Pulmonary Impairments, Traumatic Injury, and More, Including Physical Therapy, Occupational Therapy, Speech/Language Therapy, Massage Therapy, Dance Therapy, Art Therapy, and Recreational Therapy

Along with Information on Assistive and Adaptive Devices, a Glossary, and Resources for Additional Help and Information

Edited by Dawn D. Matthews. 519 pages. 2000. 978-0-7808-0236-0.

"This is an excellent resource for public library reference and health collections."
—*American Reference Books Annual, 2001*

"Recommended reference source."
—*Booklist, May '00*

Respiratory Disorders Sourcebook, 2nd Edition

Basic Consumer Health Information about Infectious, Inflammatory, and Chronic Conditions Affecting the Lungs and Respiratory System, Including Pneumonia, Bronchitis, Influenza, Tuberculosis, Sarcoidosis, Asthma, Cystic Fibrosis, Chronic Obstructive Pulmonary Disease, Lung Abscesses, Pulmonary Embolism, Occupational Lung Diseases, and Other Bacterial, Viral, and Fungal Infections

Along with Facts about the Structure and Function of the Lungs and Airways, Methods of Diagnosing Respiratory Disorders, and Treatment and Rehabilitation Options, a Glossary of Related Terms, and a Directory of Resources for Additional Help and Information

Edited by Sandra L. Judd. 638 pages. 2008. 978-0-7808-1007-5.

"A great addition for public and school libraries because it provides concise health information . . . readers can start with this reference source and get satisfactory answers before proceeding to other medical reference tools for more in depth information . . . A good guide for health education on lung disorders."
—*ARBAonline, Nov '08*

SEE ALSO *Lung Disorders Sourcebook*

Sexually Transmitted Diseases Sourcebook, 4th Edition

Basic Consumer Health Information about Chlamydial Infections, Gonorrhea, Hepatitis, Herpes, HIV/AIDS, Human Papillomavirus, Pubic Lice, Scabies, Syphilis, Trichomoniasis, Vaginal Infections, and Other Sexually Transmitted Diseases, Including Facts about Risk Factors, Symptoms, Diagnosis, Treatment, and the Prevention of Sexually Transmitted Infections

Along with Updates on Current Research Initiatives, a Glossary of Related Terms, and Resources for Additional Help and Information

Edited by Laura Larsen. 600 pages. 2009. 978-0-7808-1073-0.

SEE ALSO *AIDS Sourcebook, 4th Edition, Contagious Diseases Sourcebook, 2nd Edition, Men's Health Concerns Sourcebook, 3rd Edition, Women's Health Concerns Sourcebook, 3rd Edition*

Sleep Disorders Sourcebook, 2nd Edition

Basic Consumer Health Information about Sleep and Sleep Disorders, Including Insomnia, Sleep Apnea, Restless Legs Syndrome, Narcolepsy, Parasomnias, and Other Health Problems That Affect Sleep, Plus Facts about Diagnostic Procedures, Treatment Strategies,

Sleep Medications, and Tips for Improving Sleep Quality

Along with a Glossary of Related Terms and Resources for Additional Help and Information

Edited by Amy L. Sutton. 567 pages. 2005. 978-0-7808-0743-3.

"This book will be useful for just about everybody, especially the 40 million Americans with sleep disorders."
—*American Reference Books Annual, 2006*

"A welcome addition to public libraries and consumer health libraries."
—*Medical Reference Services Quarterly, Summer '06*

Smoking Concerns Sourcebook

Basic Consumer Health Information about Nicotine Addiction and Smoking Cessation, Featuring Facts about the Health Effects of Tobacco Use, Including Lung and Other Cancers, Heart Disease, Stroke, and Respiratory Disorders, Such as Emphysema and Chronic Bronchitis

Along with Information about Smoking Prevention Programs, Suggestions for Achieving and Maintaining a Smoke-Free Lifestyle, Statistics about Tobacco Use, Reports on Current Research Initiatives, a Glossary of Related Terms, and Directories of Resources for Additional Help and Information

Edited by Karen Bellenir. 595 pages. 2004. 978-0-7808-0323-7.

"Provides everything needed for the student or general reader seeking practical details on the effects of tobacco use."
—*The Bookwatch, Mar '05*

"Public libraries and consumer health care libraries will find this work useful."
—*American Reference Books Annual, 2005*

SEE ALSO *Respiratory Disorders Sourcebook, 2nd Edition*

Sports Injuries Sourcebook, 3rd Edition

Basic Consumer Health Information about Sprains and Strains, Fractures, Growth Plate Injuries, Overtraining Injuries, and Injuries to the Head, Face, Shoulders, Elbows, Hands, Spinal Column, Knees, Ankles, and Feet, and with Facts about Heat-Related Illness, Steroids and Sport Supplements, Protective Equipment, Diagnostic Procedures, Treatment Options, and Rehabilitation

Along with a Glossary of Related Terms and a Directory of Resources for Additional Help and Information

Edited by Sandra J. Judd. 623 pages. 2007. 978-0-7808-0949-9.

SEE ALSO *Fitness and Exercise Sourcebook, 3rd Edition*

Stress-Related Disorders Sourcebook, 2nd Edition

Basic Consumer Health Information about Stress and Stress-Related Disorders, Including Types of Stress, Sources of Acute and Chronic Stress, the Impact of Stress on the Body's Systems, and Mental and Emotional Health Problems Associated with Stress, Such as Depression, Anxiety Disorders, Substance Abuse, Posttraumatic Stress Disorder, and Suicide

Along with Advice about Getting Help for Stress-Related Disorders, Information about Stress Management Techniques, a Glossary of Stress-Related Terms, and a Directory of Resources for Additional Help and Information

Edited by Amy L. Sutton. 608 pages. 2007. 978-0-7808-0996-3.

"Accessible to the lay reader. Highly recommended for medical and psychiatric collections."
—*Library Journal, Mar '08*

"Well-written for a general readership, the 2nd Edition of *Stress-Related Disorders Sourcebook* is a useful addition to the health reference literature."
—*American Reference Books Annual, 2008*

SEE ALSO *Mental Health Disorders Sourcebook, 4th Edition*

Stroke Sourcebook, 2nd Edition

Basic Consumer Health Information about Stroke, Including Ischemic, Hemorrhagic, and Mini Strokes, as Well as Risk Factors, Prevention Guidelines, Diagnostic Tests, Medications and

Surgical Treatments, and Complications of Stroke

Along with Rehabilitation Techniques and Innovations, Tips on Staying Healthy and Maintaining Independence after Stroke, a Glossary of Related Terms, and a Directory of Resources for Stroke Survivors and Their Families

Edited by Amy L. Sutton. 626 pages. 2008. 978-0-7808-1035-8.

"An encyclopedic handbook on stroke that is written in a language the layperson can understand. . . . This is one of the most helpful, readable books on stroke. This volume is highly recommended and should be in every medical, hospital and public library; in addition, every family practitioner should have a copy in his or her office."

—*ARBAonline Dec '08*

SEE ALSO *Hypertension Sourcebook*

Surgery Sourcebook, 2nd Edition

Basic Consumer Health Information about Common Inpatient and Outpatient Surgeries, Including Critical Care and Trauma, Gastrointestinal, Gynecologic and Obstetric, Cardiac and Vascular, Neurologic, Ophthalmologic, Orthopedic, Reconstructive and Cosmetic, and Other Major and Minor Surgeries

Along with Information about Anesthesia and Pain Relief Options, Risks and Complications, Postoperative Recovery Concerns, and Innovative Surgical Techniques and Tools, a Glossary of Related Terms, and a Directory of Additional Resources

Edited by Amy L. Sutton. 645 pages. 2008. 978-0-7808-1004-4.

"Large public libraries and medical libraries would benefit from this material in their reference collections."

—*ARBAonline Aug '08*

SEE ALSO *Cosmetic and Reconstructive Surgery Sourcebook, 2nd Edition*

Thyroid Disorders Sourcebook

Basic Consumer Health Information about Disorders of the Thyroid and Parathyroid Glands, Including Hypothyroidism, Hyperthyroidism, Graves Disease, Hashimoto Thyroiditis, Thyroid Cancer, and Parathyroid Disorders, Featuring Facts about Symptoms, Risk Factors, Tests, and Treatments

Along with Information about the Effects of Thyroid Imbalance on Other Body Systems, Environmental Factors That Affect the Thyroid Gland, a Glossary, and a Directory of Additional Resources

Edited by Joyce Brennfleck Shannon. 573 pages. 2005. 978-0-7808-0745-7.

"Recommended for consumer health collections."

—*American Reference Books Annual, 2006*

"Highly recommended pick for basic consumer health reference holdings at all levels."

—*The Bookwatch, Aug '05*

SEE ALSO *Endocrine and Metabolic Disorders Sourcebook, 2nd Edition*

Transplantation Sourcebook

Basic Consumer Health Information about Organ and Tissue Transplantation, Including Physical and Financial Preparations, Procedures and Issues Relating to Specific Solid Organ and Tissue Transplants, Rehabilitation, Pediatric Transplant Information, the Future of Transplantation, and Organ and Tissue Donation

Along with a Glossary and Listings of Additional Resources

Edited by Joyce Brennfleck Shannon. 610 pages. 2002. 978-0-7808-0322-0.

"Recommended for libraries with an interest in offering consumer health information."

—*E-Streams, Jul '02*

"This is a unique and valuable resource for patients facing transplantation and their families."

—*Doody's Review Service, Jun '02*

Traveler's Health Sourcebook

Basic Consumer Health Information for Travelers, Including Physical and Medical Preparations, Transportation Health and Safety, Essential Information about Food and Water, Sun Exposure, Insect and Snake Bites, Camping and Wilderness Medicine, and Travel with Physical or Medical Disabilities

Along with International Travel Tips, Vaccination Recommendations, Geographical Health Issues, Disease Risks, a Glossary, and a Listing of Additional Resources

Edited by Joyce Brennfleck Shannon. 619 pages. 2000. 978-0-7808-0384-8.

"Recommended reference source."

—*Booklist, Feb '01*

"This book is recommended for any public library, any travel collection, and especially any collection for the physically disabled."

—*American Reference Books Annual, 2001*

SEE ALSO *Worldwide Health Sourcebook*

Urinary Tract and Kidney Diseases and Disorders Sourcebook, 2nd Edition

Basic Consumer Health Information about the Urinary System, Including the Bladder, Urethra, Ureters, and Kidneys, with Facts about Urinary Tract Infections, Incontinence, Congenital Disorders, Kidney Stones, Cancers of the Urinary Tract and Kidneys, Kidney Failure, Dialysis, and Kidney Transplantation

Along with Statistical and Demographic Information, Reports on Current Research in Kidney and Urologic Health, a Summary of Commonly Used Diagnostic Tests, a Glossary of Related Terms, and a Directory of Resources for Additional Help and Information

Edited by Ivy L. Alexander. 621 pages. 2005. 978-0-7808-0750-1.

"A good choice for a consumer health information library or for a medical library needing information to refer to their patients."

—*American Reference Books Annual, 2006*

SEE ALSO *Prostate and Urological Disorders Sourcebook*

Vegetarian Sourcebook

Basic Consumer Health Information about Vegetarian Diets, Lifestyle, and Philosophy, Including Definitions of Vegetarianism and Veganism, Tips about Adopting Vegetarianism, Creating a Vegetarian Pantry, and Meeting Nutritional Needs of Vegetarians, with Facts Regarding Vegetarianism's Effect on Pregnant and Lactating Women, Children, Athletes, and Senior Citizens

Along with a Glossary of Commonly Used Vegetarian Terms and Resources for Additional Help and Information

Edited by Chad T. Kimball. 337 pages. 2002. 978-0-7808-0439-5.

"Organizes into one concise volume the answers to the most common questions concerning vegetarian diets and lifestyles. This title is recommended for public and secondary school libraries."

—*E-Streams, Apr '03*

"Invaluable reference for public and school library collections alike."

—*Library Bookwatch, Apr '03*

"The articles in this volume are easy to read and come from authoritative sources. The book does not necessarily support the vegetarian diet but instead provides the pros and cons of this important decision. . . . Recommended for public libraries and consumer health libraries."

—*American Reference Books Annual, 2003*

SEE ALSO *Diet and Nutrition Sourcebook, 3rd Edition*

Women's Health Concerns Sourcebook, 3rd Edition

Basic Consumer Health Information about Issues and Trends in Women's Health and Health Conditions of Special Concern to Women, Including Endometriosis, Uterine Fibroids, Menstrual Irregularities, Menopause, Sexual Dysfunction, Infertility, Cancer in Women, and Other Such Chronic Disorders as Lupus, Fibromyalgia, and Thyroid Disease

Along with Statistical Data, Tips for Maintaining Wellness, a Glossary, and a Directory of Resources for Further Help and Information

Edited by Sandra J. Judd. 600 pages. 2009. 978-0-7808-1036-5.

SEE ALSO *Breast Cancer Sourcebook, 3rd Edition, Cancer Sourcebook for Women, 3rd Edition, Healthy Heart Sourcebook for Women, Osteoporosis Sourcebook*

Workplace Health and Safety Sourcebook

Basic Consumer Health Information about Workplace Health and Safety, Including the Effect of Workplace Hazards on the Lungs,

Skin, Heart, Ears, Eyes, Brain, Reproductive Organs, Musculoskeletal System, and Other Organs and Body Parts

Along with Information about Occupational Cancer, Personal Protective Equipment, Toxic and Hazardous Chemicals, Child Labor, Stress, and Workplace Violence

Edited by Chad T. Kimball. 610 pages. 2000. 978-0-7808-0231-5.

"As a reference for the general public, this would be useful in any library."

—E-Streams, Jun '01

"Provides helpful information for primary care physicians and other caregivers interested in occupational medicine. . . . General readers; professionals."

—CHOICE, May '01

Worldwide Health Sourcebook

Basic Information about Global Health Issues, Including Malnutrition, Reproductive Health, Disease Dispersion and Prevention, Emerging Diseases, Risky Health Behaviors, and the Leading Causes of Death

Along with Global Health Concerns for Children, Women, and the Elderly, Mental Health Issues, Research and Technology Advancements, and Economic, Environmental, and Political Health Implications, a Glossary, and a Resource Listing for Additional Help and Information

Edited by Joyce Brennfleck Shannon. 597 pages. 2001. 978-0-7808-0330-5.

"Named an Outstanding Academic Title."

—CHOICE, Jan '02

"Yet another handy but also unique compilation in the extensive *Health Reference Series*, this is a useful work because many of the international publications reprinted or excerpted are not readily available. Highly recommended."

—CHOICE, Nov '01

SEE ALSO *Traveler's Health Sourcebook*

Teen Health Series

Complete Catalog

List price $69 per volume. School and library price $62 per volume.

Abuse and Violence Information for Teens

Health Tips about the Causes and Consequences of Abusive and Violent Behavior

Including Facts about the Types of Abuse and Violence, the Warning Signs of Abusive and Violent Behavior, Health Concerns of Victims, and Getting Help and Staying Safe

Edited by Sandra Augustyn Lawton. 411 pages. 2008. 978-0-7808-1008-2.

"A useful resource for schools and organizations providing services to teens and may also be a starting point in research projects."

—*Reference and Research Book News, Aug '08*

"Violence is a serious problem for teens. . . . This resource gives teens the information they need to face potential threats and get help—either for themselves or for their friends."

—*ARBAonline, Aug '08*

Accident and Safety Information for Teens

Health Tips about Medical Emergencies, Traumatic Injuries, and Disaster Preparedness

Including Facts about Motor Vehicle Accidents, Burns, Poisoning, Firearms, Natural Disasters, National Security Threats, and More

Edited by Karen Bellenir. 420 pages. 2008. 978-0-7808-1046-4.

***SEE ALSO** Sports Injuries Information for Teens, 2nd Edition*

Alcohol Information for Teens, 2nd Edition

Health Tips about Alcohol and Alcoholism

Including Facts about Alcohol's Effects on the Body, Brain, and Behavior, the Consequences of Underage Drinking, Alcohol Abuse Prevention and Treatment, and Coping with Alcoholic Parents

Edited by Lisa Bakewell. 400 pages. 2009. 978-0-7808-1043-3.

***SEE ALSO** Drug Information for Teens, 2nd Edition*

Allergy Information for Teens

Health Tips about Allergic Reactions Such as Anaphylaxis, Respiratory Problems, and Rashes

Including Facts about Identifying and Managing Allergies to Food, Pollen, Mold, Animals, Chemicals, Drugs, and Other Substances

Edited by Karen Bellenir. 410 pages. 2006. 978-0-7808-0799-0.

"This is a comprehensive, readable text on the subject of allergic diseases in teenagers. 5 Stars (out of 5)!"

—*Doody's Review Service, Jun '06*

"This authoritative and useful self-help title is a solid addition to YA collections, whether for personal interest or reports."

—*School Library Journal, Jul '06*

Asthma Information for Teens

Health Tips about Managing Asthma and Related Concerns

Including Facts about Asthma Causes, Triggers, Symptoms, Diagnosis, and Treatment

Edited by Karen Bellenir. 386 pages. 2005. 978-0-7808-0770-9.

"Highly recommended for medical libraries, public school libraries, and public libraries."

—*American Reference Books Annual, 2006*

"Although this volume is nearly 400 pages long, it is so clearly written and well organized that even hesitant readers will be able to find the facts they need, whether for reports or personal information. . . . A succinct but complete resource."

—*School Library Journal, Sep '05*

Body Information for Teens

Health Tips about Maintaining Well-Being for a Lifetime

Including Facts about the Development and Functioning of the Body's Systems, Organs, and Structures and the Health Impact of Lifestyle Choices

Edited by Sandra Augustyn Lawton. 458 pages. 2007. 978-0-7808-0443-2.

■

Cancer Information for Teens, 2nd Edition

Health Tips about Cancer Awareness, Symptoms, Prevention, Diagnosis, and Treatment

Including Facts about Common Cancers Affecting Teens, Causes, Detection, Coping Strategies, Clinical Trials, Nutrition and Exercise, Cancer in Friends or Family, and More

Edited by Karen Bellenir and Lisa Bakewell. 400 pages. 2009. 978-0-7808-1085-3.

■

Complementary and Alternative Medicine Information for Teens

Health Tips about Non-Traditional and Non-Western Medical Practices

Including Information about Acupuncture, Chiropractic Medicine, Dietary and Herbal Supplements, Hypnosis, Massage Therapy, Prayer and Spirituality, Reflexology, Yoga, and More

Edited by Sandra Augustyn Lawton. 407 pages. 2007. 978-0-7808-0966-6.

"This volume covers CAM specifically for teenagers but of general use also. It should be a welcome addition to both public and academic libraries."

—*American Reference Books Annual, 2008*

"This volume provides a solid foundation for further investigation of the subject, making it useful for both public and high school libraries."

—*VOYA: Voice of Youth Advocates, Jun '07*

■

Diabetes Information for Teens

Health Tips about Managing Diabetes and Preventing Related Complications

Including Information about Insulin, Glucose Control, Healthy Eating, Physical Activity, and Learning to Live with Diabetes

Edited by Sandra Augustyn Lawton. 410 pages. 2006. 978-0-7808-0811-9.

"A comprehensive instructional guide for teens. . . . some of the material may also be directed towards parents or teachers. 5 stars (out of 5)!"

—*Doody's Review Service, 2006*

"Students dealing with their own diabetes or that of a friend or family member or those writing reports on the topic will find this a valuable resource."

—*School Library Journal, Aug '06*

"This text is directed to the teen population and would be an excellent library resource for a health class or for the teacher as a reference for class preparation. It can, however, serve a much wider audience. The clinical educator on diabetes may find it valuable to educate the newly diagnosed client regardless of age. It also would be an excellent reference and education tool for a preventive medicine seminar on diabetes."

—*Physical Therapy, Mar '07*

■

Diet Information for Teens, 2nd Edition

Health Tips about Diet and Nutrition

Including Facts about Dietary Guidelines, Food Groups, Nutrients, Healthy Meals, Snacks, Weight Control, Medical Concerns Related to Diet, and More

Edited by Karen Bellenir. 432 pages. 2006. 978-0-7808-0820-1.

"A very quick and pleasant read in spite of the fact that it is very detailed in the information it gives. . . . A book for anyone concerned about diet and nutrition."

—*American Reference Books Annual, 2007*

SEE ALSO *Eating Disorders Information for Teens, 2nd Edition*

■

Drug Information for Teens, 2nd Edition

Health Tips about the Physical and Mental Effects of Substance Abuse

Including Information about Marijuana, Inhalants, Club Drugs, Stimulants, Hallucinogens,

Opiates, Prescription and Over-the-Counter Drugs, Herbal Products, Tobacco, Alcohol, and More

Edited by Sandra Augustyn Lawton. 468 pages. 2006. 978-0-7808-0862-1.

"As with earlier installments in Omnigraphics' *Teen Health Series, Drug Information for Teens* is designed specifically to meet the needs and interests of middle and high school students. . . . Strongly recommended for both academic and public libraries."

—*American Reference Books Annual, 2007*

"Solid thoughtful advice is given about how to handle peer pressure, drug-related health concerns, and treatment strategies."

—*School Library Journal, Dec '06*

SEE ALSO *Alcohol Information for Teens, 2nd Edition, Tobacco Information for Teens*

Eating Disorders Information for Teens, 2nd Edition

Health Tips about Anorexia, Bulimia, Binge Eating, And Other Eating Disorders

Including Information about Risk Factors, Diagnosis and Treatment, Prevention, Related Health Concerns, and Other Issues

Edited by Sandra Augustyn Lawton. 377 pages. 2009. 978-0-7808-1044-0.

SEE ALSO *Diet Information for Teens, 2nd Edition*

Fitness Information for Teens, 2nd Edition

Health Tips about Exercise, Physical Well-Being, and Health Maintenance

Including Facts about Conditioning, Stretching, Strength Training, Body Shape and Body Image, Sports Nutrition, and Specific Activities for Athletes and Non-Athletes

Edited by Lisa Bakewell. 432 pages. 2009. 978-0-7808-1045-7.

SEE ALSO *Diet Information for Teens, 2nd Edition, Sports Injuries Information for Teens, 2nd Edition*

Learning Disabilities Information for Teens

Health Tips about Academic Skills Disorders and Other Disabilities That Affect Learning

Including Information about Common Signs of Learning Disabilities, School Issues, Learning to Live with a Learning Disability, and Other Related Issues

Edited by Sandra Augustyn Lawton. 400 pages. 2006. 978-0-7808-0796-9.

"This book provides a wealth of information for any reader interested in the signs, causes, and consequences of learning disabilities, as well as related legal rights and educational interventions. . . . Public and academic libraries should want this title for both students and general readers."

—*American Reference Books Annual, 2006*

Mental Health Information for Teens, 2nd Edition

Health Tips about Mental Wellness and Mental Illness

Including Facts about Mental and Emotional Health, Depression and Other Mood Disorders, Anxiety Disorders, Conduct Disorder, Self-Injury, Psychosis, Schizophrenia, and More

Edited by Karen Bellenir. 424 pages. 2006. 978-0-7808-0863-8.

"This excellent overview of the psychological disorders that affect teens provides clear definitions and descriptions, and discusses resources, therapies, coping mechanisms, and medications."

—*School Library Journal Curriculum Connections, Fall '07*

"A well done reference for a specific, often under-represented group."

—*Doody's Review Service, 2006*

SEE ALSO *Stress Information for Teens*

Pregnancy Information for Teens

Health Tips about Teen Pregnancy and Teen Parenting

Including Facts about Prenatal Care, Pregnancy Complications, Labor and Delivery,

Postpartum Care, Pregnancy-Related Lifestyle Concerns, and More

Edited by Sandra Augustyn Lawton. 434 pages. 2007. 978-0-7808-0984-0.

SEE ALSO *Sexual Health Information for Teens, 2nd Edition*

Sexual Health Information for Teens, 2nd Edition

Health Tips about Sexual Development, Reproduction, Contraception, and Sexually Transmitted Infections

Including Facts about Puberty, Sexuality, Birth Control, Chlamydia, Gonorrhea, Herpes, Human Papillomavirus, Syphilis, and More

Edited by Sandra Augustyn Lawton. 430 pages. 2008. 978-0-7808-1010-5.

"This offering represents the most up-to-date information available on an array of topics including abstinence-only sexual education and pregnancy-prevention methods. . . . The range of coverage—from puberty and anatomy to sexually transmitted diseases—is thorough and extensive. Each chapter includes a bibliographic citation, and the three back sections containing additional resources, further reading, and the index are all first-rate. . . . This volume will be well used by students in need of the facts, whether for educational or personal reasons."

—*School Library Journal, Nov '08*

SEE ALSO *Pregnancy Information for Teens*

Skin Health Information for Teens, 2nd Edition

Health Tips about Dermatological Concerns and Skin Cancer Risks

Including Facts about Acne, Warts, Allergies, and Other Conditions and Lifestyle Choices, Such as Tanning, Tattooing, and Piercing, That Affect the Skin, Nails, Scalp, and Hair

Edited by Edited by Kim Wohlenhaus. 400 pages. 2009. 978-0-7808-1042-6.

Sleep Information for Teens

Health Tips about Adolescent Sleep Requirements, Sleep Disorders, and the Effects of Sleep Deprivation

Including Facts about Why People Need Sleep, Sleep Patterns, Circadian Rhythms, Dreaming, Insomnia, Sleep Apnea, Narcolepsy, and More

Edited by Karen Bellenir. 355 pages. 2008. 978-0-7808-1009-9.

SEE ALSO *Body Information for Teens*

Sports Injuries Information for Teens, 2nd Edition

Health Tips about Acute, Traumatic, and Chronic Injuries in Adolescent Athletes

Including Facts about Sprains, Fractures, and Overuse Injuries, Treatment, Rehabilitation, Sport-Specific Safety Guidelines, Fitness Suggestions, and More

Edited by Karen Bellenir. 429 pages. 2008. 978-0-7808-1011-2.

"An engaging selection of informative articles about the prevention and treatment of sports injuries. . . The value of this book is that the articles have been vetted and are often augmented with inserts of useful facts, definitions of technical terms, and quick tips. Sensitive topics like injuries to genitalia are discussed openly and responsibly. This revised edition contains updated articles and defines sport more broadly than the first edition."

—*School Library Journal, Nov '08*

"This work will be useful in the young adult collections of public libraries as well as high school libraries. . . . A useful resource for student research."

—*ARBAonline, Aug '08*

SEE ALSO *Accident and Safety Information for Teens*

Stress Information for Teens

Health Tips about the Mental and Physical Consequences of Stress

Including Information about the Different Kinds of Stress, Symptoms of Stress, Frequent Causes of Stress, Stress Management Techniques, and More

Edited by Sandra Augustyn Lawton. 392 pages. 2008. 978-0-7808-1012-9.

"Understanding what stress is, what causes it, how the body and the mind are impacted by it,

and what teens can do are the general categories addressed here. . . . The chapters are brief but informative, and the list of community-help organizations is exhaustive. Report writers will find information quickly and easily, as will those who have personal concerns. The print is clear and the format is readable, making this an accessible resource for struggling readers and researchers."

—School Library Journal, Dec '08

"The articles selected will specifically appeal to young adults and are designed to answer their most common questions."

—ARBAonline, Aug '08

SEE ALSO *Mental Health Information for Teens, 2nd Edition*

Suicide Information for Teens

Health Tips about Suicide Causes and Prevention

Including Facts about Depression, Risk Factors, Getting Help, Survivor Support, and More

Edited by Joyce Brennfleck Shannon. 368 pages. 2005. 978-0-7808-0737-2.

"Highly Recommended for libraries serving teenagers as well as those who work with them."

—E-Streams, Apr '06

SEE ALSO *Mental Health Information for Teens, 2nd Edition*

Tobacco Information for Teens

Health Tips about the Hazards of Using Cigarettes, Smokeless Tobacco, and Other Nicotine Products

Including Facts about Nicotine Addiction, Immediate and Long-Term Health Effects of Tobacco Use, Related Cancers, Smoking Cessation, Tobacco Use Prevention, and Tobacco Use Statistics

Edited by Karen Bellenir. 440 pages. 2007. 978-0-7808-0976-5.

"A comprehensive resource. Each chapter is written to stand alone, so students can dip in and use the information in each section for reports or to answer personal questions without having to read the entire book. . . . The book is packed full of statistics, with sources to help students look up more."

—School Library Journal, Sep '07

"Pulls together a wide variety of authoritative sources to provide a comprehensive overview of tobacco use for this age group. . . . This reasonably priced reference title should be considered a necessary purchase for all public libraries and school media centers, along with academic libraries supporting teacher education."

—American Reference Books Annual, 2008

SEE ALSO *Drug Information for Teens, 2nd Edition*

Health Reference Series

Adolescent Health Sourcebook, 2nd Edition
Adult Health Concerns Sourcebook
AIDS Sourcebook, 4th Edition
Alcoholism Sourcebook, 2nd Edition
Allergies Sourcebook, 3rd Edition
Alzheimer Disease Sourcebook, 4th Edition
Arthritis Sourcebook, 2nd Edition
Asthma Sourcebook, 2nd Edition
Attention Deficit Disorder Sourcebook
Autism & Pervasive Developmental Disorders Sourcebook
Back & Neck Sourcebook, 2nd Edition
Blood & Circulatory Disorders Sourcebook, 2nd Edition
Brain Disorders Sourcebook, 2nd Edition
Breast Cancer Sourcebook, 3rd Edition
Breastfeeding Sourcebook
Burns Sourcebook
Cancer Sourcebook, 5th Edition
Cancer Sourcebook for Women, 3rd Edition
Cancer Survivorship Sourcebook
Cardiovascular Diseases & Disorders Sourcebook, 3rd Edition
Caregiving Sourcebook
Child Abuse Sourcebook
Childhood Diseases & Disorders Sourcebook, 2nd Edition
Colds, Flu & Other Common Ailments Sourcebook
Communication Disorders Sourcebook
Complementary & Alternative Medicine Sourcebook, 3rd Edition
Congenital Disorders Sourcebook, 2nd Edition
Contagious Diseases Sourcebook
Cosmetic & Reconstructive Surgery Sourcebook, 2nd Edition
Death & Dying Sourcebook, 2nd Edition
Dental Care & Oral Health Sourcebook, 3rd Edition
Depression Sourcebook, 2nd Edition
Dermatological Disorders Sourcebook, 2nd Edition
Diabetes Sourcebook, 4th Edition
Diet & Nutrition Sourcebook, 3rd Edition
Digestive Diseases & Disorder Sourcebook
Disabilities Sourcebook
Disease Management Sourcebook
Domestic Violence Sourcebook, 3rd Edition
Drug Abuse Sourcebook, 2nd Edition
Ear, Nose & Throat Disorders Sourcebook, 2nd Edition
Eating Disorders Sourcebook, 2nd Edition
Emergency Medical Services Sourcebook
Endocrine & Metabolic Disorders Sourcebook, 2nd Edition
Environmental Health Sourcebook, 2nd Edition
Ethnic Diseases Sourcebook
Eye Care Sourcebook, 3rd Edition
Family Planning Sourcebook
Fitness & Exercise Sourcebook, 3rd Edition
Food Safety Sourcebook
Forensic Medicine Sourcebook
Gastrointestinal Diseases & Disorders Sourcebook, 2nd Edition
Genetic Disorders Sourcebook, 3rd Edition
Head Trauma Sourcebook
Headache Sourcebook
Health Insurance Sourcebook
Healthy Aging Sourcebook
Healthy Children Sourcebook
Healthy Heart Sourcebook for Women
Hepatitis Sourcebook
Household Safety Sourcebook
Hypertension Sourcebook
Immune System Disorders Sourcebook, 2nd Edition
Infant & Toddler Health Sourcebook
Infectious Diseases Sourcebook
Injury & Trauma Sourcebook